FLORIDA HOSPITAL
MEDICAL LIBRARY

REFERENCE BOOK
PLEASE DO NOT REMOVE
FROM LIBRARY.

Partial Knee Arthroplasty
Techniques for Optimal Outcomes

Partial Knee Arthroplasty Techniques for Optimal Outcomes

Keith R. Berend, MD

Associate, Joint Implant Surgeons, Inc., New Albany, Ohio;
Associate Professor, Department of Orthopaedic Surgery,
The Ohio State University, Columbus, Ohio

Fred D. Cushner, MD

Director, Insall Scott Kelly Institute;
Chairman, Orthopaedic Surgery, Southside Hospital, New York, New York

ELSEVIER
SAUNDERS

1600 John F. Kennedy Blvd.
Ste 1800
Philadelphia, PA 19103-2899

PARTIAL KNEE ARTHROPLASTY: TECHNIQUES FOR OPTIMAL OUTCOMES   ISBN: 978-1-4377-1756-3
Copyright © 2012 by Saunders, an imprint of Elsevier Inc.

All rights reserved. No part of this publication may be reproduced or transmitted in any form or by any means, electronic or mechanical, including photocopy, recording, or any information storage and retrieval system, without permission in writing from the publisher. Details on how to seek permission, further information about the Publisher's permissions policies and our arrangements with organizations such as the Copyright Clearance Center and the Copyright Licensing Agency, can be found at our website: www.elsevier.com/permissions.

This book and the individual contributions contained in it are protected under copyright by the Publisher (other than as may be noted herein).

Notices

Knowledge and best practice in this field are constantly changing. As new research and experience broaden our understanding, changes in research methods, professional practices, or medical treatment may become necessary.

Practitioners and researchers must always rely on their own experience and knowledge in evaluating and using any information, methods, compounds, or experiments described herein. In using such information or methods they should be mindful of their own safety and the safety of others, including parties for whom they have a professional responsibility.

With respect to any drug or pharmaceutical products identified, readers are advised to check the most current information provided (i) on procedures featured or (ii) by the manufacturer of each product to be administered, to verify the recommended dose or formula, the method and duration of administration, and contraindications. It is the responsibility of practitioners, relying on their own experience and knowledge of their patients, to make diagnoses, to determine dosages and the best treatment for each individual patient, and to take all appropriate safety precautions.

To the fullest extent of the law, neither the Publisher nor the authors, contributors, or editors, assume any liability for any injury and/or damage to persons or property as a matter of products liability, negligence or otherwise, or from any use or operation of any methods, products, instructions, or ideas contained in the material herein.

Library of Congress Cataloging-in-Publication Data
Berend, Keith R.
  Partial knee arthroplasty : techniques for optimal outcomes / Keith R. Berend, Fred D. Cushner.—1st ed.
    p. ; cm.
  Includes bibliographical references and index.
  ISBN 978-1-4377-1756-3 (hardback : alk. paper)
  1. Total knee replacement. 2. Arthroplasty. I. Cushner, Fred D. II. Title.
  [DNLM: 1. Arthroplasty, Replacement, Knee.   WE 870]
  RD561.B47 2011
  617.5′820592—dc23   2011017687

Acquisitions Editor: Dolores Meloni
Developmental Editor: Taylor E. Ball
Publishing Services Manager: Pat Joiner-Myers
Senior Project Manager: Joy Moore
Design Manager: Louis Forgione

Working together to grow
libraries in developing countries

www.elsevier.com | www.bookaid.org | www.sabre.org

ELSEVIER   BOOK AID International   Sabre Foundation

Printed in China

Last digit is the print number: 9 8 7 6 5 4 3 2 1

To CIPKA

KRB and FDC

Contributors

Jean-Noël Argenson, MD, PhD
Professor of Orthopaedic Surgery, Faculty of Medecine, University of the Mediterranée; Chairman of the Hospital for Arthritis Surgery, Sainte Marguerite Hospital, Universitary Hospital of Marseille, Marseille, France
Medial Unicompartmental Knee Arthroplasty:
Fixed-Bearing Techniques

Wael K. Barsoum, MD
Chairman, Surgical Operations, Vice Chairman, Orthopaedic Surgery, and Fellowship Director, Section of Adult Reconstruction, Cleveland Clinic, Cleveland, Ohio
Lateral Unicompartmental Knee Arthroplasty

Erhan Basad, MD
Assistant Professor, Giessen University Faculty of Medicine; Assistant Medical Director, Department of Orthopaedic Surgery, Giessen-Marburg University Hospital GmbH, Giessen, Germany
Spacer Devices—Old and New

Keith R. Berend, MD
Associate, Joint Implant Surgeons, Inc., New Albany; Associate Professor, Department of Orthopaedic Surgery, The Ohio State University, Columbus, Ohio
The Patella in Medial Unicompartmental Knee Arthroplasty

Michael E. Berend, MD
Volunteer, Indiana University School of Medicine, Indianapolis; Orthopaedic Biomechanical Engineering Laboratory, Rose-Hulman Institute of Technology, Terre Haute, Indiana; Orthopaedic Surgeon, St. Francis Hospital Center for Hip and Knee Surgery, Joint Replacement Surgeons of Indiana, Mooresville, Indiana
The Painful Medial Unicompartmental Knee Arthroplasty

Richard A. Berger, MD
Assistant Professor of Orthopedic Surgery, Rush University Medical Center, Chicago, Illinois
Anesthesia, Pain Management, and Early Discharge for Partial Knee Arthroplasty

Jack M. Bert, MD
Adjunct Clinical Professor, University of Minnesota School of Medicine, Minneapolis, Minnesota; Summit Orthopedics, Ltd., St. Paul, Minnesota
Failure Modes of Unicompartmental Arthroplasty

Nicholas Bottomley, MBBS, MRCS
Clinical Research Fellow, Nuffield Orthopaedic Centre, Oxford, United Kingdom
Indications for Unicompartmental Knee Arthroplasty;
Medial Unicompartmental Knee Replacement: Cementless Options; Mobile-Bearing Uni: Long-Term Outcomes

William D. Bugbee, MD
Attending Physician, Division of Orthopaedics, Scripps Clinic, La Jolla, California; Associate Professor, Department of Orthopaedic Surgery, University of California, San Diego, San Diego, California
Allografts for the Arthritic Knee

Thomas M. Coon, MD
Founder and Director, Coon Joint Replacement Institute, St. Helena Hospital, St. Helena, California
Computer-Guided Partial Knee Replacement

Fred D. Cushner, MD
Director, Insall Scott Kelly Institute; Chairman, Orthopaedic Surgery, Southside Hospital, New York, New York
Surgical Pearls for Fixed-Bearing Medial Unicompartmental Knee Arthroplasty

David F. Dalury, MD
Assistant Professor, Orthopedic Surgery, Johns Hopkins School of Medicine, Baltimore, Maryland; Chief, Adult Reconstructive Surgery, St. Joseph Medical Center, Towson, Maryland
Fixed-Bearing Uni: Long-Term Outcomes;
Practical Issues in Unicompartmental Knee Arthroplasty—The Secrets for Success

Jeffrey H. DeClaire, MD
Clinical Assistant Professor, Oakland University; Chief, Department of Surgery and Department of Orthopaedic Surgery, Crittenton Hospital Medical Center, Rochester Hills, Michigan; Bald Mountain Surgical Center, Lake Orion, Michigan
Patellofemoral Arthroplasty: Indications and Outcomes;
The Failed Uni

Craig J. Della Valle, MD
Associate Professor of Orthopaedic Surgery, and Director, Adult Reconstructive Fellowship, Rush University Medical Center, Chicago, Illinois
Long-Term Patellofemoral Progression

Allison J. De Young, BS
Clinical Research Assistant, Shiley Center for Orthopaedic Research and Education (SCORE) at Scripps Clinic, La Jolla, California
Allografts for the Arthritic Knee

Christopher Dodd, MB, ChB, FRCS
Consultant Knee Surgeon, Nuffield Orthopaedic Centre, Headington, Oxford, UK
Indications for Unicompartmental Knee Arthroplasty; Medial Unicompartmental Knee Replacement: Cementless Options; Mobile-Bearing Uni: Long-Term Outcomes

Karim Elsharkawy, MD, 7MRCS (Eng)
Resident of Orthopaedic Surgery, Cleveland Clinic Foundation, Cleveland, Ohio
Lateral Unicompartmental Knee Arthroplasty

Gerard A. Engh, MD
Director, Knee Research, Anderson Orthopaedic Research Institute, Alexandria, Virginia
Uni: History and Look to the Future

Wolfgang Fitz, MD
Clinical Instructor in Orthopaedic Surgery, Harvard Medical School; Associate Orthopaedic Surgeon, Department of Orthopaedic Surgery, Brigham and Women's Hospital, Boston, Massachusetts
Individualized Unicompartmental Knee Arthroplasty

Jared R.H. Foran, MD
Panorama Orthopedics and Spine Center, Golden, Colorado
Long-Term Patellofemoral Progression

Simon Görtz, MD
Research Fellow, Department of Orthopaedic Surgery, University of California, San Diego School of Medicine, San Diego, California
Osteochondral Allografting Plug Technique (Video)

Amrit Goyal, MBBS, MS (Ortho)
Lecturer, S.N. Medical College, Agra, India
Minimally Invasive Surgery: Medial Fixed-Bearing Onlay Unicompartmental Knee Arthroplasty

Jason M. Hurst, MD
Director, Joint Preservation Institute at Joint Implant Surgeons, Inc., New Albany, Ohio
Nonarthroplasty Treatment Options for Unicompartmental Degenerative Joint Disease

William A. Jiranek, MD
Professor of Orthopaedics and Chief of Adult Reconstruction, Department of Orthopaedic Surgery, Virginia Commonwealth University Health System, Richmond, Virginia
Incidence of Partial Knee Arthroplasty: A Growing Phenomenon?

Todd C. Kelley, MD
Assistant Professor of Orthopaedic Surgery, University of Cincinnati College of Medicine, Cincinnati, Ohio
Fixed-Bearing Uni: Long-Term Outcomes

Benjamin Kendrick, MRCS (Eng)
Clinical Research Fellow, Nuffield Orthopaedic Centre, Oxford, United Kingdom
Indications for Unicompartmental Knee Arthroplasty; Medial Unicompartmental Knee Replacement: Cementless Options; Mobile-Bearing Uni: Long-Term Outcomes

Franz Xaver Koeck, MD
Teacher for General Orthopaedics, Orthopaedic Surgery, Orthopaedic Rheumatology, and Bone and Joint Infections, Foot and Ankle Faculty, and Member of ComGen of AE (Arthroplasty Work Group of German Orthopaedic Society), University of Regensburg, Regensburg, Germany; Assistant Medical Director, Department of Orthopaedic Surgery, Asklepios Klinikum, Bad Abbach, Germany
Spacer Devices—Old and New

Adolph V. Lombardi, Jr., MD, FACS
Clinical Assistant Professor, Department of Orthopaedics and Department of Biomedical Engineering, The Ohio State University, Columbus, Ohio; President and Attending Surgeon, Joint Implant Surgeons, Inc., Mount Carmel Health System, New Albany, Ohio
Deep Vein Thrombosis Prophylaxis following Unicompartmental Knee Arthroplasty

William J. Long, MD, FRCSC
GME Committee Member, Lenox Hill Hospital, North Shore–Long Island Jewish Hospital System; Attending Orthopaedic Surgeon, Insall Scott Kelly Institute, New York, New York
Use of Biologics for Degenerative Joint Disease of the Knee

Jess H. Lonner, MD
Associate Professor of Orthopaedic Surgery, Thomas Jefferson University, Philadelphia, Pennsylvania; Bryn Mawr Hospital, Bryn Mawr, Pennsylvania
Modular Bicompartmental Knee Arthroplasty

William Macaulay, MD
Nas S. Eftekhar Professor of Clinical Orthopaedic Surgery, Columbia University; Chef, Division of Adult Reconstruction, and Director, Center for Hip and Knee Replacement, New York Presbyterian Hospital at Columbia University, New York, New York
Minimally Invasive Surgery: Medial Fixed-Bearing Onlay Unicompartmental Knee Arthroplasty

Michael J. Morris, MD
Associate, Joint Implant Surgeons, Inc., New Albany, Ohio
Unicompartmental Knee Arthroplasty: Mobile-Bearing
Techniques

David Murray, MA, MD, FRCS (Orth)
*Consultant Orthopaedic Surgeon, Nuffield Department of
Orthopaedics, Rheumatology and Musculoskeletal Sciences,
Nuffield Orthopaedic Centre, Headington, Oxford, UK*
Indications for Unicompartmental Knee Arthroplasty;
Medial Unicompartmental Knee Replacement:
Cementless Options; Mobile-Bearing Uni: Long-Term
Outcomes

Michael P. Nett, MD
*Orthopedic Surgeon, Insall Scott Kelly Institute, Southside
Hospital, Bay Shore, New York*
A Multimodal Approach to Transfusion Avoidance and
Blood Loss Management in Partial Knee Arthroplasty

Vincent Y. Ng, MD
*Clinical Instructor, Department of Orthopaedics, The Ohio
State University, Columbus, Ohio*
Deep Vein Thrombosis Prophylaxis following
Unicompartmental Knee Arthroplasty

Hemant Pandit, FRCS (Orth), DPhil (Oxon)
*Senior Research Fellow, Nuffield Department of Orthopaedics,
Rheumatology and Musculoskeletal Sciences, University of
Oxford; Orthopaedic Surgeon, Nuffield Orthopaedic Centre,
Oxford, United Kingdom*
Indications for Unicompartmental Knee Arthroplasty;
Medial Unicompartmental Knee Replacement:
Cementless Options; Mobile-Bearing Uni: Long-Term
Outcomes

Sébastien Parratte, MD, PhD
*Assistant Professor of Orthopaedic Surgery, Faculty of Medecine,
University of the Mediterranée; Consultant in the Hospital for
Arthritis Surgery, Sainte Marguerite Hospital, Universitary
Hospital of Marseille, Marseille, France*
Medial Unicompartmental Knee Arthroplasty:
Fixed-Bearing Techniques

Andrew Price, DPhil, FRCS (Orth)
*Reader in Musculoskeletal Science, Nuffield Department of
Orthopaedics, Rheumatology and Musculoskeletal Sciences,
University of Oxford; Consultant Orthopaedic Surgeon,
Nuffield Orthopaedic Centre, Oxford, United Kingdom*
Indications for Unicompartmental Knee Arthroplasty;
Medial Unicompartmental Knee Replacement:
Cementless Options; Mobile-Bearing Uni: Long-Term
Outcomes

Daniel L. Riddle, PT, PhD
*Otto D. Payton Professor, Departments of Physical Therapy
and Orthopaedic Surgery, Virginia Commonwealth University,
Richmond, Virginia*
Incidence of Partial Knee Arthroplasty: A Growing
Phenomenon?

Lindsey Rolston, MD
*University of Indiana (affiliate); Board Certified Orthopedic
Surgery (ABOS), Henry County Center for Orthopedics and
Sports Medicine, New Castle, Indiana*
Hybrid Arthroplasty: Two-Compartment Approach

Erik P. Severson, MD
*Director of Orthopaedic Outcomes, Department of Orthopaedic
Surgery, Minnesota Center for Orthopaedics (MCO), Cuyuna
Regional Medical Center and Riverwood Hospitals,
Crosby, Minnesota*
Bilateral Unicompartmental Knee Arthroplasty

Neil P. Sheth, MD
*Attending Orthopaedic Surgeon, OrthoCarolina, Charlotte,
North Carolina*
Long-Term Patellofemoral Progression

Rafael J. Sierra, MD
*Associate Professor, Mayo Clinic College of Medicine;
Consultant Orthopedic Surgeon, Mayo Clinic,
Rochester, Minnesota*
Bilateral Unicompartmental Knee Arthroplasty

Alfred J. Tria, Jr., AB, MD
*Clinical Professor of Orthopaedic Surgery, Robert Wood
Johnson Medical School; Chief of Orthopaedic Surgery,
St. Peter's University Hospital, New Brunswick, New Jersey*
Classical Patient Selection for Unicondylar Knee
Arthroplasty

Creighton C. Tubb, MD
*Adjunct Assistant Professor of Surgery, Uniformed Services
University of the Health Sciences, Bethesda, Maryland;
Orthopaedic Surgeon, Madigan Army Medical Center,
Tacoma, Washington*
Lateral Unicompartmental Knee Arthroplasty

John H. Velyvis, MD
*Director of Clinical Research, Coon Joint Replacement
Institute, St. Helena Hospital, St. Helena, California*
Computer-Guided Partial Knee Replacement

Preface

At this time, we would like to thank all of our friends and fellow partial knee zealots who have assisted not only with the production of this book but who have also supported our annual CIPKA meeting and the SOURCE Initiative. Aside from our love for acronyms, we truly give thanks for the hard work and cooperation of our orthopaedic colleagues.

Partial knee arthroplasty encompasses those treatments of knee pathology that involve treatment of the knee in a compartmental approach. Such treatments, and this book, include nonoperative arthritic modalities, arthroscopic treatments, single and double compartment replacements—anything short of a total knee arthroplasty.

CIPKA, Current Issues in Partial Knee Arthroplasty, is now celebrating its fourth year. The event is a 3-day meeting that is dedicated to the education and advancement of partial knee arthroplasty. This meeting has been successful in part because of the involvement of Adolph Lombardi, Jr., our co-chairman.

Adolph brings a wealth of knowledge, excitement, and organization to the meeting. But the success is also due to our well-known faculty who give up time from their practice and families to attend this meeting on an annual basis.

SOURCE, the Study Group of Unicompartmental Research and Continuing Education, is in its early stages and was developed to link like-minded physicians interested in further studying the area of partial knee arthroplasty. Ongoing projects include multicenter studies on the indications, outcomes, and techniques of partial knee arthroplasty.

Through this textbook, the annual CIPKA meeting, and ongoing projects through SOURCE, the authors continue to strive for improvement in the level of care readers can provide to their patients. Together, we hope to improve the science of partial knee arthroplasty.

Keith R. Berend, MD
Fred D. Cushner, MD

Contents

Video Contents

SECTION 1
Uni History

CHAPTER 1
Uni: History and Look to the Future

Gerard A. Engh

KEY POINTS

- The early clinical results with unicondylar implants often included results in which the implants were used to replace the tibio-femoral compartments of both condyles with independent components.
- The use of polyethylene less than 6 mm thick and without metal backing accounted for early failures with the Marmor implant. The FDA now requires a minimum thickness for polyethylene of greater than 6 mm.
- Factors that led to higher failure rates of unicondylar implants included younger age, male gender, and most importantly gamma-in-air sterilization. A prolonged shelf age led to oxidative degradation of the tibial polyethylene.
- Early failures with unicondylar arthroplasty are related mostly to technical errors with surgical technique and component malposition.
- Surgeons have a bias against revising a painful total knee without a known cause but little bias against revising a painful unicondylar knee.

EARLY CLINICAL EXPERIENCE WITH UNICONDYLAR IMPLANTS

The earliest nonlinked implants for the management of gonarthrosis were mostly unicompartmental implants often used to replace both the tibial and femoral compartments of the knee. The Polycentric knee was described in 1971 as an implant to restore normal knee movement.[1] The probability of success of the first 209 Polycentric implants performed at the Mayo Clinic between July 1970 and November 1971 was 66% at 10 years.[2] Results were similar when this implant was used for single-compartment replacement.[3] These devices, which were single-radius femoral components, were subsequently abandoned for treating arthritis in both single and bicompartmental arthritis of the knee.

During the same time interval, surgeons were having early clinical success when using the Marmor (Richards, Memphis,

TN) knee as a unicompartmental implant. The clinical results, however, did not appear in the literature in a timely fashion. In 1981, Scott and Santore reported early encouraging results with only three revisions in the first 100 patients with a different unicondylar implant.[4] Unfortunately, these early encouraging results were overshadowed by inferior results reported by others. In 1976, Insall and Walker had already reported a high failure rate in 19 knees with medial unicompartmental implants of a different design.[5] The authors had satisfactory outcomes with 5 lateral unicondylar arthroplasties and related that the use of unicondylar implants in the future may only be indicated for such deformities. In a subsequent report involving many of the same patients, Insall and Aglietti reported 7 conversions to another knee prosthesis and 14 fair or poor results from a group of 22 knees.[6] This implant had a coronal curved-on-curved design, and 12 of the 22 cases underwent a concomitant patellectomy. Likewise, Laskin experienced and reported discouraging results in 37 patients with unicondylar implants because of recurrent pain, prosthetic settling, and progression of arthritis.[7]

Oxford meniscal-bearing implants were introduced a decade after traditional fixed-bearing unicondylar implants. The earliest clinical results were reported in 1986 by Goodfellow and O'Connor on 125 cases with 2- to 6-year follow-up.[8] These early cases also were bicompartmental replacements with unicondylar implants similar to the earliest cases with fixed-bearing unicondylar implants. The early revision rate was 4.8% for knees that had intact anterior cruciate ligaments (ACLs). The survivorship for all osteoarthritis knees was 83% at 6 years. In a subsequent study of 301 knees followed as long as 9 years, Goodfellow and O'Connor further emphasized the need to have an intact ACL with meniscal-bearing implants.[9] Knees in which the ACL was damaged or absent had a survival rate of only 81% at 6 years. Two hundred five of the 301 cases were bicompartmental arthroplasties. In comparison, Murray et al. reported the outcome of 143 medial unicompartmental arthroplasties in which the Oxford implant was used in knees with an intact ACL.[10] In this 1998 report, the survival rate of the implants used as unicompartmental replacements was 98% at 10 years.

Swedish Knee Arthroplasty Register—Early Reports

The Swedish Knee Arthroplasty Register, initiated in 1981, has provided invaluable information as it relates to the outcome of knee arthroplasty surgery and insight into some of the problems that impacted the clinical results. Knutson et al. reported the results of a nationwide survey of over 30,000 knees operated on between 1976 and 1992.[11] Total knee components showed gradually improving survival, whereas unicompartmental prostheses did not. The authors reported that this was partly because of newly introduced inferior unicondylar designs that had high failure rates. A survey was mailed to all living patients in the Registry who were operated on between 1981 and 1995 to address the issues of reoperation and patient satisfaction.[12] Ninety-five percent of patients answered this survey. Eight percent of patients were dissatisfied. When revision was necessary, the proportion of satisfied patients was higher among patients who underwent a medial unicompartmental knee arthroplasty (UKA) revision than for patients revised following a failed total knee arthroplasty (TKA). Another review of Swedish register data compared the outcome for 699 Oxford (Biomet, Bridgend, UK) UKAs to a matched group of Marmor (Smith & Nephew Richards, Orthez, France) UKAs for unicompartmental arthroplasty.[13] After 6 years, the revision rate for the Oxford group was more than two times the revision rate of the Marmor group. Meniscal-bearing dislocation and component loosening were the two main reasons for the 50 Oxford revisions in this cohort of patients.

Unicondylar Arthroplasty in the 1990s

Unicondylar implants fell out of favor among most orthopaedic surgeons during the decade of the 1990s. In 1991, Scott et al. reported that bicompartmental arthroplasties with a condylar prosthesis done in the 1970s had a longer survivorship.[14] In this study, the survivorship of 100 consecutive UKAs was 85% at 10 years. Kozinn and Scott also reported very strict criteria for unicondylar arthroplasty to include weight less than 180 pounds, noninflammatory arthritis, an intact ACL, and no evidence of degenerative changes greater than grade II in the opposite and patellofemoral compartments.[15] The authors felt that strict selection criteria were essential to avoid failures from progression of disease and failures from implant loosening. Using such strict criteria limited the number of surgical candidates for a unicondylar arthroplasty to less than 5%. Proponents of tricompartmental arthroplasty argued that most orthopedic surgeons in the United States do less than 20 knee arthroplasty cases a year. Therefore, they would only have an opportunity to do 1 or 2 unicondylar procedures a year using strict selection criteria and would have difficulty maintaining the necessary technical proficiency for consistently good clinical results. Furthermore, Padgett et al. related that revision surgery for a failed unicondylar implant was not always a simple procedure.[16] In this series of 19 revisions, 76% had osseous defects and two cases required re-revision surgery.

A small number of surgeons advocated UKA for unicompartmental disease and continued to report the benefits of a smaller and less invasive surgical procedure in contrast to full knee arthroplasty. Benefits to the knee with a unicondylar implant included: less blood loss, better flexion in the knee, dominant use of the knee on stairs, and a lesser need for ambulatory aids. Also, patients had better pain relief with the UKA and preferred the UKA to the TKA. Such benefits were reported in studies by Cobb et al. comparing 42 patients who had a TKA in 1 knee and a UKA in the other,[17] by Rougraff et al. comparing 120 UKAs to 81 TKAs,[18] and by Laurencin et al. comparing 23 patients who had a UKA in 1 knee and a TKA in the other knee during a single hospitalization.[19] Knutson et al. had reported earlier from the Swedish Knee Arthroplasty Register data a statistically significant reduction in rate of infection by more than 50% with a unicondylar arthroplasty (0.8% with UKA vs. 2% with TKA).[20]

The use of unicondylar implants remained sparse through the 1990s. Although patient satisfaction remained high, the revision rates remained marginal. Some of these failures were design issues. As an example, the Robert Brigham implant offered a metal-backed nonmodular tibia that was 6 mm thick. The polyethylene was 4 mm thick. The original Marmor implant had an all-polyethylene tibia that was less than 6 mm thick. Such components had high early failure rates and were withdrawn from the market. As early as 1991, Knutson et al. reported that deformation and loosening occurred in one third of the 6-mm-thick unicompartmental implants placed in rheumatoid knees and one fifth of the osteoarthritic knees within 2 years.[21] The 6-mm components had a higher loosening rate. The Food and Drug Administration (FDA) subsequently set greater than 6 mm as the minimum allowable thickness for a tibial polyethylene component. Another design error with unicondylar implants was to try to reduce contact stress by creating a significant coronal curvature to both components. Insall and Aglietti's original experience featured such a configuration.[6] The PCA unicondylar device was a curved-on-curved design in a frontal plane somewhat similar to Insall's original implant. This implant had an unacceptable failure rate as reported in the Norwegian and Finnish knee arthroplasty registries.[22] Positioning the two components correctly in the coronal plane to allow full flexion and axial rotation was technically difficult.

Anderson Orthopaedic Research Institute Results

Four hundred eleven medial unicondylar implantations were performed at the Anderson Clinic between 1984 and 1998.[23] The implants were of 12 different designs from six different manufacturers. The Kaplan-Meier survivorship with an end point of revision was 80% at 9 years. Rather than abandoning unicondylar arthroplasty at this time because of this unacceptable revision rate, the risk factors for revision were identified and survivorship reexamined using multivariate data analysis to determine the role (if any) for unicondylar arthroplasty in the treatment of isolated unicondylar arthritis. The risk factors examined were patient factors, including age, weight, and gender, and implant variables, including polyethylene thickness, method of sterilization, shelf age of polyethylene, and implant design. Using Cox proportional hazards regression with revision as an end point, three variables were statistically significant; younger age ($p < .01$), thin polyethylene ($p < .01$), and shelf age ($p < .01$). Of the 411 medial unicondylar knees, 152 had a shelf age less than 1 year and polyethylene thickness of at least 8 mm. The survivorship for this subset of patients was 95%. Confidence was restored in this surgical procedure by using polyethylene of adequate thickness without the potential of oxidative degradation.

The impact of oxidation on the failure of knee implants is best documented in retrieval studies. The 42 unicondylar implants that were revised at the Anderson Clinic between 1986 and 2000 were cataloged as to reason for revision and then analyzed for wear. Seventy-one percent of the revisions were for polyethylene wear. An analysis of the retrieved components confirmed severe fatigue wear with delamination and in some instances wear-through of polyethylene to the underlying tibial baseplate. No revisions occurred in 42 of the 411 implants that were sterilized by methods other than gamma irradiation in air.[23] In another study, Blunn et al. examined 26 retrievals of Marmor unicondylar implants in situ from 1–13 years.[24] These nonirradiated tibial polyethylene components showed no delamination. In contrast, Williams et al. in 1998 identified delamination with subsurface white bands characteristic of oxidation in over 80% of gamma-in-air sterilized components.[25] In this study, 32 unicondylar implants sterilized by ethylene oxide had no delamination or evidence of oxidation. The impact of shelf age leading to polyethylene oxidation and its impact on survivorship was far greater for unicondylar implants because of infrequent usage of unicondylar implants and the frequent usage and popularity of total knee implants. Implants were manufactured and sterilized in large batches. Depleted inventory was replenished frequently with total knee implants. The shelf age on unicondylar implants at the Anderson Clinic averaged 2.0 ± 1.9 years. This was more than a year longer than total knee implants, which averaged 0.9 ± 1.0 years (AORI Knee Clinic Database). Two studies best demonstrate the impact of shelf age on implant survivorship. In the first study, 100 consecutive SCR (Osteonics, Allendale, NJ) UKA components with an average shelf age of 1.7 years after gamma irradiation in air were divided into two equal groups: shelf age greater than 1.7 versus shelf age less than 1.7 years.[26] The survivorship at 6 years was 96% for

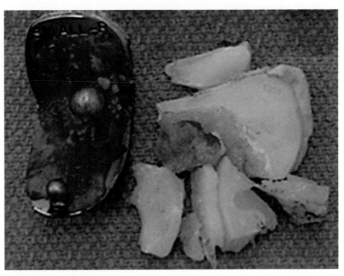

Figure 1-1 Embrittlement from prolonged shelf storage (4.5 years) of a failed UKA implant in situ only 18 months.

the shorter shelf-age group versus 71% for the group with the longer shelf age ($p < .01$). The second study was a review of 75 Duracon (Stryker Osteonics Howmedica, Rutherford, NJ) unicondylar implants (**Fig. 1–1**).[27] Seventy-three of the components had a shelf-age storage of 4.5–6.5 years. Since publication of that study, 65 of the 75 implants were revised in less than 5 years, with all revisions performed for accelerated polyethylene wear.

Unicondylar Implants That Were Successful in the 1990s

Historically, some unicondylar fixed-bearing implants that were performed in the 1980s and 1990s faired well. Squire et al. reported an 84% survivorship at 22 years using revision for any reason with the original Marmor implant with an all-polyethylene tibial component.[28] This implant was minimally congruent, and success was probably related to non-gamma sterilization (most early implants were sterilized with ethylene oxide) and precise surgical technique as this was a single senior surgeon experience. Berger et al. reported a 10-year survivorship of 98% for 51 patients with the Miller-Galante implant.[29] The method of polyethylene sterilization is not reported. The implant probably had a short shelf age if gamma irradiated in air, as this was the surgeon-designers' initial clinical experience with this implant. In another study, Pennington et al. reported 98% retained components at a mean follow-up of 11 years with the same Miller-Galante implant in young, active patients (mean age of 54 years).[30] Some early studies with mobile bearings were equally promising. Murray et al. reported a 98% survivorship at 10 years with the Oxford mobile-bearing unicondylar knee.[31] Again this was a series of cases done by surgeon-designers in a select subset of patients including only knees that had an intact ACL. In addition, better contact stresses made this implant less sensitive to fatigue modes of wear. The benefits of lower contact stress with a mobile-bearing implant probably contributed to the excellent outcome with 124 Oxford implants with a 10- to 15-year survivorship in a study by Svard and Price.[32]

Although excellent unicondylar results began appearing in the literature, survivorship from other studies and joint registry data continued to favor TKA. Once again, the reader of these reports can either accept this information at face value or take more than a cursory look at the data that led to these conclusions and determine the feasibility for unicondylar arthroplasty for unicondylar disease. As an example, in 2003 Gioe et al. reported the 10-year survivorship for 516 UKAs in comparison with 4654 TKAs from a regional joint registry.[33] The survivorship at 10 years was 88.6% for UKAs versus 94.8% for TKAs during the same time interval. Two confounding variables may have dramatically impacted these findings. First, the authors reported that two thirds of the UKAs were sterilized by gamma irradiation in air but the shelf age was not reported. More than likely, the shelf age of the unicondylar implants in this study was significantly longer than the total knee implants. The second variable was the Kirchner implant that was inserted in 34 of the 516 unicondylar cases. This implant alone accounted for 38% (15/39) of the UKA failures in the study. If the 34 Kirschner implants were excluded from the analysis, the revision rate for UKAs would be 5% (24/482); hence 95% of the implants would remain in situ after 10 years. Without the Kirschner UKA in the analysis, the survivorship of UKA implants would be similar to that of the TKA implants in this study.

MINIMALLY INVASIVE SURGERY: AN EPIPHANY FOR UKA

Minimally invasive surgery became an epiphany for the popularity of and demand for unicondylar arthroplasty. John Repicci, a dentist turned orthopaedic surgeon, reported his clinical experience performing medial compartment arthroplasties through a 3-inch incision with next-day or same-day discharge and a rapid recovery. The concept of minimally invasive surgery was attractive to orthopaedic surgeons, appealing to patients, and extremely marketable by the implant industry. Still, because the arthroplasty industry was composed of so few unicondylar procedures and mainly total knee procedures, the manufacturers' initial focus was to modify instruments that would enable surgeons to perform total knee procedures through limited incisions. Terms such as "quad-sparing approach" and "mini-midvastus approach" were created to describe such surgical approaches. Many surgeons found such TKA procedures difficult and somewhat compromising to their clinical results. Unicondylar implants were much more amenable to small incisions simply because the implants were smaller and easier to insert through a small incision, creating a rejuvenation of interest in unicondylar arthroplasty surgery.

The popularity and demand for minimally invasive techniques led to the introduction of new unicondylar implants and instruments modified for minimally invasive procedures. Surgeons were learning a new surgical procedure with new instruments and implants but with little or no previous experience with traditional unicondylar surgery. The early clinical results with unicondylar procedures reflect the impact of these variables. In some instances the complications were clearly secondary to the limited surgical exposure. Hamilton et al. reported an increase in new complications and modes of failure not previously reported.[34] Wound complications, most likely, were secondary to overzealous soft tissue retraction with small incisions. Retained cement fragments, not encountered with traditional surgical exposures, were secondary to limited surgical exposure to the back of the knee with small incisions. Femoral loosening was probably related to a change in implant design and instrumentation to accommodate implant insertion through a limited surgical approach. As an example in Hamilton et al.'s study, the single femoral peg parallel to the posterior condylar bone cut made implant insertion easier but was not optimal for femoral component fixation. Very thin bone resections were secondary to implant and instrument modifications that did not expose adequate porous bone for optimal cement penetration and contributed to the early femoral loosening. The placement of multiple small drill holes in areas of dense sclerotic bone to allow cement penetration is now advocated to address the problem of early component loosening (**Fig. 1–2**).

The impact of surgical experience is best reflected in joint registry data. The Swedish Knee Arthroplasty Register reports

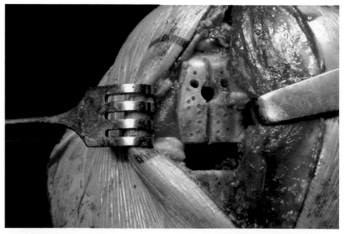

Figure 1-2 Drill holes enhance cement penetration and fixation of the femoral component.

? UKA AND EARLY REVISIONS

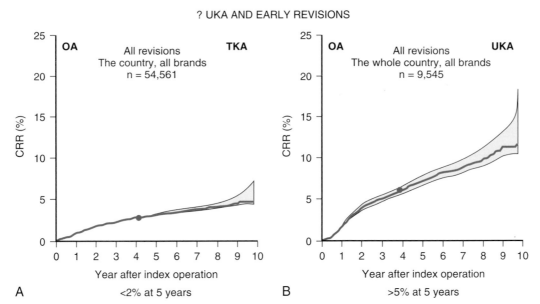

Figure 1-3 Higher failure rates in the first 4 years with unicondylar implants. (Reprinted with permission from Department of Orthopedics. The Swedish Knee Arthroplasty Registry—Annual Report 2007-Part II. Lund, Sweden: Lund University Hospital, 2007, pp 26, 29.)

a more than threefold increase in the revision rate of Oxford unicompartmental knees for institutions that perform fewer than 23 procedures per year.[35] This limited experience factor is also evident from other registries. The 2004 Australian Knee Registry report includes a revision rate of 5.9 to 7.4 for implants, with more than 100 revisions per year. The New Zealand registry for implants inserted from 2000 to 2006 documented revision rates from 3.4 to 6.4 for the most commonly used components. In essence, surgeons with little surgical experience with unicondylar arthroplasty were inserting new designs using new instruments modified for minimally invasive techniques. In the United States, where roughly 8% of knee arthroplasty cases are unicondylar implants, a surgeon doing 100 cases a year using traditional indications would perform 7 or 8 TKAs per month but only 1 UKA every other month using traditional indications for this procedure. A still unresolved question is: what volume of cases is essential to maintain adequate technical expertise with a unicondylar surgical technique?

UKA TODAY: COMPARING APPLES TO APPLES

Joint arthroplasty surgeons today must contend with the issue that the raw data from registries substantiates a higher failure rate at both 5 and 10 years with unicondylar arthroplasty procedures. In the Swedish Knee Arthroplasty Register report for 2007, the revision rate for all UKAs at 10 years was 10% as compared to 5% at 10 years for TKAs.[36] The 10-year failures somewhat reflect oxidized polyethylene with implants inserted in the 1980s and 1990s sterilized by gamma radiation in air. Implant manufacturers eliminated manufacturing and

distributing gamma sterilization in air implants in the late 1990s. This variable therefore cannot account for the early implant failures in the current joint registry reports. We can explain and address the higher early failure rates with unicondylar components inserted after the year 2000 by carefully examining knee registry data. A marked difference is noted in the slope of the curves in the first 4 years, with higher early failures for UKAs (**Fig. 1–3**). Early failures are commonly related to technical errors in the surgical procedure. The three common modes of early failure are infection, aseptic loosening, and progression of disease. Since we know that infection rates are lower with UKA, then loosening and progression of disease are the likely cause of these early failures. Early failures are most likely technical errors in surgical technique. Industry needs to focus on refined instrumentation and enhancing surgical training to resolve this problem. There is compelling support for unicondylar arthroplasty procedures in 10-year registry data, if the data are analyzed with adjustment for patient variables as well as the surgeon experience variables that are known to impact outcomes. Patient demographics are distinctly different. The most common age group for a UKA in the Swedish register is under the age of 60, with almost half the cases in this age group. The revision rate at 10 years for TKAs done in patients under the age of 60 is 13%.[37] UKAs, unlike TKAs, are not performed in patients with an inflammatory disease diagnosis. The Mayo Clinic study reported a higher survivorship in this category and a higher survivorship for female patients following TKA surgery.[38] The ratio of females to males undergoing TKA is roughly 2:1. In the 2006 Australian registry, 50% of the patients undergoing a UKA were male (ratio 1:1) and 40% were males in the 2007 Swedish

PAINFUL ARTHROPLASTY ALGORITHM

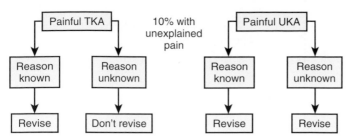

Figure 1-4 Algorithm for managing patients with unexplained pain following knee arthroplasty surgery.

Box 1-1 Controlling the Surgeon Variable in Surgical Technique

The future for knee arthroplasty will focus on controlling the surgeon variable with instruments that:
- Minimize the potential for technical errors
- Protect the soft tissues
- Control component-to-component alignment
- Optimize knee kinematics

register. Males and particularly young males have statistically higher revision rates in TKA outcome reports.[38]

One additional explanation for the continued higher failures with unicondylar surgery is that, in most outcome studies, roughly 10% of patients have fair or poor results following knee arthroplasty, without a known explanation for subjective failure. Surgeons commonly have a different bias for revision of a painful UKA than a TKA (**Fig. 1–4**). Surgeons are hesitant to revise a painful TKA without a known cause for the pain because the reported success rate with such a procedure is only 25%.[39] They are not hesitant, however, to convert a UKA to a TKA.

UKA VERSUS TKA REVISION

The conversion of a failed UKA to a TKA in the Swedish register is similar to the outcome with a primary TKA. The same is not true with revision of a failed TKA. Primary TKA components are used most of the time when a unicondylar implant is revised. The reasons for revision are quite different, with infection, wear, and osteolysis commonly the basis for a revision of a failed TKA. These are more complex revision cases that may result in poorer outcomes. Unicondylar implants are revised more frequently for unexplained pain that usually is recorded as progression of disease. Bone loss is usually not a problem with these cases, and expensive revision long-stemmed implants are not needed.

THE FUTURE FOR UKA (SEE VIDEO 1-1)

Unicondylar knee arthroplasty did not become an accepted surgical procedure for most of the orthopaedic community until the year 2000. To a certain extent UKA implants, instruments, and surgical experience are in their infancy. The results are spectacular when the procedure is properly performed and equivalent to or better than TKA, as recently reported by Newman et al. in a prospective randomized study with 15-year outcome data.[40] The literature supports excellent outcomes with both fixed- and mobile-bearing unicondylar implants

inserted with cement fixation. Correct component-to-component alignment is a variable that is not present with a TKA and comes only with surgical experience with today's traditional instrumentation. Progression of disease in the opposite compartment appears to be a rare occurrence, but overstuffing the replaced compartment to try to restore full correction of mechanical alignment is contraindicated. The status of acceptable changes in the opposite patellofemoral and tibiofemoral compartments for a successful unicompartmental arthroplasty remains controversial and requires critical prospective randomized study data. The greatest challenge, however, appears to be the surgeon variable (**Box 1–1**).

The continued early failures in registry reports will be corrected only by technologic advances in instrumentation to optimize component-to-component alignment and restore patient kinematics to allow full functional activities. To realize this goal, the preparation of the bone must be integrated with the tension in the capsular envelope of the knee in all positions of knee flexion and extension. Instruments that provide feedback to the surgeon during the procedure will integrate the relationship between bone and soft tissue tension and make knee arthroplasty a procedure that restores full functional activity to a younger and more active patient population.

Advances in imaging technology should allow for the more accurate placement of knee components during surgery. Patient-specific instruments can be designed from either computed tomography or magnetic resonance images and used to create an anatomic reconstruction of a patient's individual anatomy. Landmarks such as the epicondylar axis can be accurately and readily identified and used for creating specific instruments with imaging before surgery for performing accurate bone resections during surgery. In essence, patient-specific instruments developed with advances in imaging make surgical navigation a more accurate and user-friendly modality.

Robotics utilizes imaging technology to create a surgical plan that controls bone preparation and accurate component placement during surgery. Surgical navigation is used to register bone landmarks and to program a robotic instrument to execute the surgical plan intraoperatively. This technology adds an element of safety to the surgical procedure as the surgeon is locked out of working outside the safe zone for bone preparation.

The ultimate goal for unicondylar arthroplasty will be the development of a biologic implant for younger patients with early-onset traumatic or degenerative unicompartmental arthritis. Allograft reconstruction for degenerative lesions has proven successful particularly with unipolar lesions. The availability of satisfactory donor material remains as the main limitation to biologic reconstructions on a larger scale. A true biologic implant will incorporate chondrocytes grown in culture to populate an appropriate matrix that can be implanted to restore the surface morphology of an arthritic joint with hyaline cartilage. Techniques will be developed for the proper preparation of the degenerated articular surface, bonding of the biologic component, and protection of the biologic implant until its structural integrity and viability are complete.

REFERENCES

1. Gunston FH. Polycentric knee arthroplasty. J Bone Joint Surg [Br] 1971;53:272-277.
2. Lewallen DG, Bryan RS, Peterson LF. Polycentric total knee arthroplasty: a ten year follow-up study. J Bone Joint Surg [Am] 1984;66:1211-1218.
3. Insall JN, Ranawat CS, Aglietti P, et al. A comparison of four models of total knee-replacement prostheses. J Bone Joint Surg [Am] 1976;58:754-765.
4. Scott RD, Santore RF. Unicondylar unicompartmental replacement for osteoarthritis of the knee. J Bone Joint Surg [Am] 1981;63:536-544.
5. Insall JN, Walker P. Unicondylar knee replacement. Clin Orthop Relat Res 1976;(120):83-85.
6. Insall JN, Aglietti P. A five to seven-year follow-up of unicondylar arthroplasty. J Bone Joint Surg [Am] 1980;62:1329-1337.
7. Laskin RS. Unicompartmental tibiofemoral resurfacing arthroplasty. J Bone Joint Surg [Am] 1978;60:182-185.
8. Goodfellow JW, O'Connor J. Clinical results of the Oxford knee: surface arthroplasty of the tibiofemoral joint with a meniscal bearing prosthesis. Clin Orthop Relat Res 1986;(205):21-42.
9. Goodfellow JW, O'Connor J. The anterior cruciate ligament in knee arthroplasty: a risk factor with unconstrained meniscal prostheses. Clin Orthop Relat Res 1992;(276):245-252.
10. Murray DW, Goodfellow JW, O'Connor J. The Oxford medial unicompartmental arthroplasty: a ten-year survival study. J Bone Joint Surg [Br] 1998;80:983-989.
11. Knutson K, Lewold S, Robertsson O, et al. The Swedish Knee Arthroplasty Register: a nation-wide study of 30,003 knees 1976–1992. Acta Orthop Scand 1994;65:375-386.
12. Robertsson O, Dunbar M, Pehrsson T, et al. Patient satisfaction after knee arthroplasty: a report on 27,372 knees operated on between 1981 and 1995 in Sweden. Acta Orthop Scand 2000;71:262-267.
13. Lewold S, Goodman S, Knutson K, et al. Oxford meniscal bearing knee versus the Marmor knee in unicompartmental arthroplasty for arthrosis: a Swedish multicenter survival study. J Arthroplasty 1995;10:722-731.
14. Scott RD, Cobb AG, McQueary FG, et al. Unicompartmental knee arthroplasty: eight- to 12-year follow-up evaluation with survivorship analysis. Clin Orthop Relat Res 1991;(271):96-100.
15. Kozinn SC, Scott RD. Unicondylar knee arthroplasty. J Bone Joint Surg [Am] 1989;71:145-150.
16. Padgett DE, Stern SH, Insall JN. Revision total knee arthroplasty for failed unicompartmental replacement. J Bone Joint Surg [Am] 1991;73:186-190.
17. Cobb AG, Kozinn SC, Scott RD. Unicondylar or total knee replacement: the patient's preference. J Bone Joint Surg [Br] 1990;70:166.
18. Rougraff BT, Heck DA, Gibson AE. A comparison of tricompartmental and unicompartmental arthroplasty for the treatment of gonarthrosis. Clin Orthop Relat Res 1991;(273):157-164.
19. Laurencin CT, Zelicof SB, Scott RD, et al. Unicompartmental versus total knee arthroplasty in the same patient. Clin Orthop Relat Res 1991;(273):151-156.
20. Knutson K, Lindstrand A, Lidgren L. Survival of knee arthroplasties: a nation-wide multicentre investigation of 8000 cases. J Bone Joint Surg [Br] 1986;68:795-803.
21. Knutson K, Jonsson G, Langer Anderson J, et al. Deformation and loosening of the tibial component in knee arthroplasty with unicompartmental endoprostheses. Acta Orthop Scand 1981;52:667-673.
22. Koskinen E, Paavolainen P, Eskelinen A, et al. Unicondylar knee replacement for primary osteoarthritis: a prospective follow-up study of 1,819 patients from the Finnish Arthroplasty Register. Acta Orthop Scand 2007;78:128-135.
23. Eickmann TH, Collier MB, Sukezaki F, et al. Survival of medial unicondylar arthroplasties placed by one surgeon 1984–1998. Clin Orthop Relat Res 2006;(452):143-149.
24. Blunn GW, Joshi AB, Lilley PA, et al. Polyethylene wear in unicondylar knee prostheses: 106 retrieved Marmor, PCA, and St Georg tibial components compared. Acta Orthop Scand 1992;63:247-255.
25. Williams IR, Mayor MB, Collier JP. The impact of sterilization method on wear in knee arthroplasty. Clin Orthop Relat Res 1998;(356):170-180.
26. Collier MB, Engh CA Jr, Engh GA. Shelf age of the polyethylene tibial component and outcome of unicondylar knee arthroplasty. J Bone Joint Surg [Am] 2004:86:763-769.
27. McGovern TF, Ammeen DJ, Collier JP, et al. Rapid polyethylene failure of unicondylar tibial components sterilized with gamma irradiation in air and implanted after a long shelf life. J Bone Joint Surg [Am] 2002;84:901-906.
28. Squire MW, Callaghan JJ, Goetz DD, et al. Unicompartmental knee replacement: a minimum 15 year followup study. Clin Orthop Relat Res 1999;(367):61-72.
29. Berger RA, Nedeff DD, Barden RM, et al. Unicompartmental knee arthroplasty: clinical experience at 6- to 10-year followup. Clin Orthop Relat Res 1999;(367):50-60.
30. Pennington DW, Swienckowski JJ, Lutes WB, et al. Unicompartmental knee arthroplasty in patients sixty years of age or younger. J Bone Joint Surg [Am] 2003;85:1968-1973.
31. Murray DW, Goodfellow JW, O'Connor JJ. The Oxford medial unicompartmental arthroplasty. J Bone Joint Surg [Br] 1998;80:983-989.
32. Svard UCG, Price AJ. Oxford medial unicompartmental knee arthroplasty: a survival study. J Bone Joint Surg [Br] 2001;83:191-194.

33. Gioe TJ, Killeen KK, Hoeffel DP, et al. Analysis of unicompartmental knee arthroplasty in a community-based implant registry. Clin Orthop Relat Res 2003;(416):111-119.

34. Hamilton WG, Collier MB, Tarabee E, et al. Incidence and reasons for reoperation after minimally invasive unicompartmental knee arthroplasty. J Arthroplasty 2006;21(6 Suppl 2):98-107.

35. Department of Orthopedics. The Swedish Knee Arthroplasty Register—Annual Report 2004, Part I. Lund, Sweden: Lund University Hospital, 2004, p 6.

36. Department of Orthopedics. The Swedish Knee Arthroplasty Register—Annual Report 2007, Part II. Lund, Sweden: Lund University Hospital, 2007, pp 26-29.

37. Harrysson OLA, Robertsson O, Nayfeh JF. Higher cumulative revision rate of knee arthroplasties in younger patients with osteoarthritis. Clin Orthop Relat Res 2004;(421):162-168.

38. Rand JA, Trousdale RT, Ilstrup DM, et al. Factors affecting the durability of primary total knee prostheses. J Bone Joint Surg [Am] 2003;85:259-265.

39. Mont MA, Serna FK, Krackow KA, et al. Exploration of radiographically normal total knee replacements for unexplained pain. Clin Orthop Relat Res 1996;(331):216-220.

40. Newman J, Pydisetty RV, Ackroyd C. Unicompartmental or total knee replacement: the 15-year results of a prospective randomized controlled trial. J Bone Joint Surg [Br] 2009;91:52-57.

CHAPTER 2

Classical Patient Selection for Unicondylar Knee Arthroplasty

Alfred J. Tria, Jr.

KEY POINTS

- The patient must be able to indicate the location of the knee pain along the medial joint line in the varus knee.
- The physical examination of the knee must confirm the location of the tenderness along the medial joint line with minimal to no tenderness in all other areas.
- The varus of the knee should be correctable to neutral on valgus stress.
- The ACL should be intact to physical examination (the anterior drawer test should be negative even if the ACL is absent on an MRI examination).
- The radiograph should show no greater than 10° of deformity in all planes with no translocation of the tibia beneath the femur.

INTRODUCTION

Unicondylar knee arthroplasty (UKA) has progressed through two separate time phases since the original designs were developed in the early 1970s. The first phase was fraught with problems related to the prosthetic designs and patient selection.[1-4] The results were good to excellent for the first 10 years after the surgery in the hands of the designing surgeons. In the second decade the results did tend to taper off and were not as good as the reports of total knee arthroplasty (TKA).[5,6] It was difficult for the standard orthopaedic surgeon to reproduce the findings of the designers, and interest decreased in the late 1980s and early 1990s. Insall's data showed that only 6% of knees satisfied the criteria for UKA, and he favored TKA as the procedure of choice.[7]

Repicci introduced the limited surgical approach (minimally invasive surgery, or MIS) for UKA in the early 1990s, and interest in the procedure increased by the year 2000.[8-13] Newer designs appeared, and the Oxford mobile-bearing UKA became very popular both in Europe and in the United States.[14,15] With this new wave of interest, surgeons looked to improve the clinical results and reviewed the patient selection criteria, the surgical approach, and instruments. If the incorrect patient is chosen, the result will be compromised despite excellent surgical technique and prosthetic design. This chapter outlines the factors involved in the choice process that should lead to a more satisfactory overall result.

HISTORY

It is important to understand the patient's complaints and disability secondary to the arthritic knee. The underlying cause of the arthritis should become evident during the course of the interview. Inflammatory arthritis is not typically acceptable for UKA because the synovial reaction in the knee tends to involve all of the compartments of the knee in an equal fashion, and partial replacement will not adequately address the problem. Previous history of infection, obesity (with a body mass index > 33 or a weight > 225 pounds), and multiple ligament injury to the knee are relative contraindications. The patient should be able to identify the location of the pain on the joint line either medially or laterally. If the patient either cannot localize the pain or is confused about it, the procedure should not be considered. Patellofemoral symptoms are a relative contraindication, and if there are more symptoms with stair climbing than on level surfaces, UKA is probably not indicated. While the reports using a mobile-bearing UKA tend to ignore or deemphasize the importance of the patellofemoral joint, other authors have indicated that this area can lead to significant symptomatology and compromise of the result.

If the opposite knee has been replaced, the surgeon should evaluate the result with the patient. If the result of the previous surgery is excellent, the same procedure should certainly be considered for the other knee because the excellent result becomes the standard for comparison and will be difficult to equal and certainly more difficult to exceed. If the first result is equivocal, the choice for the second side is much easier. The pain should be localized and should be aggravated with activity and better with rest. If the pain is much worse with rest and at night during sleep, the diagnostic evaluation should be even more thorough to be sure that there is no other underlying condition, such as infection or inflammatory arthritis. If the patient has not had any previous replacements, the opposite side should also be evaluated at the same time with the same questions and discussion.

LABORATORY TESTS

There are some pertinent tests for UKA in order to better guarantee the clinical result. If the erythrocyte sedimentation rate and C-reactive protein are both elevated, the possibility of underlying infection should certainly be ruled out. Patients who are seropositive for the inflammatory arthritides (rheumatoid arthritis, lupus, and gout) should not have a UKA because of the prevalence of the synovitis in the entire joint space.

PHYSICAL EXAMINATION

The examination should include inspection of the gait and, then, the full evaluation of both lower extremities. There should be a component of antalgia to the gait, and any thrust of the femur on the tibia through the stance phase should especially be noted. As the deformity progresses either in the varus or the valgus knee, the collateral ligament on the compressed side of the joint shortens and the ligament on the tension side lengthens. This ultimately leads to shifting of the tibia beneath the femur with impingement of the lateral tibial spine against the lateral femoral condyle in the varus knee and impingement of the medial tibial spine against the medial femoral condyle in the valgus knee (**Fig. 2–1**). The shift of the tibia correlates with a lateral thrust of the femur on the tibia through the stance phase of gait in the varus knee and a medial thrust in the valgus knee (**Fig. 2–2**). This finding is a relative contraindication to UKA and should alert the examiner to correlate the physical finding with the standing anteroposterior radiograph.

The range of motion of the knee should be at least 5–105° of flexion. A flexion contracture of 5° can be partially corrected with the UKA; however, any greater degree of deformity will not be correctable and will lead to difficulty with the required flexion-extension balancing during the surgical procedure. The knee does not have to flex completely normally, but 105° will permit proper flexion exposure during the surgery and allow for functional motion afterward. UKA will not increase the preexisting motion.

The ligaments of the knee should all be intact for an ideal replacement. There will most certainly be some collateral ligament laxity as the deformity increases in either varus or valgus; however, there should be a distinct end point to the stress test for each collateral. The varus deformity should not exceed 5° and should correct to neutral on stress examination in the

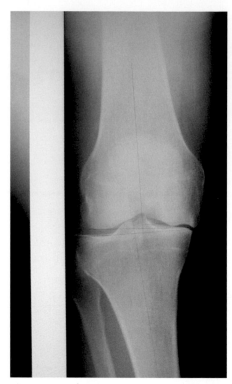

Figure 2-1 The tibia has translocated beneath the femur with impingement of the lateral tibial spine into the lateral femoral condyle.

ideal case. The standard UKA does not include collateral ligament releases as in TKA (see Videos 2-1 and 2-2).

If the deformity is fixed and greater than 5°, the tibial cut will be deeper in order to accommodate the prosthetic thickness. This deeper cut can lead to increased loss of bone and metaphyseal fracture (**Fig. 2–3**). The valgus deformity can be as great as 10° but should correct passively to 5°.

Cruciate ligament deficiency is a relative contraindication. When the posterior cruciate ligament is torn, the drop-back of the tibia beneath the femur will lead to increased wear across the polyethylene surface and an earlier failure. If the anterior cruciate ligament (ACL) is torn and there is excess motion to either the anterior drawer test or the Lachman test, UKA is once again contraindicated. However, in most cases, the ACL may be torn at the time of the surgical procedure but there will be no significant laxity to the knee on physical examination. This often occurs because the knee has progressed with arthritis and the spurs and irregularities of the joint surface prohibit excess motion. When this is the case, the absent ACL is not a contraindication.

In the varus knee, the majority of the tenderness should be along the medial joint line. In the valgus knee it should be along the lateral side. These physical findings should correlate with the patient's description of the pain. There may be a small effusion; however, if the effusion is large, the examiner should

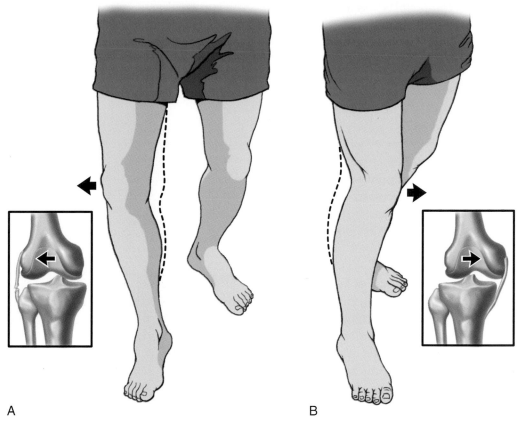

A   B

Figure 2-2 (A) In the varus knee, the femur will shift laterally on the tibia through the stance phase of gait as the deformity increases.
(B) In the valgus knee, the femur will shift medially on the tibia through the stance phase of gait as the deformity increases.

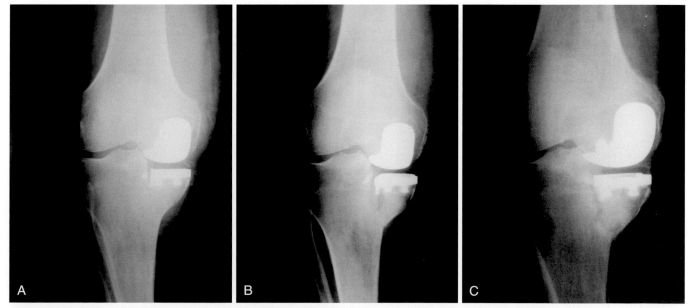

Figure 2-3 (A) The postoperative anteroposterior radiograph shows the UKA well aligned but the tibial resection level is deep secondary to the fixed deformity of 10° that was too great for the procedure. **(B)** Fracture of the tibial metaphysis with some displacement distally but without angulation. **(C)** The fracture healed without repeat surgery.

suspect more involved tricompartmental disease and be more hesitant to suggest a UKA. The extensor mechanism should be normal with no evidence of lateral patellar tracking (especially in the valgus knee). Slight patellofemoral crepitus is acceptable, but if there is marked crepitation with motion of the patella, the examiner should be more critical of the patellofemoral joint.

IMAGING STUDIES

The primary imaging tool is the standing full-length radiograph. This allows the examiner to determine the mechanical axis of the limb and the associated joint space narrowing on the medial or lateral aspect of the joint. It is valuable to measure both the anatomic axis and the mechanical axis. There should be no greater than 5° of anatomic varus and 10° of valgus (**Fig. 2–4**). This should correlate with the physical examination findings. Translocation of the tibia beneath the femur on the standing view indicates that the disease is progressing with involvement of the opposite compartment (see Fig. 2–1). As such, it is a relative contraindication. The anteroposterior flexed view will show more detail of the posterior femoral condyles within the notch, and the posteroanterior flexed view will give more details about the loss of joint space on either the medial or lateral side. The lateral view will show the extent of patellofemoral disease, and if there is more than mild involvement, the patient should be examined and interviewed again to be sure that there are minimal symptoms attributable to this joint. In a similar fashion, there should be limited involvement of the opposite femorotibial joint on the radiograph, and this should also correlate with the history and

physical examination. There is no doubt that there will always be a certain degree of arthritic disease in the entire knee; however, the primary involvement should be the medial or lateral femorotibial joint.

Magnetic resonance imaging (MRI) has become a very common tool for evaluation of the knee. Oftentimes, this

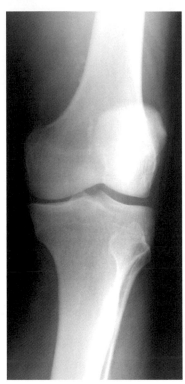

Figure 2-4 The ideal varus knee with medial narrowing and deformity less than 5°.

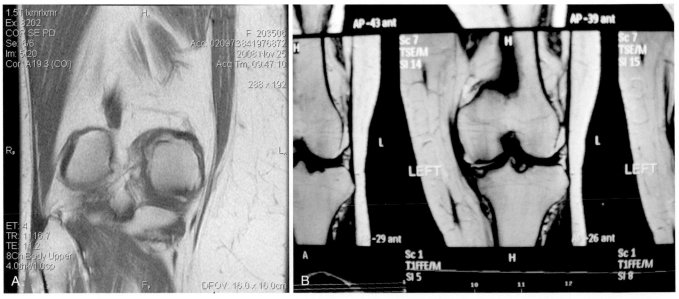

Figure 2-5 (A) Avascular necrosis of the medial femoral condyle in the resolving phase. **(B)** Avascular necrosis of the medial tibial plateau in the resolved phase.

study is requested before any radiographs are completed, and this is a mistake in the diagnostic chain. However, there are times when the MRI is valuable in combination with the appropriate radiographs. Sudden onset of distinct pain on the medial aspect of the knee often correlates with avascular necrosis, and it is important to make this diagnosis. If the event is recent, there will be hemorrhage into the medial femoral condyle or (less commonly) into the medial tibial metaphyseal area (**Fig. 2–5**). It is important to allow this early event to progress and mature with protected weight bearing before considering any UKA. If the hemorrhage is in the early phases, surgical intervention may lead to extensive loss of bone in the involved area and may require a TKA with complex augments to make up for the bone loss. After the avascular necrosis has matured, the remaining defect will be quite evident and it is usually surrounded by sclerotic bone that is much more amenable to UKA. On occasion, the patient may present with joint line pain medially and instability that may be secondary to pathology in the opposite lateral compartment. The author does not favor routine arthroscopy at the time of the UKA and does not favor routine MRI studies. However, MRI is a good tool to evaluate the lateral compartment and the lateral meniscus when there is a significant clinical suspicion. If the lateral meniscus is torn and the lateral compartment is also arthritic on the MRI, the surgeon should rethink the UKA and consider TKA.

Computed tomography or arthrography of the knee are both infrequent studies but may be considered when a patient has a pacemaker and cannot undergo MRI evaluation. Technetium scans of the knee are sometimes valuable to pinpoint the area of primary arthritic involvement and also allow a visual comparison to the other areas of the knee (**Fig. 2–6**).

CONCLUSIONS

The results of UKA can be equally successful as TKA if the correct indications are followed.[10] In a busy practice, UKA can represent 10–15% of the operative knee arthroplasty cases. It is extremely important to combine all three arms of the evaluation: history, physical examination, and imaging. If any one

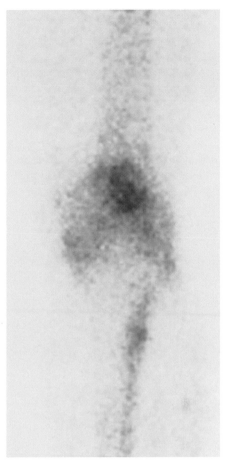

Figure 2-6 A technetium scan of a varus knee showing greater involvement of the patellofemoral joint than the medial joint, making UKA less desirable.

of these is questionable, it is best to abandon the UKA and consider TKA. However, if there are only relative contraindications in each of the three areas, the UKA can be performed with excellent results. The hesitant surgeon will often find reasons to abandon the UKA when the patient may very well be an excellent case for the surgery. The author has never abandoned the UKA during the operative procedure, and all decisions should be made well before the surgical procedure so that both the surgeon and the patient will be well prepared for the postoperative management and therapy.

REFERENCES

1. Marmor L. Marmor modular knee in unicompartmental disease: minimum four-year follow-up. J Bone Joint Surg [Am] 1979;61: 347-353.
2. Insall J, Walker P. Unicondylar knee replacement. Clin Orthop Relat Res 1976;(120):83-85.
3. Laskin RS. Unicompartment tibiofemoral resurfacing arthroplasty. J Bone Joint Surg [Am] 1978;60:182-185.
4. Goodfellow J, O'Connor J. The mechanics of the knee and prosthesis design. J Bone Joint Surg [Br] 1978;60:358-369.
5. Marmor L. Unicompartmental arthroplasty of the knee with a minimum of 10-year follow-up. Clin Orthop Relat Res 1988;(228): 171-177.
6. Scott RD, Cobb AG, McQueary FG, Thornhill TS. Unicompartmental knee arthroplasty: eight to twelve year follow-up with survivorship analysis. Clin Orthop Relat Res 1991;(271):96-100.
7. Stern SH, Becker MW, Insall J. Unicompartmental knee arthroplasty: an evaluation of selection criteria. Clin Orthop Relat Res 1993;(286):143-148.

8. Repicci JA, Eberle RW. Minimally invasive surgical technique for uni-condylar knee arthroplasty. J South Orthop Assoc 1999;8(1):20-27.

9. Romanowski MR, Repicci JA. Minimally invasive unicondylar arthroplasty: eight year follow-up. J Knee Surg 2002;15:17-22.

10. Berger RA, Nedeff DD, Barden RN, et al. Unicompartmental knee arthroplasty. Clin Orthop Relat Res 1999;(367):50-60.

11. Svard UCG, Price AJ. Oxford medial unicompartmental knee arthroplasty: a survival analysis of an independent series. J Bone Joint Surg [Br] 2001;83:191-194.

12. Price AJ, Webb J, Topf H, et al, and the Oxford Hip and Knee Group. Rapid recovery after Oxford Unicompartmental Arthroplasty through a short incision. J Arthroplasty 2001;16:970-976.

13. Gesell MW, Tria AJ. MIS unicondylar knee arthroplasty: surgical approach and early results. Clin Orthop Rel Res 2004;(428): 53-60.

14. Beard DJ, Pandit H, Gill HS, et al. The influence of the presence and severity of pre-existing patellofemoral degenerative changes on the outcome of the Oxford medial unicompartmental knee replacement. J Bone Joint Surg [Br] 2007;89:1597-1601.

15. Beard DJ, Pandit H, Ostlere S, et al. Pre-operative clinical and radiological assessment of the patellofemoral joint in unicompartmental knee replacement and its influence on outcome. J Bone Joint Surg [Br] 2007;89:1602-1607.

CHAPTER 3

Indications for Unicompartmental Knee Arthroplasty

Hemant Pandit, Benjamin Kendrick, Nicholas Bottomley, Andrew Price, David Murray, and Christopher Dodd

KEY POINTS

- Unique design features of the Oxford UKA minimize wear and make the implant "patella friendly."
- Principal indications for medial UKA are anteromedial osteoarthritis and avascular necrosis (also called spontaneous osteonecrosis of the knee).
- There should be "bone-on-bone" contact in the affected medial compartment with a functionally intact ACL and varus correctible if present.
- Contraindications described by Kozinn and Scott are unnecessary for the Oxford UKA.

INTRODUCTION

This chapter provides an overview of the indications and contraindications for unicompartmental knee arthroplasty (UKA), with specific reference to the Oxford UKA. The Oxford UKA has a fully congruent, freely mobile meniscal bearing that is free to slide and rotate between the congruent surfaces of the spherical femur and flat tibia, and this congruency is maintained in all positions throughout the range of movement of the knee joint.[1] These unique design features help in minimizing wear[2] and also make the implant "patella friendly." Therefore, the indications outlined in this chapter have a specific reference to (or evidence for) the Oxford UKA, and generalization of all these indications for any other design of UKA may not be possible.

INDICATIONS

The principal indications for a medial Oxford UKA are anteromedial osteoarthritis (AMOA)[3] (**Fig. 3–1**), and avascular necrosis (also known as spontaneous osteonecrosis of the knee, or SONK)[1] (**Fig. 3–2**). AMOA, the most common indication for UKA, is a distinct entity, and it can be recognized by a consistent association between the clinicoradiologic signs and the pathologic lesions that cause them.[1]

Principal Physical Signs

The patient usually presents with a painful knee, pain being mainly noted when the patient stands and/or on walking. This may or may not be associated with swelling. Examination reveals that the leg is in varus alignment (usually 5–15°), and this deformity cannot be corrected in extension (as near-full extension as possible). However, this deformity can be corrected by valgus stress with the knee flexed 20° or more, and the deformity corrects spontaneously with the knee flexed to 90°.

Principal Anatomic Features

At surgery, knees with the above physical signs almost always demonstrate functionally normal cruciate ligaments, though the anterior cruciate ligament (ACL) may have suffered surface damage. In addition, the articular cartilage on the tibia is eroded, and eburnated bone is exposed, in an area that extends from the anteromedial margin of the medial plateau for a variable distance posteriorly but never as far as the posterior margin. An area of full-thickness cartilage is always present, preserved at the back of the plateau. Similarly, the cartilage on the distal articular surface of the medial femoral condyle is eroded, and eburnated bone is exposed. The posterior surface of the femoral condyle retains its full-thickness cartilage. The articular cartilage of the lateral compartment, although often fibrillated, preserves its full thickness. The medial collateral ligament (MCL) is of normal length and the posterior capsule is shortened.

Correlations

Intact cruciate ligaments and MCL can explain the symptoms and physical signs.[1] Cruciate ligaments maintain the normal pattern of roll-back ("physiological roll-back") of the femur on the tibia in the sagittal plane and thereby preserve the distinction between the damaged contact areas in extension (the anterior tibial plateau and the distal surface of the medial femoral condyle) and the intact contact areas in flexion (the posterior tibial plateau and the posterior surface of the femoral condyle). The shortened posterior capsule causes the flexion deformity. The varus deformity of the extended leg is caused by loss of cartilage and bone from the contact areas in extension. The angle of varus will depend on the amount of bone loss. To expose bone on both surfaces, the total thickness of cartilage lost is about 5 mm, causing about 5° of varus. At least this degree of deformity is usual on presentation because pain seldom becomes severe until there is bone-on-bone contact

during weight bearing. Thereafter, each millimeter of bone eroded will increase the deformity by about 1°.

The varus deformity corrects spontaneously at 90° as the cartilage is intact in the area of contact in flexion. Therefore, the MCL is drawn out to its normal length every time the patient bends the knee, and structural shortening of the ligament does not occur. Thus, an intact ACL ensures a normal-length MCL as demonstrated by manual correction of varus when the posterior capsule is relaxed by flexing the knee 20°.

A diagnosis of AMOA is usually based on clinical findings as described above, although supportive evidence from radiographs is useful. Good-quality weight-bearing anteroposterior and lateral radiographs of the knee will help establish the presence of bone-on-bone appearance in the medial compartment and a varus deformity, which is usually present. If for some reason the radiograph does not confirm the presence of bone on bone in the affected medial compartment—that is, there is full-thickness cartilage loss (FTCL) over the femur as well as the tibia in the affected compartment—one can confirm the same by other investigations such as a varus stress view (**Fig. 3–3A**). In this view, the surgeon (or his or her assistant/radiographer) gives a varus stress to the knee under examination and takes an anteroposterior radiograph with the knee flexed to 20° to allow relaxation of the posterior capsule. After performing the varus stress radiograph, it is a good practice to obtain a valgus stress view (**Fig. 3–3B**). The valgus stress view allows confirmation of the presence of full-thickness cartilage in the lateral compartment, which is a prerequisite before proceeding to UKA. Some surgeons prefer to perform a Rosenberg view, which is equally useful in confirming the presence of FTCL in the medial compartment. If

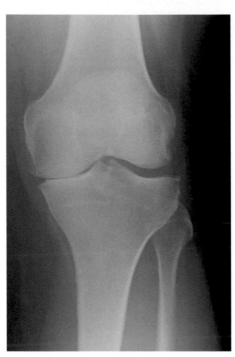

Figure 3-1 Preoperative radiograph of a patient with anteromedial osteoarthritis.

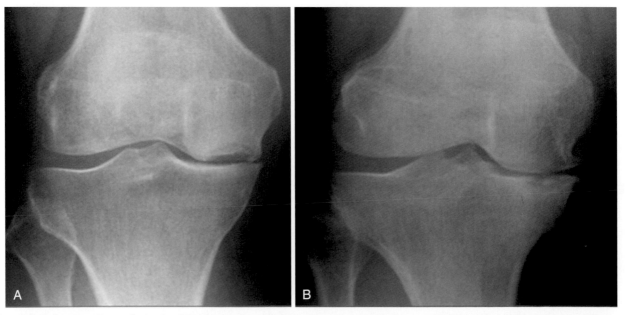

Figure 3-2 Preoperative radiograph of SONK showing **(A)** femoral condyle involvement and **(B)** medial tibial plateau involvement.

all these investigations fail to confirm the presence of FTCL in the affected medial compartment, the surgeon should perform an arthroscopy of the affected knee. If any of these investigations confirmed FTCL on both femur and tibia and the patient's symptoms are bad enough to undergo knee replacement, then the surgeon can proceed to perform a UKA. If, indeed, this is not the case, then one should not perform UKA as the results are unreliable. We have not found other investigations (e.g., magnetic resonance imaging, computed tomography, or bone scan) to be of any specific value to confirm the presence of FTCL in the medial compartment; however, with improving imaging technology, this remains a possibility.

Anterior Cruciate Ligament

The anatomic state of the ACL at the time of surgery is an important determinant in the long-term outcome of UKA, as shown by Goodfellow et al. in 1992.[1] They reported a sixfold difference in the 7-year cumulative survival of the Oxford UKA between knees with or without a functioning ACL at the time of surgery, irrespective of the primary disease and of all the other variables measured. In patients with AMOA, the ACL is invariably intact. White et al. described 46 medial tibial plateaus excised sequentially from a series of osteoarthritic knees treated by Oxford UKA, all of them with an intact ACL and with cartilage erosion exposing bone (Ahlbäck stages 2, 3, and 4).[3] The erosions were all anterior and central. These rarely extended to the posterior quarter of the plateau and never reached the posterior joint margin. Similar findings

have been confirmed by other investigators. Harman et al.[4] examined the tibial plateau excised from 143 osteoarthritic knees during operations for total knee arthroplasty (TKA). They found that wear in ACL-deficient knees was located a mean 4 mm more posterior on the medial plateau than wear in ACL-intact knees. The ACL-deficient knees also exhibited more severe varus deformity. The site and extent of the tibial erosions can be reliably determined from lateral radiographs. Based on this, Keyes et al.[5] studied the preoperative lateral radiographs of 50 osteoarthritic knees in which the state of the ACL had been recorded at surgery. Using four blind observers, they found a 95% correlation between preservation of the posterior part of the medial tibial plateau on radiograph and an intact ACL at surgery, and a 100% correlation of erosion of the posterior plateau on the radiograph with an absent or badly damaged ACL. These correlations show that, as long as the ACL remains intact, the tibiofemoral contact areas in flexion remain distinct from the areas of contact in extension. Progressive loss of bone causes the varus deformity in extension to increase but, while the ACL continues to function, this deformity corrects spontaneously in flexion and structural shortening of the MCL does not occur. If not treated in time, the deterioration observed in the ACL usually progresses via the following sequence[1]: normal → loss of synovial covering, → usually starting distally, → longitudinal splits in the substance of the exposed ligament, → stretching and loss of strength of the collagen bundles, which results in the ligament becoming "friable and fragmented." The ACL will eventually rupture and disappear.

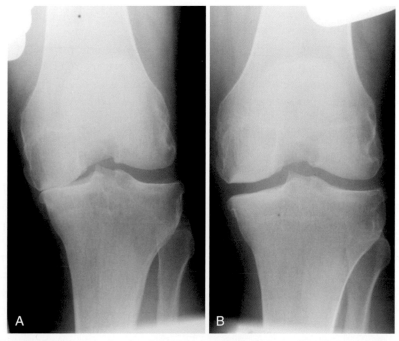

Figure 3-3 Varus **(A)** and valgus **(B)** stress views showing full-thickness cartilage loss in the affected medial compartment and intact cartilage in the lateral compartment **(B)**.

For the purpose of performing an Oxford UKA, we believe that, as long as the ACL is functionally intact (i.e., normal ACL or ACL with loss of synovial covering or longitudinal splits in the substance of the exposed ACL), an Oxford UKA may be safely performed. If the ACL is functionally impaired, this event will cause the transition from AMOA to the postero-medial form of the disease, with posterior subluxation of the femur and structural shortening of the MCL. Deschamps and Lapeyre[6] observed that the absence of the ACL in an osteo-arthritic knee was associated with the posterior subluxation of the femur on the tibia in extension. This subluxation results in the abrasion of the cartilage at the back of the tibial plateau by the exposed bone on the inferior surface of the femoral condyle. Thereafter, in flexion the cartilage on the posterior surface of the femoral condyle gets destroyed by abrasion on the tibial plateau, which is now devoid of any cartilage. The varus deformity is also therefore present in flexion as well as in extension and the MCL shortens structurally.

"CONTRAINDICATIONS"

We believe that there is virtually no contraindication for performing Oxford UKA in a patient with AMOA. This may sound contentious, but we will try to provide evidence for the same. Any patient with bone-on-bone AMOA and significant pain can be offered a UKA and patient's age, activity level, extent of obesity, chondrocalcinosis, patellofemoral arthritis, and/or preoperative site of pain can be safely ignored. This is contradictory to the recommendations made by Kozinn and Scott back in 1989.[7] They suggested that patients who were younger than 60, patients with weight greater than 82 kg, patients with exposed bone in the patellofemoral compartment, or patients who are physically active or perform heavy labor should not be offered a UKA. They also suggested chondrocalcinosis to be a relative contraindication. It must be pointed out that these strict selection criteria were based on their experience with fixed-bearing UKAs and in general are thought to be more intuitive rather than evidence based. The Oxford Group have ignored these so-called contraindications over the past 25 years, and our data presented here support our stance. Since 1998, when the Phase III Oxford UKA was introduced (implanted using minimally invasive surgical technique), we have collected preoperative and subsequent follow-up clinical and radiologic data on a cohort of 1000 Oxford UKAs.

Exposed Bone in Patellofemoral Joint

In the consecutive series of 1000 UKAs, nearly one quarter of patients had the presence of exposed bone in the patellofemoral joint (PFJ) either on the patella or on the trochlea or on both sides. When compared to the patients without the presence of FTCL in the PFJ, no significant difference was noted in the clinical scores or in survivorship. In 2007, our group published its experience of Oxford UKA with specific reference to the intraoperative status of the PFJ in a cohort of 824 consecutive knees.[8,9] In that series we had noted the presence of FTCL on the trochlea surface in 13% of cases, on the medial facet of the patella in 9%, and on the lateral facet in 4% of cases. No significantly worse outcome was noticed in these cases as compared to those without any patellofemoral arthritis. Similarly, the presence of preoperative anterior knee pain and/or radiologic evidence of degeneration of the PFJ was also assessed in a separate cohort of 100 consecutive knees. Fifty-four percent of patients had preoperative anterior knee pain. The clinical outcome in these patients was independent of the presence or absence of preoperative anterior knee pain. The presence of degenerative changes seen on the preoperative radiographs (in the PFJ as seen on skyline radiographs) did not show any significant difference in the clinical outcome. This was particularly evident in patients with medial patellofemoral degeneration. However, for some outcome measures in patients with lateral femoral patellofemoral degeneration, the Oxford knee score (OKS) tended to be 38 (lateral PFJ arthritis) versus 41 (normal lateral PFJ). We therefore recommend that, if there is severe damage to the lateral part of the PFJ with bone loss, grooving, or subluxation, a TKA should be performed.

Age

Some surgeons may consider the young age (age < 60) or old age (age > 80) of a patient as a contraindication to UKA. Wear and component loosening are concerns in the young while unnecessary risk of revision surgery is a concern in the old. The unique design features of the Oxford UKA minimize the wear, and the wear is independent of bearing thickness. This means that one can use a bearing as thin as 3 mm without any added risks of catastrophic wear or bearing fracture. This ensures the surgery to be bone conserving, which is an important advantage especially in the young. Various studies involving national joint registries have shown significantly lower complication rates with the use of UKA as compared to TKA, with particular reference to lower mortality, lower infection rate, and reduced need for blood transfusion. Hospital stay is reduced, range of movement is better, and faster recovery makes UKA an ideal implant in the elderly. In our cohort of 1000 UKAs, 25% of patients were younger than 60 at the time of the index procedure. At the last follow-up, no statistically significant difference was noted in the clinical or functional outcome or the failure rate between patients in this group and those over 60 years of age at the time of index procedure. In addition, Price et al. in 2005 compared the results of the Oxford UKA in patients younger and older than 60.[10] The survival for the younger group of patients was 91% (95% confidence interval [CI], 12) while in the older group it was 96% (95% CI, 3). These results are comparable to those achieved with TKA in patients younger than 60 at the time of surgery and, in addition, the Hospital for Special Surgery score at 10-year follow-up was 94/100 for the younger patients as compared to 86/100 for the older patients.

Obesity

Fixed-bearing (particularly the all-polyethylene tibia) UKAs have not performed well in obese patients. This is due to the associated risk of catastrophic failure and/or tibial component loosening. The Oxford UKA has a fully congruent bearing with minimal wear and therefore wear is not an issue. Provision of a metal baseplate reduces the risk of tibial loosening. In the Oxford cohort, nearly 50% of patients' weight was greater than 82 kg and therefore according to Kozinn and Scott's criteria[7] these patients would be considered as "less than ideal." When this cohort of patients was compared to patients weighing less than 82 kg, no significant difference was noticed in any clinical or functional outcome or in the failure rate.[11] Berend et al. retrospectively reviewed the early results of a consecutive series of fixed-bearing UKAs implanted via minimally invasive surgery using two implant designs (EIUS, Stryker Orthopaedics; and Repicci II, Biomet).[12] At an average follow-up of 40.2 months, the authors had 16 failures from a consecutive series of 79 UKAs, with the most common reason for failure being tibial loosening in six cases. The authors concluded that a body mass index (BMI) greater than 32 increased the failure rate. More recently, the authors have published their results of the Oxford UKA and found that BMI greater than 32 did not increase the failure rate.[12]

Recently, we presented the impact of BMI on a consecutive series of nearly 600 Oxford UKAs with a minimum 5-year follow-up.[13] The patients were divided into four groups: group 1 = BMI less than 25, group 2 = BMI 25–30, group 3 = BMI 30–35, and group 4 = BMI of 35 or greater. There was no significant difference in the 10-year survivorship among the four groups, although the numbers in group 4 were relatively small. Patients in groups 3 and 4 tended to have a lower preoperative OKS and lower OKS at the last follow-up, although the change in the OKS was similar to that in the other groups. Similarly, the functional American Knee Society score (AKSS) was lower in groups 3 and 4, although the change in the functional score was not significantly different. These results suggest that, for the Oxford UKA, obesity should not be considered a contraindication.

Chondrocalcinosis

Thirteen percent of cases from our Oxford UKA cohort showed the presence of chondrocalcinosis as evident on radiography and/or histology. Again no difference was noted in any of the clinical or functional outcomes or in the survivorship.[11] Woods et al. in 1995 published the results of chondrocalcinosis in patients undergoing Oxford UKA.[14] The survival rates between patients with and without chondrocalcinosis were not significantly different. Again there was no significant difference in clinical outcomes or radiologic outcomes.

Activity Level

It continues to be a contentious issue as to what activity levels are safe for patients undergoing knee arthroplasty. It obviously depends upon the type and frequency of activity as well as the type of implant. Nearly 10% of patients in our cohort have a Tegner activity level of 5 or more. (Tegner 5 activity level means that they are regularly involved in either heavy labor [building/forestry] or competitive [cycling/cross-country skiing] or recreational [jogging on uneven ground at least twice per week] sports). In this cohort of patients, the OKS and AKSS functional scores are superior with a lower failure rate, and the only failure we have noticed in this patient subgroup is in a patient who ruptured his ACL, which required subsequent reconstruction. If all these unnecessary contraindications (for the Oxford UKA) were adhered to (as suggested by Kozinn and Scott[9]), nearly 70% of these patients would not have been considered to be ideal candidates to undergo a UKA. There is, however, no difference in their functional outcome or failure rate as compared to the so-called ideal candidates, with survivorship being 96% at 12 years in those with or without accepted contraindications (not statistically different).

Spontaneous Osteonecrosis of the Knee

UKA is well suited to treat SONK, and various studies have shown excellent functional outcome and survivorship in these patients. From a technical point of view, implantation of the UKA can be demanding, and certain considerations must be taken into account when using the implant for osteonecrosis. The classic defect in the medial femoral condyle occurs in the weight-bearing area in extension: failure to identify the presence of a crater may result in the unwary surgeon recessing the spigot too deeply and thereby milling too much bone from the medial femoral condyle. This could then cause problems in balancing the extension gap. In addition, because of surrounding bony sclerosis, an attempt should be made to completely excavate any craters in the femoral condyle or to completely remove the osteonecrotic lesion in the medial tibial plateau so that normal bone can be used as a base for cement impregnation. It may be necessary for large craters to be filled with autologous bone graft harvested from the bone removed at surgery. Langdown et al. assessed the outcome of the Oxford UKA in 29 patients with end-stage SONK and compared the results with a matched group of patients with an Oxford UKA for AMOA.[15] The clinical and functional outcomes were noted to be similar in these two groups.

Previous High Tibial Osteotomy

Rees et al. showed that the cumulative 10-year survivorship after a UKA in patients with previous high tibial osteotomy (HTO) is 66%, and this is significantly lower than in those with AMOA (96%).[16] The authors noted persistent pain and/or early progression of osteoarthritis to the lateral compartment as the most common reasons for failure. We believe that the reason for the pain, lateral wear, and subsequent failure is that a medial UKA for primary AMOA results in correction of the varus deformity within the joint, restoring the leg to its predisease alignment. However, if the varus deformity has already been fully or partially corrected extra-articularly by an HTO, then any further change in alignment from a UKA can cause an overcorrection, which will increase loading of the lateral compartment. We therefore recommend that a previous HTO should be considered to be a contraindication to the use of an Oxford UKA. Knees in which symptoms recur after a previous HTO may be more effectively treated by TKA.

ACL Deficiency

The options for treatment of the young active patient with isolated symptomatic osteoarthritis of the medial compartment and preexisting deficiency of the ACL are limited. The potential longevity of the implant and the activity level of the patient may preclude TKA, and tibial osteotomy and UKA are unreliable because of the ligamentous instability. UKAs tend to fail because of wear or tibial loosening resulting from eccentric loading. In cases of primary traumatic ACL rupture with secondary arthritis of the medial compartment, the cartilage defect and bony erosion tend to be central and posterior on the tibia (posteromedial osteoarthritis). This is likely to be due to recurrent episodes of giving way, in which posterior femoral subluxation in the medial compartment places a heavy load on the posterior meniscus and posterior articular cartilage of the tibia, producing meniscal tears and the development of arthritis. In some cases the rest of the knee joint remains essentially intact, with no shortening of the MCL. This is probably because, in extension, the intact distal femoral cartilage is in contact with intact anterior tibial cartilage, so the varus deformity is corrected and the MCL is of normal

length. It is in these patients, who are often young, that we would perform a combined ACL reconstruction followed by UKA.[17] Depending on the presenting symptoms, the combined procedure can be done in one or two stages. The majority of patients present primarily with pain, and we tend to perform a combined single-stage procedure of ACL reconstruction and UKA under the same anesthetic, while in patients presenting with instability we tend to do a staged surgery—the first stage comprising ACL reconstruction followed by a subsequent UKA after a few months if the pain becomes a significant issue.

We have performed more than 50 cases with combined ACL reconstruction and UKA, and these patients have excellent clinical and functional outcomes with survivorship not dissimilar to those with AMOA and an intact ACL. We have also assessed in vivo functional kinematics, including bearing movement and femoral roll-back, in patients with an Oxford UKA with an intact ACL and an Oxford UKA with a reconstructed ACL. The kinematic patterns were similar in both groups and closely mimicked normal (native) knee kinematics.[18]

SUMMARY

The indications and contraindications for UKA are design dependent and, for the Oxford UKA, virtually any patient with significant pain and bone-on-bone AMOA can undergo a UKA. In particular, one can ignore the age, activity level, presence of chondrocalcinosis, patellofemoral damage, preoperative site of pain, and obesity in these patients. If one uses the selection criteria recommended by Kozinn and Scott,[7] UKA can only be offered to 2–10% of patients undergoing knee replacement, and this means that the surgeon is unable to gain experience and increase his or her skill in performing UKAs. When UKA is performed on an infrequent basis, the results may be suboptimal. In contrast, with the Oxford philosophy one can offer a UKA to about one in three patients undergoing a knee replacement (and maybe even higher, as suggested by some groups); this will allow the surgeon to gain experience and the patients to benefit from UKA.

REFERENCES

1. Goodfellow J, O'Connor J. The anterior cruciate ligament in knee arthroplasty: a risk factor with unconstrained meniscal prosthesis. Clin Orthop 1992;276:245-252.
2. Psychoyios V, Crawford RW, O'Connor JJ, Murray DW. Wear of congruent meniscal bearings in unicompartmental knee arthroplasty: a retrieval study of 16 specimens. J Bone Joint Surg [Br] 1998;80:976-982.
3. White SH, Ludkowski PF, Goodfellow JW. Anteromedial osteoarthritis of the knee. J Bone Joint Surg [Br] 1991;73:582-586.
4. Harman MK, Markovich GD, Banks SA, Hodge WA. Wear patterns on tibial plateaus from varus and valgus osteoarthritic knees. Clin Orthop 1998;325:149-158.
5. Keyes GW, Carr AJ, Miller RK, Goodfellow JW. The radiographic classifications of medial gonarthrosis. Correlation with operation methods in 200 knees. Acta Orthop Scand 1992;63:497-501.
6. Deschamps G, Lapeyre B. Rupture of the anterior cruciate ligament: a frequently unrecognised cause of failure of unicompartmental knee prostheses. Fr J Orthop Surg 1987;1:323-330.

7. Kozinn SC, Scott R. Unicondylar knee arthroplasty. J Bone Joint Surg [Am] 1989;71:145-150.

8. Beard DJ, Pandit H, Gill HS, et al. The influence of the presence and severity of pre-existing patellofemoral degenerative changes on the outcome of the Oxford medial unicompartmental knee replacement. J Bone Joint Surg [Br] 2007;89:1597-1601.

9. Beard DJ, Pandit H, Ostlere S, et al. Pre-operative clinical and radiological assessment of the patellofemoral joint in unicompartmental knee replacement and its influence on outcome. J Bone Joint Surg [Br] 2007;89:1602-1607.

10. Price AJ, Dodd CA, Svard UG, Murray DW. Oxford medial unicompartmental knee arthroplasty in patients younger and older than 60 years of age. J Bone Joint Surg [Br] 2005;87:1488-1492.

11. Pandit H, Jenkins C, Gill HS, et al. Unnecessary contraindications for mobile bearing unicompartmental knee replacement. Accepted for publication in J Bone Joint Surg Jan 2011.

12. Berend KR, Lombardi AV Jr, Adams JB. Total knee arthroplasty in patients with greater than 20 degrees flexion contracture. Clin Orthop Relat Res 2006;(452):83-87.

13. Ferguson J, Pandit H, Price AJ, et al. The impact of body mass index on the outcome of the unicompartmental knee arthroplasty. BASK, Oxford, March 2010.

14. Woods DA, Wallace DA, Woods CG, et al. Chondrocalcinosis and medial unicompartmental knee arthroplasty. Knee 1995;2:117-119.

15. Langdown AJ, Pandit H, Price AJ, et al. Oxford medial unicompartmental arthroplasty for focal spontaneous osteonecrosis of the knee. Acta Orthop 2005;76:688-692.

16. Rees JL, Price AJ, Lynskey TG, et al. Medial unicompartmental arthroplasty after failed high tibial osteotomy. J Bone Joint Surg [Br] 2001;83:1034-1036.

17. Pandit H, Beard DJ, Jenkins C, et al. Combined anterior cruciate reconstruction and Oxford unicompartmental knee arthroplasty. J Bone Joint Surg [Br] 2006;88:887-892.

18. Pandit H, Van Duren BH, Gallagher JA, et al. Combined anterior cruciate reconstruction and Oxford unicompartmental knee arthroplasty: in vivo kinematics. Knee 2008;15:101-106.

CHAPTER **4**

Spacer Devices—Old and New

Franz Xaver Koeck and Erhan Basad

KEY POINTS

- Bone and joint preservation are the main goals of treatment of unicompartmental osteoarthritis, especially in younger patients.
- The primary surgical options include osteotomy and unicompartmental arthroplasty.
- Knee osteotomies provide the adjustment of leg axis malalignment, but do not address rebuilding the worn cartilage surface of the compartment.
- Unilateral knee arthroplasty calls for bone resection and has shown shorter durability than total knee arthroplasty.
- Early unilateral implants such as the McKeever tibial hemiarthroplasty have addressed this problem without bone resection, with single-surface tibial resurfacing, and with reasonable long-term results. Later the UniSpacer, a self-centering mobile unilateral interpositional metal implant, was introduced, but failed because of inadequate alignment and its tendency for dislocation.
- Recently, based on the principles of the nonfixed implants, the iForma, an individual metal interpositional device, was developed using patients' individual magnetic resonance imaging data, mimicking the shape of the affected joint compartment. The iForma device can provide improvement in knee function and reduction in pain within a narrow indication of patients with unicompartmental knee arthritis, but with a significantly higher risk of early revision compared to traditional unicompartmental arthroplasty.

INTRODUCTION

Hemiarthroplasty is an option for the treatment of unicompartmental osteoarthritis. The implants designed by McKeever and MacIntosh more than 50 years ago provided the intellectual and clinical basis for interpositional hemiarthroplasty. Although these approaches had generally good clinical outcomes, the technical difficulty associated with their use and the advent of very successful total knee arthroplasty led to their general abandonment among most orthopaedic surgeons. However, the challenges of treating younger, more active patients and the desire to adopt minimally invasive and bone-preserving techniques have given rise to the development of interpositional devices (iPDs) that represent an evolutionary change from the early versions of such devices. This chapter gives an overview of spacer devices designed for the operative treatment of unicompartmental osteoarthritis. The design and conceptual approach of each of the current options are reviewed.

EARLY DEVELOPMENT OF HEMIARTHROPLASTY

For patients with osteoarthritis limited to a single femoral-tibial compartment, the concept of a metallic hemiarthroplasty has a long history. The genesis of the concept of using an iPD, in which a material is placed between the condyles within the joint to reduce wear or prevent adhesion, goes back almost 150 years, when it was first suggested by Verneuil.[1] Over the ensuing years, a wide variety of materials were tried, ranging from chromicized pig bladder in 1918 to vitallium in 1940. In 1960, McKeever[2] described a metallic prosthesis that was designed to be placed in the femorotibial compartment and fixed to the tibial condyle (Howmedica, Rutherford, NJ) (**Fig. 4–1**). This design was subsequently modified by MacIntosh. Metallic hemiarthroplasty was introduced into orthopaedic practice in the 1950s and 1960s by McKeever[2] and MacIntosh.[3] MacIntosh and Hunter described the hemiarthroplasty approach as follows: "The aims of hemiarthroplasty are to correct the varus or valgus deformity by inserting a tibial plateau prosthesis of appropriate diameter and thickness to build up the worn side of the joint and thus to restore normal stability of the knee, to relieve pain and to improve function and gait. The collateral ligaments usually maintain their own length in spite of long-standing varus and valgus deformity, and stability is maintained by a prosthesis that is thick enough to correct the deformity and to take up the slack of the collateral ligaments."[4]

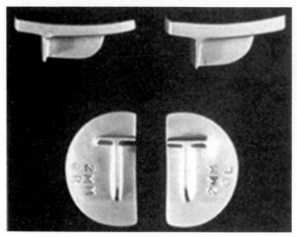

Figure 4-1 McKeever hemiarthroplasty implant. (Courtesy of Howmedica, Rutherford, NJ.)

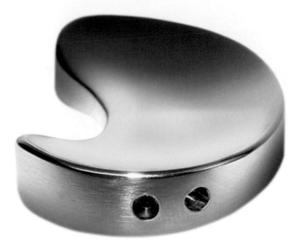

Figure 4-2 UniSpacer implant. (Courtesy of Zimmer, Warsaw, IN.)

Reports of early experience with both of these devices were generally encouraging. The two approaches differed primarily in the method of fixation. The McKeever implant had a keel that was inserted into the tibial condyle to provide mechanical fixation. In contrast, the MacIntosh implant was "held in position by the anatomy of the knee joint, and stability depends upon the taut collateral ligaments. No additional fixation is necessary. The top of the prosthesis has a contoured surface with rounded edges to provide the condyle with a permanent low-friction area. The undersurface is flat with multiple serrations to ensure a snug fit and stability."[4] In a series reporting 10-year follow-up for 75 MacIntosh implants, Wordsworth et al. found that 11 (14.7%) had been revised to arthroplasty and concluded that, although "greater angular deformities pre-operatively reduced the chance of success in the medium term, late failure of the arthroplasty after five years was very rare."[5] In a more recent clinical report on 44 McKeever implants followed for an average of 8 years, Scott et al. noted that, at final follow-up, 70% of the knees were rated as good or excellent.[6] Similarly, Emerson and Potter also reported good results in 61 McKeever implants followed for up to 13 years (average, 5 years), in which 72% were rated as having good to excellent results.[7] The most recent report of long-term results, published by Springer et al. in 2006, continued to show excellent long-term results with tibial hemiarthroplasty using the McKeever device.[8] In spite of reports of early experience with these prostheses that were generally encouraging, the approach gained only limited use within the orthopaedic community due to its invasive nature and the subsequent development of total knee arthroplasty.

RECENT DEVELOPMENTS

UniSpacer

Decades after being set aside, the fundamental concept of hemiarthroplasty reemerged several years ago. The first such

iPD to come to market was the UniSpacer (Zimmer, Warsaw, IN). The UniSpacer (**Fig. 4–2**) is a mobile iPD that does not achieve fixation to the tibial plateau using a keel, as did the McKeever device, or by means of a roughened undersurface, as did the MacIntosh prosthesis. The UniSpacer is designed to move freely on the tibial plateau as determined by the conforming articulation of its top surface with the femoral condyle. The UniSpacer is intended for use only in the medial compartment, primarily because, in the lateral compartment, roll-back could cause prosthetic dislocation, soft tissue impingement, or both. The design of the UniSpacer permits insertion using a minimally invasive approach.[9] In a peer-reviewed article, Sisto and Mitchell reported on a series of 37 UniSpacer cases followed for an average of 26 months.[10] In this series, the mean Knee Society Function Score was 69 and the Knee Score was 72. There were 12 revisions (35.4%), 6 as a result of device dislocation (17.6%) and 6 for pain or other reasons (17.6%). Friedman reported on an initial series of 23 cases in which there was an overall revision rate of 34% with an 8% dislocation rate.[11] The results of these surgeons are consistent with early reports from the implant's developers.

OrthoGlide

Another recently introduced hemiarthroplasty iPD is the OrthoGlide (Advanced Bio-Surfaces, Inc., Minnetonka, MN). The OrthoGlide implant (**Fig. 4–3**) is available only for use in the medial compartment, where it is placed between the tibial plateau and the femoral condyle by means of a minimally invasive surgical approach. The device is intended "to improve the alignment of the knee, with the aim of returning the joint to a more valgus position. Realignment of the knee tends to distribute the weight-bearing forces across the joint and thus helps restore the normal relationships of the articular surfaces and the surrounding capsular, ligamentous and muscular structures. The device is designed to relieve pain by providing an articulating surface with a low coefficient of friction and

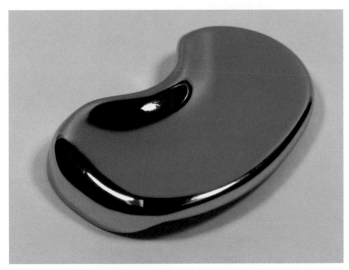

Figure 4-3 OrthoGlide implant. (Courtesy of Advanced Bio-Surfaces, Inc., Minnetonka, MN.)

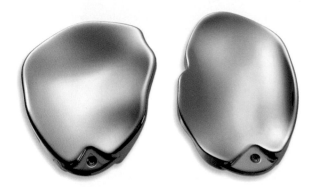

Figure 4-4 iForma medial and lateral implants. Note: product is no longer offered by the manufacturer. (Courtesy of ConforMIS, Burlington, MA.)

high durability."[12] The device geometry and ligament tension combine to keep the implant in place along with a posterior "lip" or overhang designed to prevent excessive movement of the device.

iForma

The iForma (ConforMIS, Burlington, MA) is a patient-specific iPD that replicates the tibial articular surface and uses functional fixation to maintain implant stability with minimal implant motion (**Fig. 4–4**). Each implant is unique, matching the patient's articular anatomy and developed from a standard magnetic resonance imaging scan using a novel technology that converts the topography of the patient's articular cartilage and subchondral bone to a patient-specific implant. The top surface of the implant conforms to the shape of the femoral condyle while the bottom surface conforms to the shape of the tibial plateau. Because the iForma is designed to replicate the patient's unique anatomy, it can be designed for either the medial or the lateral condyle (**Fig. 4–5**).

One of the stated aims of treatment using interpositional or hemiarthroplasty prostheses is the restoration or improvement of alignment. The ability of such a device to actually achieve improvement in alignment has been evaluated in a formal study of the iForma. Koeck et al.[13] evaluated changes in leg axis in a clinical study of 27 patients who received a patient-specific iForma implant. All patients had early to moderate-stage osteoarthritis of the knee (Kellgren-Lawrence grade 3 or less). A single surgeon implanted a total of 27 iForma prostheses (23 medial, 4 lateral) in sequential cases. The average age of the patients (15 women and 12 men) was 55.3 years (range, 38–67 years). Standardized preoperative and postoperative standing long-leg radiographs were obtained and the deviation from the load axis of the surgically treated knee joint under stress was determined twice by two independent evaluators. The preoperative objective was to correct the leg axis to 0° and/or to a slight undercorrection of up to 2°. This was achieved in 23 of 27 cases (85.2%). The correlation coefficient between the implant offset as determined by the design algorithm and the extent of the axis correction was 0.838.

A multicenter study to report safety and efficacy of the iForma patient–specific interpositional device was performed from June 2005 to June 2008.[14] Seventy-eight subjects (42 men, 36 women) received an iForma implant. The mean age was 53 years, the mean body mass index 29.0. The WOMAC scores, the visual analog pain scale and the Knee Society Scores were surveyed. The mean follow-up was 16.4 months. The mean WOMAC knee scores increased from 48.3 before surgery to 71.3 after 24 months. A reduction in pain was achieved for all five pain measures using a standard visual analog scale (VAS). Knee Society Knee Score improved from 39.2 before to 61.9 24 months after surgery. The Knee Society Function Scores improved from preoperative 64.5 to 82.5 2 years postoperative. The preoperative range of motion could be restored. The overall revision rate was 24%. Fifteen implants were removed early, 4 knees were revised without implant removal. Within a narrow indication of patients with unicompartmental disease, the iForma device can provide improvement in knee function and reduction in pain, however, with a significantly higher risk of early revision compared to traditional arthroplasty. Respecting this limitation, it may be an alternative option for arthritic patients with unicompartmental disease who have contraindications to high tibial osteotomy or are too young for knee replacement; the iForma device further has the distinct advantage of time and cost-saving compared to those procedures.

DISCUSSION

Hemiarthroplasty has undergone a renaissance, and the insights of McKeever and MacIntosh have evolved into several new alternatives for the treatment of unicompartmental femorotibial osteoarthritis. Mobile interpositional implants have shown a lack of adjustment and a tendency for roll-back and dislocation. The introduction of an individualized mobile

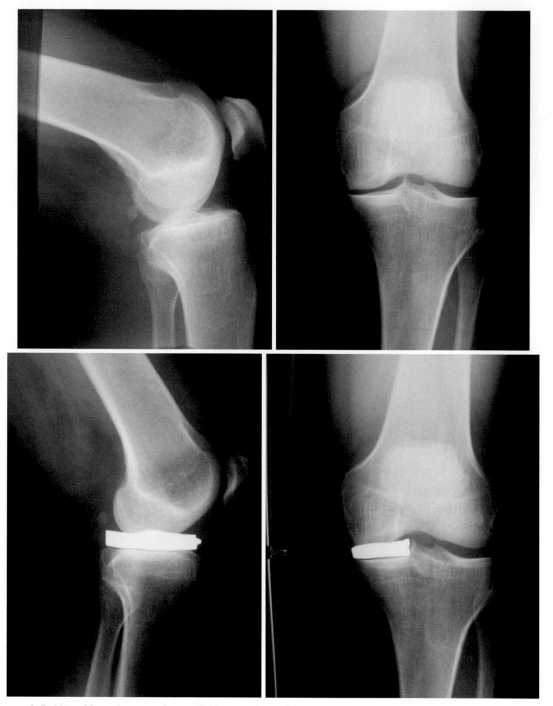

Figure 4-5 AP and lateral x-rays of a medial knee arthritis following iForma implantation in a 52-year-old woman.

interpositional implant has provided better functional fixation because of an accurate anatomic fit, even improving the anatomic axis. Therefore, individual mobile implants provide a minimally invasive alternative treatment option for a range of patients with unilateral osteoarthritis (see Video 4-1). Against the backdrop of high early revision rates, biomechanical testings on implant stability and pressure distribution within the treated compartment are required as well. Longer follow-ups must be investigated to evaluate clear indications and the relevance of the latest generation of spacers. **Table 4–1** presents a comparison of some of the features of the currently available devices.

Table 4-1	**Comparison of Characteristics of Currently Available Interpositional Hemiarthroplasty Devices**				
Device	FDA Cleared?	Material	Patient-Matched Design?	Mechanical Fixation?	Lateral Use?
iForma	Yes	Cobalt chrome alloy	Yes	No	Yes
OrthoGlide	Yes	Cobalt chrome alloy	No	Yes, partial	No
UniSpacer	Yes	Cobalt chrome alloy	No	No	No

FDA, U.S. Food and Drug Administration.

REFERENCES

1. Verneuil AS. De la création d'une fausse articulation par section ou resection partielle de l'os maxillaire inférieur, comme moyen de rémedier a l'ankylose vraie ou fausse de la machoire inférieure. Arch Gen Med 1860;15:174-179.
2. McKeever DC. Tibial plateau prosthesis. Clin Orthop Relat Res 1960;(18):86-95.
3. MacIntosh DL. Hemi-arthroplasty of the knee using a space occupying prosthesis for painful varus and valgus deformities. Proceedings of the Joint Meeting of Orthopaedic Associations of the English Speaking World. J Bone Joint Surg [Am] 1958;40:1431.
4. MacIntosh DL, Hunter GA. The use of the hemiarthroplasty prosthesis for advanced osteoarthritis and rheumatoid arthritis of the knee. J Bone Joint Surg [Br] 1972;54:244-255.
5. Wordsworth BP, Shakespeare DT, Mowat AG. MacIntosh arthroplasty for the rheumatoid knee: a 10-year follow up. Ann Rheum Dis 1985;44:738-741.
6. Scott RD, Joyce MS, Ewald FC, Thomas WH. McKeever metallic hemiarthroplasty of the knee in unicompartmental degenerative arthritis. J Bone Joint Surg [Am] 1985;67:203-207.
7. Emerson R, Potter T. The use of the McKeever metallic hemiarthroplasty for unicompartmental arthritis. J Bone Joint Surg [Am] 1985;67:208-212.
8. Springer BD, Scott RD, Sah AP, Carrington R. McKeever hemiarthroplasty of the knee in subjects less than sixty years old. J Bone Joint Surg [Am] 2006;88:366-371.
9. Scott RD. The UniSpacer: insufficient data to support its widespread use. Clin Orthop Relat Res 2003;(416):164-166.
10. Sisto DJ, Mitchell IL. UniSpacer arthroplasty of the knee. J Bone Joint Surg [Am] 2005;87:1706-1711.
11. Friedman MJ. Unispacer. Arthrosc 2003;19(Suppl):120-121.
12. Pre-Market Notification. 510(k) Summary, Advanced Bio-Surfaces, Inc. OrthoGlide® (Medial Knee Implant, K053094), Feb. 6, 2006. Available at: www.accessdata.fda.gov/scripts/cdrh/cfdocs/cfPMN/pmn.cfm?ID=19941
13. Koeck FX, Perlick L, Luring C, et al. Leg axis correction with ConforMIS iForma (interpositional device) in unicompartmental arthritis of the knee. Int Orthop 2009;33:955-960.
14. Koeck FX, Luring C, Goetz J, et al. Prospective single-arm, multicenter trial of a patient-specific interpositional knee implant: Early clinical results. Open Orthop J 2011;5:37-43.

CHAPTER 5
Incidence of Partial Knee Arthroplasty: A Growing Phenomenon?

William A. Jiranek and Daniel L. Riddle

KEY POINTS

- Between 1998 and 2005, the incidence of partial knee replacement in the United States grew by over three times.
- As of 2005, partial knee replacement comprised approximately 9% of all knee arthroplasties in the United States.
- Most recent estimates for other countries providing public data indicate a utilization rate ranging from 8% of all arthroplasties in Great Britain and Canada to a high of 19% in Australia.
- Partial knee replacement appears to be a viable and potentially underutilized procedure worldwide.

INTRODUCTION

Because osteoarthritis of the knee is one of the most common disease processes in humans, data concerning the incidence of knee arthroplasty are important to estimate the societal cost of treatment for this condition. While utilization in countries that sponsor joint registries is well delineated, few data are available in the United States due to the lack of a national implant registry. While the Medicare databases give some idea of utilization of knee arthroplasty, partial versus total cannot be differentiated, and only patients covered by Medicare (generally greater than 65 years of age) are captured. Utilization of partial knee replacement can be considered in several ways, including as a percentage of total knee arthroplasties as well as the percentage of patients who have isolated unicompartmental arthritis. There have been previous spikes in the utilization of partial knee replacement that usually corresponded to an increase in the number of surgeons performing partial knee replacement, usually followed by a pullback related to an increase in the failure rate.

While the number of patients with symptomatic osteoarthritis has continued to grow significantly, it appears that the percentage of patients in which the osteoarthritis is confined to predominantly one compartment (and thus amenable to

partial knee replacement) has remained relatively constant, and has been estimated at 30%. This chapter reports the incidence of partial knee arthroplasty (PKA) in all countries that have an existing registry. For the United States, which does not have a registry, we have estimated the incidence of unicondylar arthroplasty by indirect methods, using implant sales data from the major manufacturers.[1] We have estimated market share by utilizing commercial databases that track market share.[2]

GROWTH OF PKA IN THE UNITED STATES

To estimate the number of PKAs performed each year, we utilized a retrospective cross-sectional design. We solicited sales data from the four major PKA orthopaedic manufacturers in the U.S. market, which included Biomet (Warsaw, IN), Zimmer (Warsaw, IN), Depuy Orthopaedics (Warsaw, IN), and Stryker Corporation (Mahwah, NJ). Stryker Corporation elected not to contribute sales figures. We multiplied each company's market share based on determinations of a market analyst firm (DataMonitor, New York, NY) by the number of unicompartmental arthroplasty implants sold, and this allowed us to determine total units sold. Sales data and market share were used to estimate total unicondylar implants implanted for 2003 (83% market share), 2004 (74% market share), and 2005 (87% market share). We used regression analysis to estimate the sales numbers for the years 1998–2002. We then used the National Hospital Discharge Survey (NHDS) to provide data for the total amount of knee arthroplasties performed in the United States during the study years, and subtracted our estimates of unicondylar knee arthroplasties (UKAs) from those to arrive at an estimate of the number of total knee replacements (TKRs) performed each year. The estimated number of unicondylar arthroplasties increased from 6570 in 1998 to 44,990 in 2005, whereas the number of total knee arthroplasties increased from 259,000 in 1998 to 441,000 in 2004 (no NHDS data available for 2005). As a percentage of all knee arthroplasties, the number of unis increased from 2.5% in 1998 to 9.8% in 2005. Between 1998 and 2005, the incidence of PKA increased by an average of 30% a year.

INCIDENCE OF PKA IN SCANDINAVIA

The Swedish Knee Arthroplasty Register has made annual reports for the period 1998–2005.[3] Between 2002 and 2005, UKAs represented between 9.4% and 11.7% of all arthroplasties. In 1998, 4400 TKRs were performed and approximately 1000 UKAs, and in 2006 the number of TKRs had grown to 9700, and the number of UKAs in relative terms declined to 900. During this period the register published several reports of a relatively high failure rate, and this may have affected the growth of UKA, because a different experience existed in Finland and Norway, and a higher rate of growth was seen. The Norwegian registry reported in their 2008 report that the number of UKAs increased from 87 in 1998 to 455 in 2005, an increase of 400%.[4] During the same period the number of total knees implanted in Norway increased from 1320 in 1998, to 2800 in 2005. The Finnish joint registry does not report their finding on the Internet, but has some data in published papers. Between 1988 and 1995, 540 UKAs were performed as compared to 12,480 TKRs, and between 1996 and 2003 the number of UKAs increased to 1251 as compared to 34,132 TKRs.

INCIDENCE OF PARTIAL KNEE REPLACEMENT IN OTHER COUNTRIES

The Australian Joint Registry reported that the annual use of unicondylar knee replacement increased four times from 6700 unis implanted in 2000 to 28,822 unis in 2008.[5] During this same time period, the number of TKRs increased fivefold from 36,442 to 197,301. The percentage of unis relative to all knee arthroplasties went from 19% to 16% during the same period.

The New Zealand Arthroplasty Registry reported that unicondylar arthroplasty utilization doubled from 2000 to 2003, with a moderate decrease from 2004 to 2008.[6] Nonetheless, in 2000, of the 3015 knee arthroplasty procedures, unicondylar arthroplasty represented 11% of all knee arthroplasty procedures, and in 2008 unicondylar procedures represented 10% of all knee arthroplasty procedures. The British arthroplasty register in 2009 reported that unicondylar arthroplasty represented 8% of all knee replacements done between 2000 and 2009.[7] In 2008, there were 71,527 primary knee arthroplasties reported to the U.K. registry. Of these, 5573 were unicondylar arthroplasties (8% of the total amount of procedures), and 1030 were patellofemoral arthroplasties (1% of the total). Consequently, 9% of knee arthroplasties were partial knee replacements, and this percentage has remained stable since 2000.

The Canadian Arthroplasty Register reported that the total number of knee arthroplasty procedures per year increased from 16,709 in 1998 to 38,922 in 2008, a change of 125%.[8] Of this figure, partial knee replacement represented about 8% of the TKR procedures in 2004, 9% in 2005, and 8% in 2007.

CONCLUSION

The use of partial knee replacement increased steadily during the 1990s, but has remained relatively stable in the first decade of the 21st century across the world. In round numbers this percentage approaches 10% of all knee arthroplasties. Those registries that have recorded a decline in the relative utilization of PKA have also reported a higher early failure rate of partial replacements, and this may have impacted surgeon utilization of PKA in these countries. The stability of incidence of PKA across the world indicates that it remains a viable option for patients with unicompartmental arthritis of the knee.

REFERENCES

1. Riddle DL, Jiranek WA, McGlynn FJ. Yearly incidence of unicompartmental knee replacement in the United States. J Arthroplasty 2008; 23:408-412.
2. DataMonitor. Hip and knee replacement market: overview of the US and European markets—growth in a mature market, 2006.
3. The Swedish Knee Arthroplasty Register, Annual report 2006. http://www.knee.nko.se/english/online/thePages/contact.php
4. The Norwegian Arthroplasty Register. 2008 Annual report. http://nrlweb.ihelse.net/eng/
5. Hip and Knee Arthroplasty National Joint Replacement Registry. 2008 Annual report. www.aoa.org.au/ or www.dmac.adelaide.edu.au/aoanjrr/
6. New Zealand National Joint Register. http://www.cdhb.govt.nz/njr/
7. National Joint Registry. http://www.njrcentre.org.uk/njrcentre/default.aspx
8. Canadian Joint Replacement Registry. www.cihi.ca/cjrr

SECTION 2
Biologic Options

CHAPTER **6**

Use of Biologics for Degenerative Joint Disease of the Knee

William J. Long

KEY POINTS

- Current cartilage-based techniques provide improved clinical outcomes when addressing full-thickness cartilage lesions of the knee.
- Newer techniques promise further refinements, with less invasive techniques, though only short-term outcome studies exist.
- There is no current technique that reproduces the native hyaline surface of the knee joint.

INTRODUCTION

Significant advances have been achieved at the two ends of the spectrum in addressing knee pathology: at one end with the arthroscopic management of knee injuries and at the other, with arthroplasty options for end-stage arthritis. The management of articular defects sits at the crossroads between these two settings. The goals of treatment for articular defects are to achieve a stable, durable, hyaline-like scaffold while correcting any instability or alignment disorder that may have contributed to the creation of the lesion. Treatment allows patients to return to their desired level of function, though patient education regarding the repaired knee and some degree of activity modification are almost always helpful.

Classification

Options available for addressing cartilage lesions can be classified as palliative, enhanced intrinsic repair, whole-tissue (allo- or auto-) transplantation, scaffold-based repair, cell-based repair, and combined techniques. The individual strategy selected should take into consideration the specific risks, benefits, and objectives of each technique in a patient-specific manner.

Natural History

Approximately 60% of knees undergoing surgical arthroscopy for knee pain have articular cartilage changes.[1] Many of these injuries are only partial thickness and are of indeterminate

significance in terms of their association with symptoms and their long-term progression to full-thickness chondral defects. Those with full-thickness lesions undergo approximately 400,000 cartilage procedures per year in the United States.[2] It is these cases that form the basis for the treatment options reviewed in this chapter.

TREATMENT OPTIONS

Palliative: Débridement

Irrigation and débridement is designed to address patient symptoms over the short term. Inflammatory mediators and loose fragments of cartilage are removed by the irrigation process. Débridement of the chondral defect removes any flaps of cartilage that may have been creating a mechanical block or irritation during range of motion. This technique is primarily palliative, and does not provide any basis for cartilage repair or regrowth.

Enhanced Intrinsic Repair: Microfracture

Due to the avascular nature of cartilage beyond the tidemark, there is limited to no regenerative potential. By breaking through this barrier, blood and associated healing and inflammatory mediators are exposed to the lesion. This reparative process, similar to the process of healing an injury in a non-articular location, proceeds through clot formation, metaplasia, and remodeling. An area of scar or nonhyaline cartilage is produced, providing some cushioning, structural support, and symptomatic relief.

Current microfracture techniques are based on this endogenous potential for regeneration, first proposed by Purdie,[3] and first described by Steadman and colleagues.[4]

Indications

Symptomatic full-thickness chondral defects of the knee can be treated with microfracture techniques.

Technique

Appropriate visualization of the lesion must be achieved. Meticulous débridement of any thin overlying fibrous tissue and calcified cartilage exposes a healthy defect bed. A vertical stable shouldered border must be created to shield the healing area. A microfracture awl is then inserted and holes are made beginning in the periphery and moving centrally. Spacing of approximately 3 mm with lesions to a depth of 3 mm should be achieved. Arthroscopic inflow is occluded and holes can be visualized for bony bleeding, indicating an appropriate depth of penetration.

Postoperative Management

Classical training dictates a strict protocol of touch-down weight bearing and continuous passive motion (CPM) for 6 weeks.[5] Animal models demonstrate an extended healing period up to 12 weeks, thus suggesting a potential benefit to a longer period of restricted load bearing. In contrast, a clinical study by Marder et al. compared this protocol to one of unrestricted weight bearing and no CPM for femoral chondral lesions less than 2 cm^2. At a mean 4.2-year follow-up (2–9 years) there was no difference in Lysholm and Tegner scores between groups.[6]

Outcomes

At early,[7] midterm,[8] and long-term[9] follow-up, good results have been reported in clinical function and pain relief with microfracture. Good fill grades, low body mass index, younger age, lack of associated meniscal and ligamentous injuries, and shorter duration of preoperative symptoms are predictive of improved outcomes.

Traditional Cell-Based Technique: Autologous Chondrocyte Implantation
Indications

Lesions from 2 to 10 cm^2 in any area in the knee can be treated with this technique.

Technique

Originally described by Brittberg et al.[10] in 1994, autologous chondrocyte implantation (ACI) is a two-stage technique that requires harvesting, culturing, and implantation of autologous chondrocytes. In the initial stage, surgical arthroscopy is used to assess whether or not the patient is a candidate for ACI; to address any associated meniscal pathology; to template the size, location, and dimensions of the defect; to locate any other cartilage lesions; and to obtain cartilage for culture. Typically the lateral edge of the notch, at the site of an anterior cruciate ligament notchplasty, is a good location for cartilage harvesting. A small curette or gouge can be used to harvest two to three small samples of cartilage, each about 3–5 mm in size. Samples are sent to a central lab. There these autologous cells are cultured to expand the cell count by up to 50 times. Chondrocytes are stored until appropriate time for implantation.

Using information gathered at the time of arthroscopy, an appropriately sized and positioned mini-arthrotomy is planned. The skin incision must be made while considering the need for a well-positioned arthrotomy, the periosteal patch harvest, and any future surgical management. Thus a midline incision is most often used. Following exposure of the lesion, it is débrided to stable borders and down to, but not through, the subchondral plate. The cross-sectional dimensions are measured and traced onto a sterile piece of paper. This is then used to harvest a periosteal flap approximately 2 mm larger than the defect. The outer layer should be marked so that the deep or cambium layer is placed facing the defect.

The periosteal patch is sutured into place with a 6-0 Vicryl stitch. An initial polar stitch in all four quadrants is helpful to appropriately position the graft, followed by interrupted simple sutures at 2- to 3-mm intervals. A small superior 5-mm opening is left to allow insertion of the cultured chondrocytes. The edges of the remainder of the patch are reinforced with fibrin glue, and the watertight nature is tested with saline. Appropriate reinforcements are made. The cultured chondrocytes are then inserted. Final sutures are tied and fibrin glue is applied. The knee is taken through a range of motion to ensure that the patch is stable and watertight.

Postoperative Management

Restricted weight bearing combined with early range of motion and CPM are begun immediately following surgery. Gradual progression of weight bearing and strengthening activities should be individually dictated by the size and location of the lesion. Impact activities are typically restricted for 6–9 months following ACI.

Outcomes

Long-term outcomes demonstrate durable results with ACI at 10–20 years postprocedure.[11] At a mean 12.8-year follow-up, 92% of patients were satisfied with results and would have the procedure again. Vasiliadis et al. examined the long-term magnetic resonance imaging appearance of lesions at 9–18 years. Though some degeneration was noted, the quality of the repair tissue was similar to that of surrounding normal cartilage.[12] In a double-blind trial, Knutsen et al. did not note any difference between short-term outcomes with ACI and microfracture, with both techniques demonstrating good results.[13]

EMERGING AND DEVELOPING TECHNOLOGIES

Despite clinical success with current conventional techniques, limitations exist. Inferior biomechanical properties of the reparative tissue,[14] and progressive degeneration of the mixed reparative tissue created,[15] limit success with a microfracture technique. Osteochondral autografts are limited by the availability of transplantable tissue. ACI is costly and time consuming and requires two surgeries, harvesting of a periosteal flap and an open arthrotomy. New technologies are currently in varied stages of development, and will seek to expand the options available for addressing cartilage lesions. These techniques are broadly categorized as cell based, and non–cell based. It is important to note that the Food and Drug Administration (FDA) has yet to approve any of these new techniques. Carticel (Genzyme, Cambridge, MA), approved by the FDA in 1995 for ACI, remains the only approved implant system in this field. As with any novel technology, long-term data do not exist to support their use. A few selected devices and techniques are reviewed.

Modifed ACI Techniques: Matrix-Associated Chondrocyte Implantation (MACI) and Hyalograft

These techniques involve placing the harvested cells in a porcine collagen membrane (MACI; Genzyme, Cambridge, MA) or a scaffold of hyaluronan derivatives (Hyalograft; Fidia Advanced Biopolymers, Abano Terme, Italy). The benefits to these modifications are a more uniform cell distribution; a smaller arthrotomy, as suturing is not required; and no need for periosteal harvest.

Postoperative Management

The rehabilitation protocol is similar to those of the traditional ACI technique. Midterm experience with a more intensive protocol in competitive athletes has demonstrated an earlier return to sport, and improved 5-year follow-up.[16]

Outcomes

In an early randomized trial comparing traditional ACI with a periosteal flap to MACI, Zeifang et al. found no difference in efficacy between the two groups.[17] In a 2- to 7-year follow-up with Hyalograft, good results were achieved with isolated lesions. However, less successful outcomes were noted with complex and salvage cases, highlighting the limitations of these techniques.[18]

Scaffold-Based Techniques
TruFit Osteobiologic Plugs

TruFit bone graft substitute plugs (Smith and Nephew, Andover, MA) were designed to fill defects created during osteochondral autografting of lesions in the knee. The plugs consist of a synthetic polymer combining polylactide-co-glycolide, polyglycolide fibers, and calcium sulfate. A plug placed in a defect provides a scaffold for marrow elements and surrounding chondrocytes to migrate into. These plugs are not approved by the FDA for the treatment of primary cartilage lesions, though they have been used outside the United States, particularly in Europe, in this manner.

Indications

As noted, the approved indication for this device is to backfill autologous sites, though they have been used elsewhere to address cartilage lesions. This is not an FDA-approved technique.

Technique

When addressing a primary cartilage lesion of the femoral condyle during arthroscopy, the size and location of the lesion are defined (**Fig. 6–1**). A perpendicular approach must be obtained to seat the plug flush with surrounding cartilage. Tamps of increasing diameter are inserted to determine the appropriate-diameter plug (**Fig. 6–2**). An obturator is secured

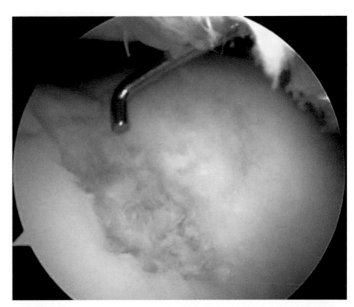

Figure 6-1 A large full-thickness cartilage lesion of the trochlea.

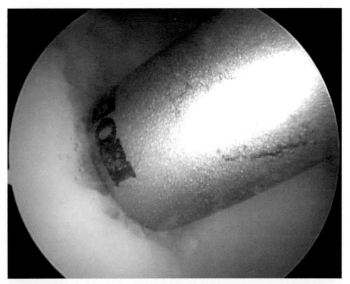

Figure 6-2 An appropriately sized tamp used as a template for sizing of the defect.

in the cutting tube and it is placed into the lesion. The obturator is removed, and the cutting tube is firmly held in place while it is malleted to a depth of 10–12 mm (**Fig. 6–3**). Care must be taken to ensure that the cutting tube remains perpendicular to the lesion. Failure to do so can damage surrounding cartilage, create a nontubular defect, and break the cutting tube. Hand reaming is performed until the reamer is flush with the cutting tube. The cutting tube is removed and the defect created is examined.

Measurements are taken from the base of the lesion to the chondral surface, in four quadrants (**Fig. 6–4**). A plug is cut to match this depth, attempting to achieve a flush position with surrounding cartilage. The plug is inserted and adjustments can be made with the appropriately sized tamp. Care must also be taken to ensure a perpendicular insertion of the plug, as it can be crushed or fractured if it is not in line with the hole. A similar open technique can be used to address patellar lesions. For larger or oblong-shaped lesions, more than one plug can be used. A narrow bony bridge (2–3 mm) should be maintained between plugs, to prevent collapse (**Fig. 6–5**).

Postoperative Management

Management is modified based on the size and location of the lesion. Following treatment of femoral condylar lesions, patients are allowed to partially bear weight with crutches. A CPM machine is used for 3 weeks, and active range of motion is encouraged on a stationary bike, without resistance. For trochlear and patellar lesions, full weight bearing may be initiated immediately following surgery.

Outcomes

Limited successful early follow-up exists with TruFit plugs[19] (**Fig. 6–6**). Some caution must be used, as case reports have noted failure of the plugs to incorporate and giant cell reactions requiring revision surgery.[20] A prolonged course of physical therapy and rehabilitation may be necessary when addressing large lesions.[21]

Cartilage Repair Device Plugs

The Cartilage Repair Device (CRD) (Kensey Nash, Exton, PA) is a biphasic scaffold comprised of type I collagen in the chondral region, and β-tricalium phosphate and polylactic acid, with interconnected pores, in the subchondral bone region (**Fig. 6–7**).

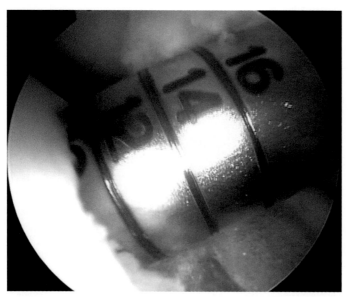

Figure 6-3 Final depth of the cutting tube perpendicular to the defect.

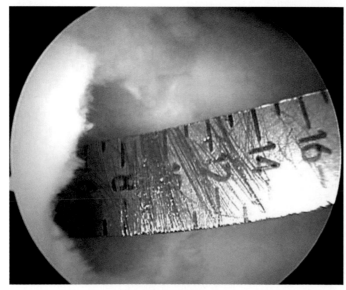

Figure 6-4 Four-quadrant depth measurement of the defect.

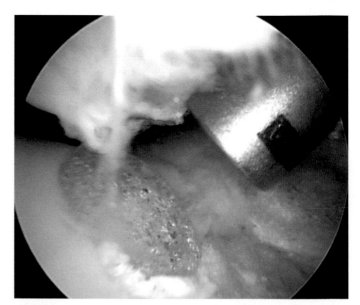

Figure 6-5 Three plugs visible with a tamp completing the impaction of the third plug.

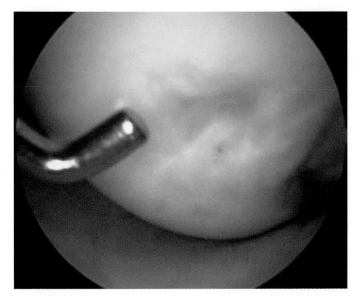

Figure 6-6 Follow-up arthroscopy of a condylar lesion treated with a TruFit plug.

Indications

These plugs are intended for the treatment of primary full-thickness cartilage lesions of the knee.

Technique

The technique for the CRD is similar to that of the TruFit plugs. Technical modifications include a guide pin for the insertion of the cutting tube, and the application of marrow elements to the plug via a bone marrow aspiration. This provides an initial cell base for repair.

Outcomes

Good clinical results have been obtained in goat and horse models (**Fig. 6–8**). IDE approval was obtained in the United States in 2010, and clinical studies are underway comparing this CRD to microfracture for full-thickness cartilage lesions.

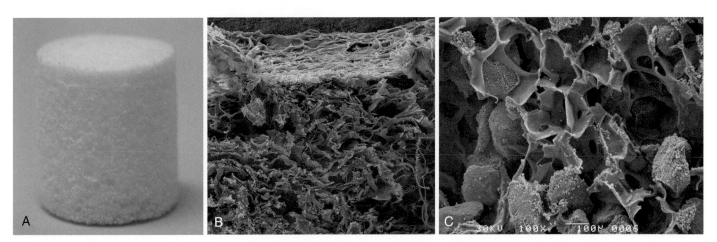

Figure 6-7 A CRD implant **(A)** with electron micrographs **(B** and **C)** demonstrating the biphasic nature of the plugs. (Courtesy of Kensey Nash Corporation, Exton, PA.)

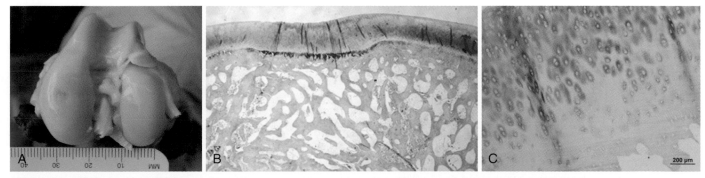

Figure 6-8 (A) A 12-month follow-up of a goat model with a cartilage plug. **(B)** Histologic examination with Safranin-O demonstrating proteoglycan. **(C)** Repair tissue staining strongly for type II collagen. (Courtesy of Kensey Nash Corporation, Exton, PA.)

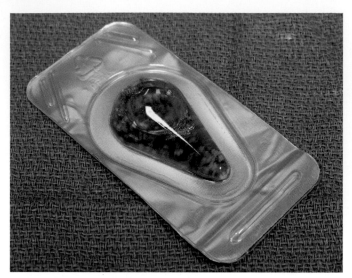

Figure 6-9 DeNovo NT in suspension. (Courtesy of Zimmer, Warsaw, IN; and ISTO Technologies, St. Louis, MO.)

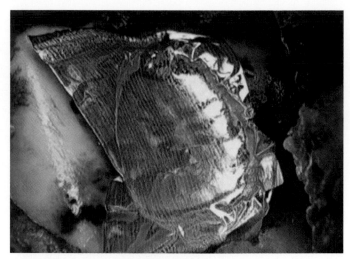

Figure 6-10 A foil template in a trochlear defect. (Coutesy of Zimmer, Warsaw, IN; and ISTO Technologies, St. Louis, MO.)

Cell-Based Techniques
DeNovo Natural Tissue (NT) Grafting

The DeNovo NT (Zimmer, Warsaw, IN; and ISTO Technologies, St. Louis, MO) graft is derived from juvenile allograft cartilage. Fragments are minced and then placed in suspension (**Fig. 6–9**). Its use is not subject to FDA approval as it is considered an allograft tissue product similar to osteochondral allografts and ligament allografts used in knee reconstructions.

Indications

DeNovo NT grafts are indicated for symptomatic full-thickness cartilage defects of the knee.

Technique

Surgical arthroscopy is used to identify the lesion, and to address any associated meniscal pathology. A mini-arthrotomy is then performed, exposing the lesion. Débridement of overlying fibrous and calcified tissue is performed to isolate a healthy bed with a stable shoulder of surrounding cartilage. The surgeon should avoid violating the subchondral bone layer. The defect is irrigated and a thin layer of fibrin glue is applied to stop bleeding. The cross-sectional area of the defect is measured with a ruler. One pack of graft is required per square inch (2.5 cm²) of defect. Simultaneously, the supplied suspension of cartilage fragments is opened and storage fluid is removed with a large angiocatheter. Foil is pressed into the lesion to create a matching mold (**Fig. 6–10**). This mold is then used to create a fibrin gel suspension of the cartilage fragments. Fragments are evenly spread in the foil defect. A layer of fibrin glue is then carefully applied to fill the defect to three fourths of the depth of the mold (**Fig. 6–11**). The construct is then left for up to 10 minutes to allow the fibrin to

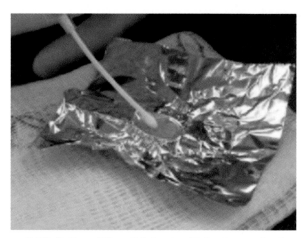

Figure 6-11 DeNovo NT graft following fibrin glue application. (Coutesy of Zimmer, Warsaw, IN; and ISTO Technologies, St. Louis, MO.)

fully set. The defect is once again irrigated and dried. A further thin fresh layer of fibrin glue is then applied to the base of the defect, followed by the DeNovo construct (**Fig. 6–12**). It should be even to slightly countersunk. Time must be allowed for the fibrin to once again set. The knee is then cycled to ensure that the implant is stable.

DeNovo Engineered Tissue (ET) Grafting

DeNovo ET (Zimmer, Warsaw, IN; and ISTO Technologies, St. Louis, MO) also employs juvenile allograft cartilage. Chondrocytes are isolated from the allograft cartilage and expanded in a cell bank. A hyaline-like cartilage graft is created from these cells by placing them in a matrix that is both chondro-inductive and chondro-conductive (**Fig. 6–13**).

Indications

Indications for DeNovo ET grafts are as noted above for DeNovo NT grafts.

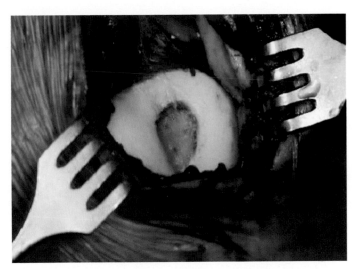

Figure 6-12 DeNovo NT graft inserted into the defect. (Coutesy of Zimmer, Warsaw, IN; and ISTO Technologies, St. Louis, MO.)

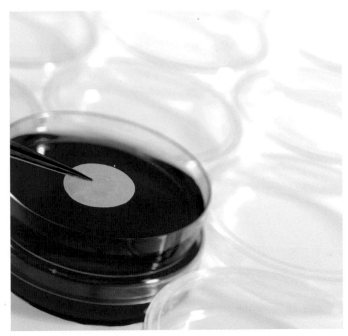

Figure 6-13 DeNovo ET graft. (Coutesy of Zimmer, Warsaw, IN; and ISTO Technologies, St. Louis, MO.)

Technique

Similar to DeNovo NT grafts, a mini-arthrotomy is required. Following site preparation, the defect is measured or an outline can be made on paper as a template. The graft product is cut to fit into the lesion. The defect is irrigated and dried. The graft is then fixed into the defect using fibrin glue. It is allowed to dry and then the knee is cycled, ensuring that the DeNovo membrane is well fixed.

Outcomes

Preclinical trials demonstrated the ability of DeNovo ET to integrate into host defects, while retaining hyaline cartilage properties.[22] Clinical trials with this product and with DeNovo NT are currently underway.

Combined Procedures

Osteochondral transplantation is reviewed in Chapter 7 in this text. A study by Lonner et al. demonstrated good early results with the use of autologous osteochondral allografts to the femoral condyles at the time of patellofemoral arthroplasty.[23] In a similar fashion, the option exists to combine partial knee arthroplasty with one of the cartilage procedures reviewed in this chapter, to address less advanced lesions in the remaining compartments. Long-term outcomes do not exist with these developing techniques.

Associated Procedures

Osteotomies about the knee are performed in conjunction with cartilage restorative procedures to address associated malalignment. Failure to correct a structural deformity will result in overload to the affected compartment, and early failure. Distal femoral, proximal tibial, and tibial tubercle osteotomies are all used to unload a specific compartment, and

improve weight-bearing kinematics across the knee.[24] Ligament reconstructions are necessary to provide a stable articulation following injury, and reduce the incidence of recurrent cartilage injury.[25] Other soft tissue reconstructions, including a proximal realignment, can also improve patellar kinematics, thus reducing stress on patellofemoral surfaces.

PATIENT EDUCATION

All patients should be educated regarding appropriate knee health. Knees bear significant multiples of body weight in day-to-day activities. Thus appropriate weight management and nonimpact conditioning are important in reducing pain and improving function.[26] Muscle strengthening, focusing on the entire lower extremity,[27] can significantly decrease pain scores in patients with arthritic knees. We encourage all patients with symptomatic cartilage lesions and arthritis of the knee toward a self-directed nonimpact conditioning program focused on a stationary bike and/or an elliptical trainer for a minimum 30 minutes, 5 days per week.

CONCLUSIONS

Existing biologic techniques used to address full-thickness cartilage lesions provide a durable, successful solution in the appropriate candidate. In the future, less invasive techniques that create a long-lasting true hyaline layer, restoring optimal function, and preventing disease progression, are the ultimate goals in this field.

REFERENCES

1. Widuchowski W, Widuchowski J, Trzaska T. Articular cartilage defects: study of 25,124 knee arthroscopies. Knee 2007;14:177-182.

2. McNickle AG, Provencher MT, Cole BJ. Overview of existing cartilage repair technology. Sports Med Arthrosc 2008;16:196-201.

3. Insall JN. Intra-articular surgery for degenerative arthritis of the knee: a report of the work of the late K. H. Pridie. J Bone Joint Surg [Br] 1967;49:211-228.

4. Blevins FT, Steadman JR, Rodrigo JJ, Silliman J. Treatment of articular cartilage defects in athletes: an analysis of functional outcome and lesion appearance. Orthopedics 1998;21:761-767.

5. Mithoefer K, Williams RJ 3rd, Warren RF, et al. Chondral resurfacing of articular cartilage defects in the knee with the microfracture technique: surgical technique. J Bone Joint Surg [Am] 2006;88(Suppl 1 Pt 2):294-304.

6. Marder RA, Hopkins G Jr, Timmerman LA. Arthroscopic microfracture of chondral defects of the knee: a comparison of two postoperative treatments. Arthroscopy 2005;21:152-158.

7. Mithoefer K, Williams RJ 3rd, Warren RF, et al. The microfracture technique for the treatment of articular cartilage lesions in the knee: a prospective cohort study. J Bone Joint Surg [Am] 2005;87: 1911-1920.

8. Asik M, Ciftci F, Sen C, et al. The microfracture technique for the treatment of full-thickness articular cartilage lesions of the knee: midterm results. Arthroscopy 2008;24:1214-1220.

9. Steadman JR, Briggs KK, Rodrigo JJ, et al. Outcomes of microfracture for traumatic chondral defects of the knee: average 11-year follow-up. Arthroscopy 2003;19:477-484.

10. Brittberg M, Lindahl A, Nilsson A, et al. Treatment of deep cartilage defects in the knee with autologous chondrocyte transplantation. N Engl J Med 1994;331:889-895.

11. Peterson L, Vasiliadis HS, Brittberg M, Lindahl A. Autologous chondrocyte implantation: a long-term follow-up. Am J Sports Med 2010;38:1117-1124.

12. Vasiliadis HS, Danielson B, Ljungberg M, et al. Autologous chondrocyte implantation in cartilage lesions of the knee: long-term evaluation with magnetic resonance imaging and delayed gadolinium-enhanced magnetic resonance imaging technique. Am J Sports Med 2010;38:943-949.

13. Knutsen G, Engebretsen L, Ludvigsen TC, et al. Autologous chondrocyte implantation compared with microfracture in the knee: a randomized trial. J Bone Joint Surg [Am] 2004;86:455-464.

14. Buckwalter JA, Martin JA, Olmstead M, et al. Osteochondral repair of primate knee femoral and patellar articular surfaces: implications for preventing post-traumatic osteoarthritis. Iowa Orthop J 2003;23: 66-74.

15. Kreuz PC, Steinwachs MR, Erggelet C, et al. Results after microfracture of full-thickness chondral defects in different compartments in the knee. Osteoarthritis Cartilage 2006;14:1119-1125.

16. Della Villa S, Kon E, Filardo G, et al. Does intensive rehabilitation permit early return to sport without compromising the clinical outcome after arthroscopic autologous chondrocyte implantation in highly competitive athletes? Am J Sports Med 2010;38:68-77.

17. Zeifang F, Oberle D, Nierhoff C, et al. Autologous chondrocyte implantation using the original periosteum-cover technique versus matrix-associated autologous chondrocyte implantation: a randomized clinical trial. Am J Sports Med 2010;38:924-933.

18. Nehrer S, Dorotka R, Domayer S, et al. Treatment of full-thickness chondral defects with Hyalograft C in the knee: a prospective clinical case series with 2 to 7 years' follow-up. Am J Sports Med 2009;37(Suppl 1):81S-87S.

19. Melton JT, Wilson AJ, Chapman-Sheath P, Cossey AJ. TruFit CB bone plug: chondral repair, scaffold design, surgical technique and early experiences. Expert Rev Med Devices 2010;7:333-341.

20. Sgaglione NA, Florence AS. Bone graft substitute plug failure with giant cell reaction in the treatment of osteochondral lesions of the distal femur: a report of 2 cases with operative revision. Arthroscopy 2009;25:815-819.

21. Carmont MR, Carey-Smith R, Saithna A, et al. Delayed incorporation of a TruFit plug: perseverance is recommended. Arthroscopy 2009;25:810-814.

22. Lu Y, Adkisson HD, Bogdanske JP, et al. In vivo transplantation of neonatal ovine neocartilage allografts: determining the effectiveness of tissue transglutaminase. J Knee Surg 2005;18:31-42.

23. Lonner JH, Mehta S, Booth RE Jr. Ipsilateral patellofemoral arthroplasty and autogenous osteochondral femoral condylar transplantation. J Arthroplasty 2007;22:1130-1136.

24. Gardiner A, Gutiérrez Sevilla GR, Steiner ME, Richmond JC. Osteotomies about the knee for tibiofemoral malalignment in the athletic patient. Am J Sports Med 2010;38:1038-1047.

25. Granan LP, Bahr R, Lie SA, Engebretsen L. Timing of anterior cruciate ligament reconstructive surgery and risk of cartilage lesions and meniscal tears: a cohort study based on the Norwegian National Knee Ligament Registry. Am J Sports Med 2009;37:955-961.

26. Fransen M, McConnell S. Land-based exercise for osteoarthritis of the knee: a metaanalysis of randomized controlled trials. J Rheumatol 2009;36:1109-1117.

27. Thorp LE, Wimmer MA, Foucher KC, et al. The biomechanical effects of focused muscle training on medial knee loads in OA of the knee: a pilot, proof of concept study. J Musculoskelet Neuronal Interact 2010;10:166-173.

CHAPTER 7

Allografts for the Arthritic Knee
William D. Bugbee and Allison J. De Young

KEY POINTS

- Biologic joint restoration should be considered as an alternative to arthroplasty in young, active individuals.
- Careful patient selection is important.
- Osteochondral allografts are particularly suited for treatment of osteochondritis dissecans, osteonecrosis, and posttraumatic periarticular deformities.
- Correction of malalignment and instability is critical to success.
- Single-surface (unipolar) grafts have better outcome than bipolar or multicompartment grafts.

INTRODUCTION

Osteochondral allografts have become an integral part of articular cartilage restoration and repair. The use of osteochondral allografts for the treatment of focal, chondral, and osteochondral lesions in the knee is well supported by clinical experience and peer-reviewed literature.[1-3] However, the use of allografts in the treatment of more advanced diseases, such as that seen in arthritis, is not as well established. Nonetheless, the need for a biologic treatment option for young individuals with degenerative conditions of the knee is clear. While this chapter describes the technical components of osteochondral allograft surgery, it is more important to understand the indications for using allografts as opposed to traditional implants.

Fundamentally, biologic joint restoration may be appropriate in any patient considered too young or active for conventional arthroplasty. While these criteria are often vague, our practice is to evaluate any patient younger than 50 years for potential biologic reconstruction. In our experience with over 500 knee allografts, we have found that successful clinical outcome is predicated on defining specific patient indications, including a definitive preoperative diagnosis (e.g., postmeniscectomy arthritis or posttraumatic arthritis vs. idiopathic osteoarthritis), with attention to all other confounding patient variables such as limb alignment and ligament status. Common indications for osteochondral allografting are listed in **Box 7–1**. This list defines a broad spectrum of clinical conditions; however, it is important to note that, as the extent of disease progresses into the realm of arthritis, the use of allografts becomes more controversial and the technical aspects more difficult, often including adjunct procedures such as osteotomy and ligament reconstruction or meniscal transplant.

In treatment of the "arthritic" patient who is considered for biologic restoration, the following diagnostic categories are relevant: osteonecrosis of the femoral condyle, either spontaneous or steroid-associated[4]; posttraumatic arthritis secondary to tibial plateau fracture malunion,[5,6] femoral condyle fracture, or patella fracture; and cases of unicompartmental arthrosis of either the tibiofemoral joint[7] or the patellofemoral joint.[8,9] These conditions may be idiopathic but, in young patients, are more likely secondary to some underlying condition such as a remote meniscectomy or long-standing chondral injury. The allografting procedure may involve a single surface, such as the femoral condyle or tibial plateau, or a multifocal reconstruction such as the femoral condyle and trochlea or both medial and lateral femoral condyles or a so-called bipolar allograft, which includes resurfacing the tibia and femoral condyle in a single compartment. There are technical aspects of each of these allografts, but they are generally classified into plug or shell grafts. A plug graft is, essentially, a round graft prepared by commercially available instruments that form grafts between 15 and 35 mm in diameter. Shell grafts are more complex geometric shapes that must be prepared by hand. These are utilized for resurfacing the femoral condyle (particularly large or difficult to reach areas, such as the posterior condyle), patella, and tibial plateau. **Table 7–1** outlines common diagnoses and allograft patterns.

SETUP AND EQUIPMENT

The setup for osteochondral allografting of the knee is very similar to a unicompartmental arthroplasty.[10,11] We prefer the use of regional blocks for postoperative pain management;

Box 7-1	Indications for Osteochondral Allografts in Complex Knee Reconstruction

- Large, focal chondral defect
- Osteochondritis dissecans
- Salvage of previous cartilage surgery
- Osteonecrosis of the femoral condyle
- Posttraumatic reconstruction
- Multifocal chondral disease
- Unicompartmental arthritis

Table 7-1   Specific Allograft Reconstruction Options for Degenerative Knee Conditions

Condition	Reconstruction Option
1. Spontaneous osteonecrosis of the medial femoral condyle	Focal allograft, with or without high tibial osteotomy
2. Steroid-associated osteonecrosis	Multiple plugs or shell graft
3. Tibial plateau fracture malunion	Combined tibial plateau allograft and meniscal transplantation, with or without osteotomy
4. Unicompartmental, tibiofemoral arthrosis (secondary to meniscectomy or repetitive chondral trauma)	- Realignment osteotomy, if indicated - Bipolar allograft (tibial plateau with meniscus and plug or shell femoral allograft)
5. Patellofemoral arthrosis	Bipolar plug or shell allograft, with or without tibial tubercle osteotomy

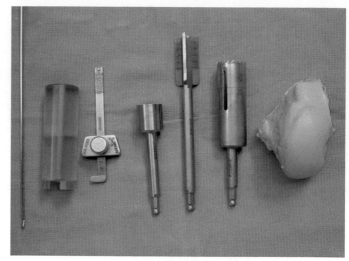

Figure 7-1 Standard, commercially available instruments used for plug allograft. A medial femoral hemicondyle allograft is also shown.

however, the anesthesia is at the discretion of the surgeon and the anesthesiologist. A tourniquet is used in all cases, and the leg positioner is set so the knee can be placed in varying degrees of flexion (70–130°), which is critical for access to the pathologic lesion(s).

The key equipment issue regarding osteochondral allografting is the availability of the allograft tissue. Osteochondral allografts are size matched to the patient and obtained from an accredited tissue bank that is experienced in the recovery, testing, and processing of fresh osteochondral allografts. We prefer fresh, as opposed to frozen allografts, in order to maximize chondrocyte viability and, therefore, to maintain viable cartilage in the allograft in vivo.[12,13] Prior to incision, the surgeon should inspect the allograft to ensure that it is the appropriate size and anatomic part for the proposed procedure. Commercially available instruments can be utilized for performing large, dowel-type allografts, typically on the femoral condyle (**Fig. 7–1**). However, in larger, degenerative conditions, the allograft must often be shaped in the freehand fashion, utilizing power equipment such as saws and burrs. Therefore, the surgeon should have the typical instrumentation utilized for a knee arthroplasty. Fluoroscopy is useful, particularly for tibial plateau allografts or for large femoral condyle allografts. Fixation of a dowel graft is achieved

with press-fit, with or without the use of bioabsorbable pins or screws. Small screws, such as cannulated 3.0- or 3.5-mm screws, should be available to provide fixation for larger shell grafts.

APPROACH

The surgical approach for osteochondral allografting typically utilizes a midline incision and small retinacular mini-arthrotomy, either medial or lateral to the patella depending on the compartment. Care should be taken to protect the meniscus, unless a meniscal transplant is planned. Once the knee is exposed, the patella must be mobilized, which can be done by sequentially extending the arthrotomy proximally, as needed. Retractors are placed in the notch (with care taken not to injure the cruciate ligaments or tibial cartilage) and along the articular margin to expose the knee joint. The knee is then flexed to the appropriate angle in order to best expose the joint surface to be grafted (see Video 7-1).

TECHNICAL DESCRIPTION

Femoral Condyle Plug Graft (Figs. 7-2 through 7-6)

Allografts of the femoral condyle can include either multiple plug grafts or a single shell allograft. In the case of plug allografts, with the femoral condyle lesion exposed, sizing dowels are used to map out the reconstruction of the diseased femoral condyle. Often this requires two or even three grafts to effectively reconstruct the entire femoral condyle. Prior to preparing the surface, the surgeon plans out the size and location of these dowels and begins in a sequential fashion, either anterior to posterior or posterior to anterior. A guide pin is

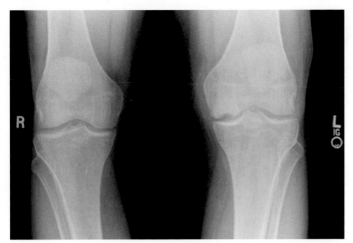

Figure 7-2 A 48-year-old man with spontaneous osteonecrosis of the left medial femoral condyle.

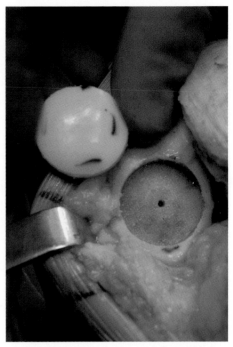

Figure 7-4 After preparation of the lesion and allograft, prior to insertion. Note healthy subchondral bone and relatively shallow depth (7 mm).

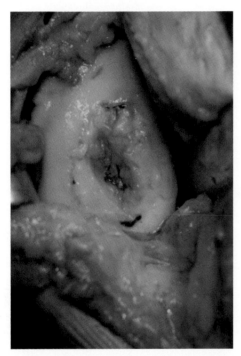

Figure 7-3 Intraoperative photo of necrotic lesion.

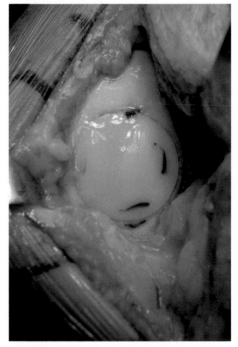

Figure 7-5 Allograft in place. No additional fixation is used.

drilled over the sizing dowel and the lesion is drilled to a depth of 5–7 mm. The depth of the preparation should be minimal and only deeper than 10 mm in cases of marked bone destruction, such as seen in osteonecrosis. The guide pin is then removed and measurements are taken to determine the depth of the preparation, and the first graft is harvested from the allograft. The measurements of the recipient site are transferred to the allograft and the excess bone is resected. The graft is then lavaged copiously. Next, the graft is seated into the prepared site and gently tamped in place either utilizing range of motion to apply joint force or impacted with a tamp. Care should be taken so as to not impact too hard to avoid chondrocyte injury. With the first graft in place, the second graft is inserted juxtaposed or overlapping the first graft. If necessary, fixation with either a bioabsorbable screw or chondral darts can aid in the fixation. However, care should

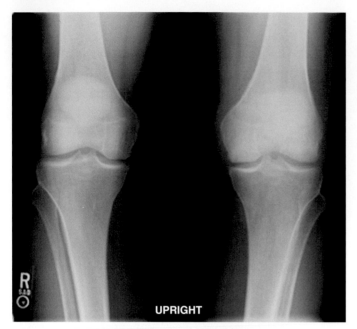

UPRIGHT

Figure 7-6 Postoperative radiograph showing reconstruction of medial femoral condyle.

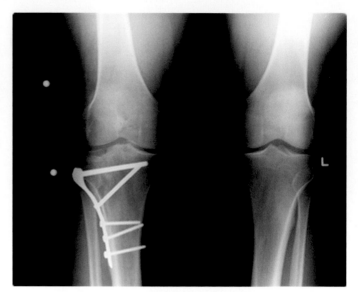

Figure 7-7 A 41-year-old man with symptomatic malunion and posttraumatic arthritis of the lateral tibial plateau.

be taken not to dislodge the first graft when preparing for the second graft. The second graft is placed in a similar fashion and at this point, if the condyle has been reconstructed, the wound is irrigated and a routine closure over a drain is performed.

Femoral Condyle Shell Graft

In cases where utilizing multiple dowel grafts is not appropriate or technically impossible (i.e., in the posterior femoral condyle), a shell graft is created. This is done utilizing a saw or burr to create a flat surface, very similar to either a posterior or a distal cut performed during a knee arthroplasty. However, in allografting, it is performed using a freehand technique and, once the cut is made, the prepared surface is then measured in length and width. These measurements are transferred to the allograft and, after marking the graft, another freehand cut is made to resect the portion of the condyle necessary for reconstruction. A series of preliminary fittings are performed and further trimming of the graft, as necessary, is done. It is important in this setting to reconstruct not only both the length and width, but also the femoral condyle height. This may require fluoroscopic imaging. With minimal fixation, a range of motion can be performed to confirm that the graft is not overstuffing the compartment and that it is relatively stable prior to fixation. Because these are uncontained grafts, they require more fixation, and typically bioabsorbable or 3.0-mm cannulated screws can be used from an extra-articular position to avoid complications of the screws on the articular surface.

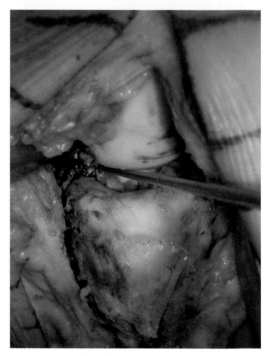

Figure 7-8 Intraoperative photo demonstrating collapse and defect of central plateau.

Tibial Plateau Allografts (Figs. 7-7 through 7-13)

Tibial plateau allografts are particularly useful for reconstruction of posttraumatic problems, such as tibial plateau fractures.[6] In this setting, the procedure is very similar to resurfacing of the tibial plateau in unicompartmental arthroplasty. After exposing the knee, it must be determined if the meniscus should be replaced. Most often, we replace the meniscus with the tibial plateau graft because meniscus pathology is almost

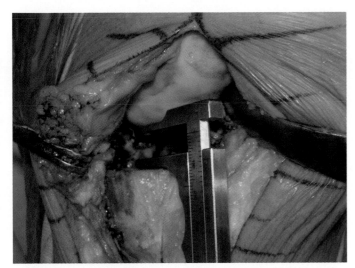

Figure 7-9 After resection of the plateau, the gap is measured to determine preliminary allograft thickness.

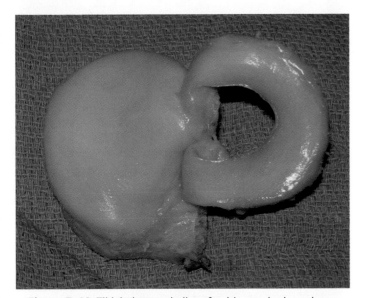

Figure 7-10 Tibial plateau shell graft with attached meniscus.

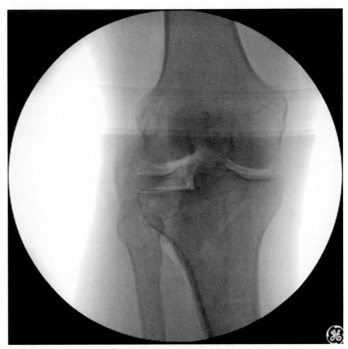

Figure 7-11 Fluoroscopic image, confirming position and height of allograft and restoration of joint line, prior to graft fixation.

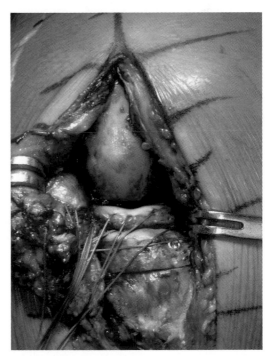

Figure 7-12 Intraoperative photo with graft in place.

universal in cases of posttraumatic or degenerative arthritis. After excising the meniscus remnant and determining the amount of bone loss from the involved plateau, the reciprocating saw is used to make a vertical cut and then, using either a unicompartmental knee jig or a freehand technique, a limited resection of the tibial plateau is made. This is important to consider, because frequently bone loss has led to a loss of plateau height that will be restored with the allograft. Over-resection of the tibial plateau should be avoided.

Once the resection is made and the meniscal remnant is removed, the knee is brought into extension and the gap between the femoral condyle and the resected tibial surface is measured. This gives the surgeon a preliminary measurement of the thickness of the tibial plateau graft that needs to be

prepared. The length and width of the prepared tibial surface should also be measured and any bone defects curetted and grafted. The length, width, and thickness measurements obtained are then transferred to the tibial plateau allograft. The graft is harvested, taking care to include the meniscus attachments with the graft. The graft is then measured and

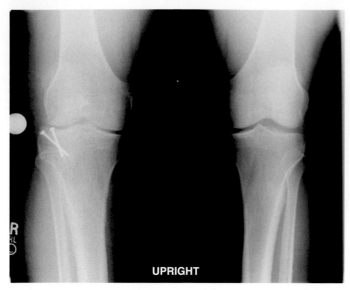

Figure 7-13 One-year postoperative radiograph showing healed lateral plateau allograft.

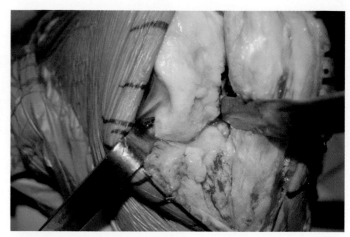

Figure 7-14 A 29-year-old woman with advanced lateral compartment arthritis.

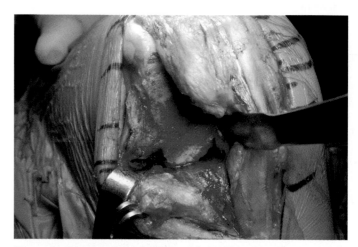

Figure 7-15 Resection of tibial and femoral surfaces for placement of bipolar shell allograft.

recut as necessary. The meniscus is seated under the femoral condyle with great care and range of motion is utilized to determine the balancing of the involved compartment. Fluoroscopic images should also be obtained to ensure that the tibial plateau height and varus-valgus angulation have been restored. Typically, multiple small revisions of the graft or the recipient plateau are performed to obtain an excellent fit with the appropriate kinematics. Once this is accomplished, typically screw fixation is used from the anterior and midcoronal line to fix the graft to the tibial plateau, and meniscus repair is performed in standard fashion.

Bipolar Grafts (Figs. 7-14 through 7-19)

Single-compartment, reciprocal bipolar grafts for the treatment of unicompartmental arthritis or when both femoral and tibial surfaces are diseased are technically very challenging and should be used with great care.[7,14] The technical aspects of each allograft have been outlined above. The sequence of events would be as follows: resection of the tibial surface, allowing for more access to the femoral side; preliminary preparation of the tibial graft, followed by allografting of the femoral condyle; and finally, insertion of the tibial allograft.

SPECIAL CONSIDERATIONS

The surgical techniques involved in osteochondral allografting are fairly straightforward, but the nuances of the biologic restoration can be daunting for inexperienced surgeons. It is important to have one or two scrubbed assistants to maintain the leg in an appropriate position for reconstruction and access to the lesions. It is important to confirm that the

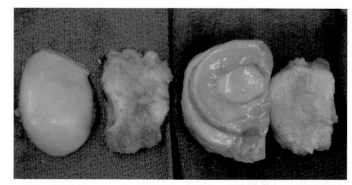

Figure 7-16 Comparison view of resected joint surfaces and prepared shell allografts.

appropriate allograft material is on hand. The least amount of allograft material necessary for reconstruction should be used, and it should be noted that unipolar grafts (i.e., single-surface grafts) are far easier and have better outcomes than bipolar grafts.[10] For this reason, in cases such as osteonecrosis of the

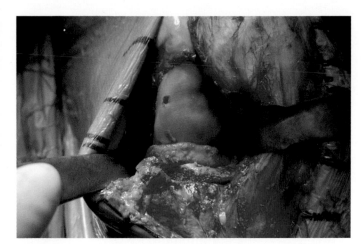

Figure 7-17 Intraoperative view of reconstructed lateral joint compartment. Grafts are fixed with bioabsorbable compression screws.

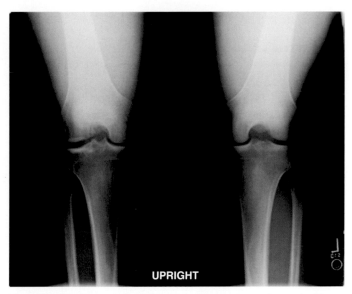

Figure 7-19 Same patient, 2-year postoperative radiograph. Note restoration of lateral joint space and healing of allograft. (Patient was not considered a candidate for osteotomy due to normal limb alignment.)

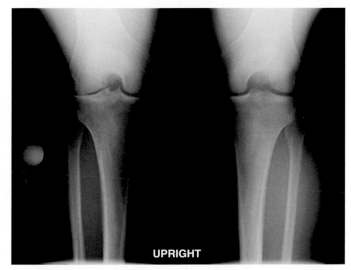

Figure 7-18 Preoperative radiograph of a 39-year-old man with post-meniscectomy arthritis.

femoral condyle, even if there is some articular cartilage disease of the tibial plateau, we would choose not to resurface the plateau. Conversely, in cases of tibial plateau disease with only modest femoral condyle articular cartilage disease, we would choose to reconstruct only the tibial plateau, rather than perform a bipolar graft. However, in those cases where exposed bone is present on both joint surfaces, it is appropriate to perform a bipolar allograft. In situations where malalignment or ligament deficiency is present, it is important to consider correction of these pathologies.

Osteochondral allografts, like artificial knee implants, are adversely affected by harsh mechanical environment. Care should be taken to avoid performing an osteotomy on the same side of the joint as the allograft (i.e., femoral condyle allografts should not be accompanied by a distal femoral

osteotomy; tibial plateau allografts should not be accompanied by a proximal tibial osteotomy). Fortunately, the most common combination procedures are (1) medial femoral condyle allograft with a high tibial valgus osteotomy or (2) lateral tibial plateau allograft with a distal femoral varus osteotomy. Ligament reconstruction and mensical transplantation can be performed in the same setting and do not severely affect rehabilitation for the allograft.

POSTSURGICAL FOLLOW-UP

Postoperative care includes a period of protective weight bearing. This depends on the size and extent of grafting, but for large grafts and advanced disease states as described here, a minimum 6 weeks of touch-down weight bearing followed by a minimum of 6 weeks of protective weight bearing is used. In cases where meniscus transplantation is performed, range of motion should be limited initially to protect the meniscus repair. At the time of surgery, the surgeon can identify specific criteria; that is, if grafts have any amount of instability, then the postoperative management should be modified. We generally try to encourage early range of motion to restore functional knee joint function and to begin closed-chain exercises, such as cycling, at 4–6 weeks. Large grafts require prolonged protective weight bearing, up to 3 months, and increases in activity should be supported by radiographic evidence of healing. Radiographs are obtained at 4–6 weeks, 3 months, 6 months, and yearly thereafter to follow the course of these patients.

TIPS AND PEARLS

- Proper indication for the allograft procedure is critical.
- Pay careful attention to limb alignment, knee stability, and meniscal status.
- Unipolar, single-surface grafts perform better than bipolar or multifocal grafts.
- Prior to surgical incision, ensure the allograft tissue is appropriate for the planned procedure.
- Whenever possible, use commercial instruments for placing large-diameter plug grafts.
- Limit the amount of bone transplanted to less than 10 mm, unless restoration of a bone defect is necessary.
- Use fluoroscopy to confirm graft position, particularly in tibial reconstruction.
- Be prepared to use screws for proper graft fixation and stability.
- Early motion but delayed weight bearing are the cornerstones of postoperative rehabilitation.

REFERENCES

1. Emmerson BC, Gortz S, Jamali AA, et al. Fresh osteochondral allografting in the treatment of osteochondritis dissecans of the femoral condyle. Am J Sports Med 2007;35:907-914.
2. Gortz S, Bugbee WD. Allografts in articular cartilage repair. J Bone Joint Surg [Am] 2006;88:1374-1384.
3. Sgaglione NA, Chen E, Bert JM, et al. Current strategies for nonsurgical, arthroscopic, and minimally invasive surgical treatment of knee cartilage pathology. Instruct Course Lect 2010;59: 157-180.
4. Gortz S, De Young AJ, Bugbee WD. Fresh osteochondral allografting for steroid-associated osteonecrosis of the femoral condyles. Clin Orthop Relat Res 2010;(468):1269-1278.
5. Gross AE, Kim W, Las Heras F, et al. Fresh osteochondral allografts for posttraumatic knee defects: long-term followup. Clin Orthop Relat Res 2008;(466):1863-1870.
6. Shasha N, Krywulak S, Backstein D, et al. Long-term follow-up of fresh tibial osteochondral allografts for failed tibial plateau fractures. J Bone Joint Surg [Am] 2003;85(Suppl 2):33-39.
7. Görtz S, De Young A, Bugbee WD. Fresh osteochondral allograft transplantation for biopolar cartilage lesions of the knee. Paper No 513, presented at the annual meeting of the American Academy of Orthopaedic Surgeons, Las Vegas, NV, February 25–28, 2009.
8. Jamali AA, Emmerson BC, Chung C, et al. Fresh osteochondral allografts: results in the patellofemoral joint. Clin Orthop Relat Res 2005;(437):176-185.
9. Torga Spak R, Teitge RA. Fresh osteochondral allografts for patellofemoral arthritis: long-term followup. Clin Orthop Relat Res 2006;(444):193-200.
10. Görtz S, Bugbee WD. Osteochondral grafts: diagnosis, operative techniques, clinical outcomes. In Noyes FR, Barber-Westin SD (eds): Knee Disorders: Surgery, Rehabilitation, Clinical Outcomes. Philadelphia: Elsevier, 2010, pp 948-960.
11. Dietrick TB, Bugbee WD. Fresh osteochondral allografting. In Scott WN (ed): Insall & Scott Surgery of the Knee, 4th ed (Vol 2). Philadelphia: Elsevier, 2006, pp 405-419.
12. Czitrom AA, Keating S, Gross AE. The viability of articular cartilage in fresh osteochondral allografts after clinical transplantation. J Bone Joint Surg Am 1990;72(4):574-581.
13. Williams SK, Amiel D, Ball ST, et al. Analysis of cartilage tissue on a cellular level in fresh osteochondral allograft retrievals. Am J Sports Med 2007;35:2022-2032.
14. Park DY, Chung DB, Bugbee WD. Fresh osteochondral allografts for younger, active individuals with osteoarthrosis of the knee. Presented at the International Cartilage Repair Society (ICRS) Meeting, San Diego, CA, January 9–11, 2006.

CHAPTER **8**

Nonarthroplasty Treatment Options for Unicompartmental Degenerative Joint Disease

Jason M. Hurst

KEY POINTS

- Joint preservation is a multimodal approach to treatment of arthritis.
- Arthroscopy is successful at treating mechanical complaints but not the generalized pain of arthritis.
- Cartilage restoration is often contraindicated in significant degenerative disease.
- Osteotomy is better for younger, active patients.

INTRODUCTION

Joint preservation is a conceptual approach to arthritis treatment using various surgical and nonsurgical modalities in a patient-specific manner. The cornerstone of joint preservation is taking into account the severity of arthritis symptoms, degree of disease, and patient expectations while developing this multimodal approach to treatment. While there is no fixed algorithm for joint preservation, it typically begins with nonoperative treatments. Oral analgesics, nonsteroidal anti-inflammatory medications, and physical therapy are known to alleviate the discomfort associated with unicompartmental arthritic disease. Unloader bracing is a good option for unicompartmental disease in the more active and athletic patient. Injection treatments with corticosteroid solutions and viscosupplementation have also been shown to be effective in alleviating pain and improving knee function. However, there are certain situations when nonarthroplasty procedures are indicated and may provide more reliable relief of pain and dysfunction than continued nonoperative treatments. These techniques are typically best suited for younger, active patients with unicompartmental disease whose age and activity level contraindicate them for a unicompartmental arthroplasty. The common nonarthroplasty options for unicompartmental disease include arthroscopic débridement, cartilage restorative techniques, high tibial osteotomy, and distal femoral osteotomy.

ARTHROSCOPIC DÉBRIDEMENT

Mechanical symptoms associated with meniscal or chondral lesions are the clearest indication for arthroscopic débridement. However, patient expectations need to be clearly defined, and patients should be cautioned that a significant portion of their knee pain might be attributed to the existing arthritis. Multiple authors have shown improvement in knee rating score, improved knee function, decreased anti-inflammatory use, and high patient satisfaction in osteoarthritic knees treated with arthroscopic lavage and débridement.[1-4] Steadman et al.'s systematic arthroscopic approach to the degenerative knee included the expansion of joint space through the release of joint contractures, removal of loose bodies, limited chondroplasty, meniscectomy of unstable tears, thermal ablation of synovitis, and excision of osteophytes blocking full extension.[4] Their published results on a consecutive series of patients with severe arthritis who underwent the procedure showed that greater than 70% of them had significant gains in knee function scores, satisfaction, and delay of arthroplasty at a minimum of 3 years postoperatively.[4]

The most cited predictors of failure of arthroscopic intervention include malalignment greater than 5°, age greater than 60, persistent symptoms greater than 1 year, history of prior surgery, and joint space less than 2 mm.[5-9] Steadman et al. added the presence of "kissing" grade 4 lesions and severity of joint contracture as additional independent predictors of failure. The preoperative presence of a symptomatic mechanical lesion seems to be the most reproducible predictor of success from arthroscopic débridement. Multiple authors have shown persistent symptomatic benefit in patients with combined meniscal pathology and degenerative changes treated with partial meniscectomy, but better results are seen if the meniscal component is acute rather than degenerative.[9-13]

In contrast to the multiple reports of success with arthroscopic débridement in osteoarthritis, Moseley et al. and Kirkley et al. demonstrated equal efficacy between a focused physical therapy program and arthroscopic débridement.[14,15]

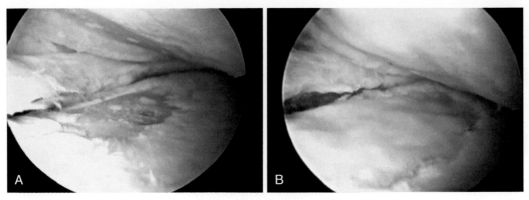

Figure 8-1 Degenerative chondral defects before microfracture **(A)** and after microfracture **(B)**. (Photos courtesy of Dr. William Sterett, Steadman-Hawkins Clinic, Vail, CO.)

Moseley et al. also reported similar outcomes with a "sham-operation" highlighting the power of the placebo effect.[14] Their interpretation of these results has caused many clinicians to question the utility of arthroscopy in the setting of osteoarthritis.[14,15] However, some surgeons criticize these studies for lacking a specific patient cohort with arthritis but predominating mechanical symptoms. The randomized nature of these two studies does demonstrate that the blind application of arthroscopic débridement to osteoarthritis is unlikely to produce successful outcomes greater than nonsurgical treatments and highlights the importance of critically analyzing the patient's symptomatology and applying strict patient selection criteria.

While the use of arthroscopy in the setting of osteoarthritis remains controversial, success from arthroscopic débridement seems to be linked to the predominance of mechanical symptoms, younger age, and neutral alignment. Steadman attributes his success with arthroscopy of degenerative disease in part to the treatment of the associated synovitis and arthrofibrosis. The patient's expectations and desire to remain active are intangibles that are difficult to quantify but should undoubtedly play a roll in the decision to offer arthroscopic débridement in the setting of osteoarthritis.

CARTILAGE RESTORATION

There are multiple, well-studied restorative options for the treatment of acute full-thickness articular cartilage defects. The most common options include microfracture, osteochondral transfer, and autologous chondrocyte transplantation. Despite the continued debate surrounding the appropriate indications and expected longevity for these procedures, one can expect good to excellent results when these restorative options are applied appropriately to the acute full-thickness lesion. On the contrary, most attempts at cartilage restoration will fail in the setting of significant degenerative disease. It is thought that the osteoarthritic environment is not conducive

to these techniques and that either the cartilage at the periphery of the degenerative lesion is too thin to contain the repair or the surrounding cartilage will continue to degenerate. In a review of microfracture in the degenerative knee, there were significant gains in Lysholm scores but the improvement in function was less when compared to their "traumatic" counterpart (**Fig. 8–1**).[16] Larger lesions, older patients, those lesions defined as "degenerative" rather than "traumatic," and bipolar lesions all were associated with less improvement in knee function scores.[16] Andres et al.'s review of osteochondral autograft transplantation demonstrated significantly greater improvements in the pain relief and function of the "isolated lesion" group compared to the "degenerative lesion" group.[17] In a diverse group of patients treated with autologous chondrocyte implantation, McNickle et al. found that age was an independent predictor of postoperative Lysholm score, with less improvement in older patients.[18]

Despite the mounting evidence against cartilage restorative attempts in significant degenerative disease, some advocate these techniques as an adjunct to other joint-preservative procedures such as high tibial osteotomy and meniscal allograft. Gomoll et al. reported on successful outcomes at 2 years postoperatively using the "Triad of Cartilage Restoration": meniscal allograft transplantation, cartilage repair, and osteotomy.[19] Marrow stimulation techniques have been shown to improve early outcomes of osteotomy, and second-look arthroscopy has demonstrated maintenance of the reparative tissue.[20-22] However, Matsunaga et al. questioned the utility of adjunctive marrow stimulation with osteotomy when they showed no significant difference in 5-year clinical outcome between the marrow stimulation and nonreparative groups.[22] Successful treatment of unicompartmental disease with current restorative techniques remains a challenge. The development of biologic scaffolds, platelet-rich gels, stem cell augmentation, and articular allografts are promising potential solutions for unicompartmental arthrosis, but their current use remains controversial and investigational.

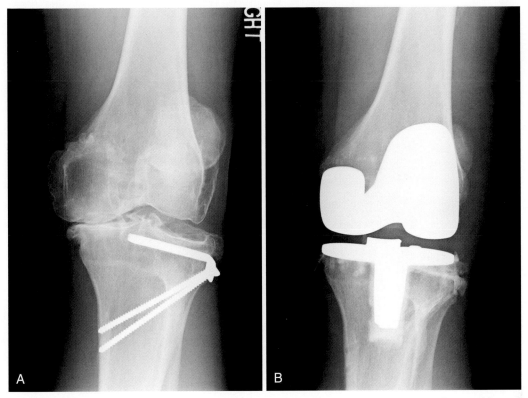

Figure 8-2 Preoperative **(A)** and postoperative **(B)** radiographs of a high tibial osteotomy converted to total knee arthroplasty.

HIGH TIBIAL OSTEOTOMY

High tibial osteotomy is indicated in patients with significant medial osteoarthritis and concomitant varus deformity. The improvement in medial unicompartmental arthroplasty design and clinical outcomes has significantly decreased the popularity of high tibial osteotomy. In addition, the conversion of a high tibial osteotomy to a total knee arthroplasty is complicated by multiple factors, including the presence of hardware, changes in the patellofemoral anatomy, scarring, and previous incisions (**Fig. 8–2**). Therefore, the indications for high tibial osteotomy have narrowed to younger, active patients with isolated medial arthrosis for whom arthroplasty is contraindicated. High tibial osteotomy is also indicated in patients who need medial compartment off-loading secondary to concomitant medial compartment cartilage restoration or meniscal allograft.

Multiple long-term studies of the clinical results of high tibial osteotomy demonstrate reproducible improvement in Lysholm knee scores, decrease in pain scores, and high patient satisfaction.[20,21,23-31] Survivorship and percentage of good to excellent results at 5 years tend to be between 80% and 90%; however, there is a steady deterioration of the survivorship to between 50% and 60% at 10 years.[20,23-27] This consistent decline in efficacy suggests that high tibial osteotomy postpones the need for total knee arthroplasty rather than actually preventing it.

Multiple different tibial osteotomy techniques have been described, including lateral closing wedge, medial opening wedge, and dome osteotomies. In addition, the fixation types have also varied between casting, external fixation, and plate fixation. Regardless of the technique, the ultimate goal of the procedure is to shift the mechanical axis from the diseased medial compartment to the preserved lateral compartment. It is commonly accepted to shift the mechanical axis into slight valgus so that the anatomic valgus angle is approximately 8–10°.[23,28] Fujisawa et al. found that postoperative success correlated with a postoperative mechanical axis that crossed the lateral compartment at a point 30–40% of the distance between the center and lateral edge of the plateau (see Fig. 8–2A).[28] The accuracy of the correction is of paramount importance because excessive overcorrection and undercorrection have been shown to be intimately associated with suboptimal satisfaction and durability of the procedure.[29-31] Other factors that have been shown to contribute to the deterioration of high tibial osteotomy include age older than 60, ligamentous instability, obesity, concomitant lateral compartment disease, poor preoperative range of motion, and greater than 12° of preoperative angular deformity.[26,31]

Conversion of high tibial osteotomy to total knee arthroplasty is technically more demanding than a primary total knee arthroplasty. An oblique medial opening wedge osteotomy at the level of the tibial tubercle has been shown to

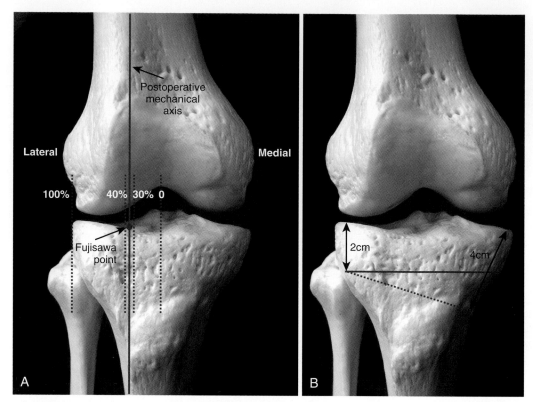

Figure 8-3 Optimizing the results of high tibial osteotomy relies on slight overcorrection of the weight-bearing line to the Fujisawa point **(A)** and performing an oblique osteotomy to limit patella baja **(B)**. (Images reproduced courtesy of Joint Implant Surgeons, Inc.)

have less of an effect on patellar height and tibial slope than a traditional horizontal osteotomy and should conceivably allow for easier conversion to total knee arthroplasty (see Fig. 8–1B).[32] However, it is important to aim the oblique osteotomy toward the lateral metaphyseal flare approximately 2–3 cm below the lateral joint line because failure is associated with osteotomies that are too distal on the lateral cortex (**Fig. 8–3**).[32] The use of external fixation with or without distraction osteogenesis can eliminate the hardware concerns, but pin tract infections are a significant problem especially when a future implant is likely. Biocompatible hardware options with PEEK (polyether ether ketone) or trabecular metals could obviate hardware concerns during conversion; however, there are no such implants currently available.

The relative indications for high tibial osteotomy have changed in recent years, making it difficult to draw accurate comparisons between high tibial osteotomy and unicompartmental arthroplasty. In addition, the ideal patient for each procedure is vastly different despite the common diagnosis of medial osteoarthritis. Typical candidates for an osteotomy tend to be younger and extremely active in high-impact sports or manual labor, and their satisfaction is dependent on their ability to continue with their active high-impact lifestyle. On the contrary, the classic unicompartmental arthroplasty candidate tends to be middle-aged or older, and his or her activity

is less impact-oriented. In these patients, the moderate activity level is not a contraindication for the implant and the main goal of treatment is pain relief rather than returning to high-impact activities. Therefore, while both procedures are valid treatment options for isolated medial compartment arthrosis, postsurgical outcomes can be optimized by focusing on the age of the patient, desired activity level, and expectations with regard to pain relief and postsurgical activity level.

DISTAL FEMORAL OSTEOTOMY

Varus-producing distal femoral osteotomy is indicated in patients with lateral compartment disease and concomitant valgus malalignment. Similar to high tibial osteotomy, distal femoral osteotomy is indicated in younger patients for whom a unicompartmental arthroplasty is contraindicated due to young age or high activity level. Medial closing wedge or lateral opening wedge are the most common surgical techniques, and larger deformities are best treated with the lateral opening wedge osteotomy. Like the high tibial osteotomy, the results are excellent in the first 5 years, but the survivorship has a predictable decline after 10 years.[33,34] Subsequent conversion to total knee arthroplasty is a challenge, and the results are inferior to that of primary knee arthroplasty.[35] Outside of the hardware complications and difficulty with intramedullary guidance, the most common problems encountered are instability necessitating a constrained prosthesis and the tendency to place the femoral component into varus angulation.[34] Therefore, extramedullary guidance, computer-assisted technology, or axial image-based systems may be of considerable utility when converting a distal femoral osteotomy to total knee arthroplasty.

SUMMARY

The nonarthroplasty treatment of unicompartmental arthritis is challenging. The initial focus of treatment is symptom management and activity modification. Arthroscopic surgery has limited benefit without the presence of mechanical symptoms or symptoms associated with synovitis and arthrofibrosis, and cartilage restoration is unpredictable in the setting of significant degenerative disease. Osteotomy procedures provide reliable improvement in function and pain scores; however, the procedure lacks durability past 10 years and may complicate future arthroplasty options. In order to optimize success from joint preservation, it is essential to focus on the age of the patient, severity of the disease, and expectations with regards to activity and pain relief.

REFERENCES

1. Livesley PJ, Doherty M, Needoff M, Moulton A. Arthroscopic lavage of osteoarthritic knees. J Bone Joint Surg [Br] 1991;73:922-926.
2. Edelson R, Burks RT, Bloebaum RD. Short-term effects of knee washout for osteoarthritis. Am J Sports Med 1995;23:345-349.
3. Merchan EC, Galindo E. Arthroscope-guided surgery versus nonoperative treatment for limited degenerative osteoarthritis of the femorotibial joint in patients over 50 years of age: a prospective comparative study. Arthroscopy 1993;9:663-667.
4. Steadman JR, Ramappa AJ, Maxwell RB, Briggs KK. An arthroscopic treatment regimen for osteoarthritis of the knee. Arthroscopy 2007;23:948-955.
5. Salisbury RB, Nottage WM, Gardner V. The effect of alignment on results in arthroscopic debridement of the degenerative knee. Clin Orthop Relat Res 1985;(198):268-272.
6. Harwin SF. Arthroscopic debridement for osteoarthritis of the knee: predictors of patient satisfaction. Arthroscopy 1999;15:142-146.
7. Wouters E, Bassett FH 3rd, Hardaker WT Jr, Garrett WE Jr. An algorithm for arthroscopy in the over-50 age group. Am J Sports Med 1992;20:141-145.
8. Ogilvie-Harris DJ, Fitsialos DP. Arthroscopic management of the degenerative knee. Arthroscopy 1991;7:151-157.
9. Aichroth PM, Patel DV, Moyes ST. A prospective review of arthroscopic debridement for degenerative joint disease of the knee. Int Orthop 1991;15:351-355.
10. Rand JA. Arthroscopic management of degenerative meniscus tears in patients with degenerative arthritis. Arthroscopy 1985;1:253-258.
11. McBride GG, Constine RM, Hofmann AA, Carson RW. Arthroscopic partial medial meniscectomy in the older patient. J Bone Joint Surg [Am] 1984;66:547-551.
12. Barrett GR, Treacy SH, Ruff CG. The effect of partial lateral meniscectomy in patients > or = 60 years. Orthopedics 1998;21:251-257.
13. Jackson RW, Rouse DW. The results of partial arthroscopic meniscectomy in patients over 40 years of age. J Bone Joint Surg [Br] 1982;64:481-485.
14. Moseley JB, O'Malley K, Petersen NJ, et al. A controlled trial of arthroscopic surgery for osteoarthritis of the knee. N Engl J Med 2002;347:81-88.
15. Kirkley A, Birmingham TB, Litchfield RB, et al. A randomized trial of arthroscopic surgery for osteoarthritis of the knee. N Engl J Med 2008;359:1097-1107 [published erratum appears in N Engl J Med 2009;361:2004].
16. Miller BS, Steadman JR, Briggs KK, et al. Patient satisfaction and outcome after microfracture of the degenerative knee. J Knee Surg 2004;17:13-17.
17. Andres BM, Mears SC, Somel DS, et al. Treatment of osteoarthritic cartilage lesions with osteochondral autograft transplantation. Orthopedics 2003;26:1121-1126.
18. McNickle AG, L'Heureux DR, Yanke AB, Cole BJ. Outcomes of autologous chondrocyte implantation in a diverse patient population. Am J Sports Med 2009;37:1344-1350.
19. Gomoll AH, Kang RW, Chen AL, Cole BJ. Triad of cartilage restoration for unicompartmental arthritis treatment in young patients: meniscus allograft transplantation, cartilage repair and osteotomy. J Knee Surg 2009;22:137-141.
20. Sterett WI, Steadman JR, Huang MJ, et al. Chondral resurfacing and high tibial osteotomy in the varus knee: survivorship analysis. Am J Sports Med 2010;38:1420-1424.
21. Miller BS, Joseph TA, Barry EM, et al. Patient satisfaction after medial opening high tibial osteotomy and microfracture. J Knee Surg 2007;20:129-133.
22. Matsunaga D, Akizuki S, Takizawa T, et al. Repair of articular cartilage and clinical outcome after osteotomy with microfracture or abrasion arthroplasty for medial gonarthrosis. Knee 2007;14:465-471.
23. Hernigou P, Medevielle D, Debeyre J, Goutallier D. Proximal tibial osteotomy for osteoarthritis with varus deformity: a ten to thirteen-year follow-up study. J Bone Joint Surg [Am] 1987;69:332-354.
24. Insall JN, Joseph DM, Msika C. High tibial osteotomy for varus gonarthrosis: a long-term follow-up study. J Bone Joint Surg [Am] 1984;66:1040-1048.
25. Sprenger TR, Doerzbacher JF. Tibial osteotomy for the treatment of varus gonarthrosis: survival and failure analysis to twenty-two years. J Bone Joint Surg [Am] 2003;85:469-474 [published erratum appears in J Bone Joint Surg [Am] 2003;85:912].
26. Berman AT, Bosacco SJ, Kirshner S, Avolio A Jr. Factors influencing long-term results in high tibial osteotomy. Clin Orthop Relat Res 1991;(272):192-198.
27. Rinonapoli E, Mancini GB, Corvaglia A, Musiello S. Tibial osteotomy for varus gonarthrosis: a 10- to 21-year follow-up study. Clin Orthop Relat Res 1998;(353):185-193.
28. Fujisawa Y, Masuhara K, Shiomi S. The effect of high tibial osteotomy on osteoarthritis of the knee: an arthroscopic study of 54 knee joints. Orthop Clin North Am 1979;10:585-608.

29. Matthews LS, Goldstein SA, Malvitz TA, et al. Proximal tibial osteotomy: factors that influence the duration of satisfactory function. Clin Orthop Relat Res 1988;(229):193-200.

30. Coventry MB, Ilstrup DM, Wallrichs SL. Proximal tibial osteotomy: a critical long-term study of eighty-seven cases. J Bone Joint Surg [Am] 1993;75:196-201.

31. Pfahler M, Lutz C, Anetzberger H, et al. Long-term results of high tibial osteotomy for medial osteoarthritis of the knee. Acta Chir Belg 2003;103:603-606.

32. Matar WY, Boscariol R, Dervin GF. Open wedge high tibial osteotomy: a roentgenographic comparison of a horizontal and an oblique osteotomy on patellar height and sagittal tibial slope. Am J Sports Med 2009;37:735-742.

33. Kosashvili Y, Safir O, Gross A, et al. Distal femoral varus osteotomy for lateral osteoarthritis of the knee: a minimum ten-year follow-up. Int Orthop 2010;34:249-254.

34. Aglietti P, Menchetti PP. Distal femoral varus osteotomy in the valgus osteoarthritic knee. Am J Knee Surg 2000;13:89-95.

35. Nelson CL, Saleh KJ, Kassim RA, et al. Total knee arthroplasty after varus osteotomy of the distal part of the femur. J Bone Joint Surg [Am] 2003;85:1062-1065.

SECTION 3
Techniques

CHAPTER 9
Surgical Pearls for Fixed-Bearing Medial Unicompartmental Knee Arthroplasty

Fred D. Cushner

KEY POINTS

- Easier to open the door than look through the keyhole; exercise caution with MIS approach.
- Avoid uni if ACL instability exists.
- Good cement technique is key.
- Tibia cut: closer to perfection, closer to perfection.

INTRODUCTION

It is hard to summarize surgical pearls since this text is dedicated to pearls and techniques for successful partial knee arthroplasty. Many of these pearls may be discussed elsewhere by experienced authors and surgeons, but I will elaborate on pearls that I believe help facilitate the unicompartmental procedure for fixed-bearing designs. While much of this information is discussed and expanded elsewhere, this chapter should serve as a summary of surgical tips and pearls to improve these outcomes, not only patient outcomes, but may translate into making the procedure a bit easier for the surgeon.

SKIN INCISION

The first pearl is regarding the skin incision. In the early 1990s, a resurgence in unicompartmental arthroplasty occurred largely due to the newer minimally invasive surgery (MIS) techniques introduced. Certainly, the size of the incision should be directly proportional to the experience of the operating surgeon. Under no circumstances should a small incision be used that results in a surgical compromise. The incision must be large enough to allow for adequate visualization so proper bone cuts can be made, flexion and extension gaps are balanced, other compartments may be visually inspected and anterior cruciate ligament (ACL) integrity evaluated, and proper femoral and tibial sizing can occur without overhang or impingement.

The ACL can be visualized at the time of the arthrotomy, but visualization of an intact ACL is not always required.

Certainly more important appears to be the stability of the knee. An examination under anesthesia can be performed and stability of the ACL assessed. A nonfunctioning ACL with an unstable knee increases the sliding forces that can eventually lead to early polyethylene wear and joint failure. Engh and Ammeen reported on the results of unicompartmental knee arthroplasty without an intact ACL, and good results can be obtained if functional instability is not present.[1] This differs from the classic article by Goodfellow and O'Connor that showed a higher failure rate without an intact ACL. Therefore, the emphasis is on knee stability, not ACL integrity.[2] Visualization at the ACL does not answer completely the status of the ACL. Cushner et al. not only described significant loss of the ACL at the time of indicated total knee arthroplasty, but pathologic changes in the "viable" ACL were also noted.[3] Mullaji et al. recently evaluated tibial cartilage wear in patients undergoing total knee arthroplasty and found that the articular wear pattern can provide clues to the functional status of the ACL.[4] Posterior-half involvement of the medial plateau was more commonly seen when a functional ACL was not present. This is a helpful pearl since studies from Trompeter et al. showed that the clinical appearance of the ACL was not a good predictor of severity on microscopic examination.[5]

Certainly, the size of the incision should not compromise results. Hamilton et al. reviewed 221 unicompartmental arthroplasties performed using the MIS technique.[6] This cohort was compared to a cohort of 514 standard-incision unicompartmental knee arthroplasty patients. In the MIS group, 9 of 221 were revised for loosening. Of the remaining 212 patients, 16 patients required 18 nonrevision reoperations. In other words, 25 of 221 required at least one reoperation (11.3%). This compared to 8.6% for the standard-incision group, with a higher aseptic loosening rate also noted in the MIS group (3.7% vs. 1%).

DECREASING BLOOD LOSS

Once a skin incision is made, a surgical pearl to decrease blood loss is to inject the knee arthrotomy site with a lidocaine (Marcaine)/epinephrine solution. Thirty milliliters injected along the arthrotomy site did result in a significant decrease in blood loss in our total knee arthroplasty patients.[7] While this procedure was initially described in a total knee arthroplasty patient, it could be also performed in unicompartmental arthroplasty patients. We have extended the use of lidocaine with epinephrine to all arthrotomy patients with the goal of not only less bleeding and fewer transfusions but overall less hematoma in the joint postoperatively. Our thoughts are that less blood in the joint improves the patient's function. Periarticular steroid injections can also be used to improve outcomes following unicondylar knee replacement. Pang et al. recently performed a prospective randomized study comparing 90 knees over a 2-year period where injection with triamcinolone acetonide, bupivacaine, and epinephrine was compared to a control group in which only bupivacaine and epinephrine injections were performed. Improvement was noted in midterm and short-term results with no increase in infection or tendon failures reported.[8]

SOLID REPAIR OF THE ARTHROTOMY

Another pearl utilized at our institution is a solid repair of the arthrotomy. If a solid repair is not performed, this can result in late patella instability and subluxation. We believe that a more watertight seal can not only improve knee appearance but also result in less wound drainage in the immediate postoperative period. We currently utilize a bidirectional barbed suture design to facilitate arthrotomy closure (Quill Suture; Angiotec, Vancouver, British Columbia). Our initial studies showed that not only did we achieve a shorter operating time secondary to a quicker closure of the arthrotomy, but a more watertight closure was also described in the laboratory setting[9,10] (**Fig. 9–1**).

TIBIAL BONE CUTS

There are numerous pearls when it comes to completing the tibial bone cuts. As with all knee procedures, the accuracy of the tibial cut must be stressed. In several ways, a tibial cut for unicompartmental knee is a bit more difficult since mis-cuts or malaligned cuts can be less forgiving during the postoperative period. For example, Hernigou and Deschamps demonstrated that extreme tibial slope could increase failure rates and concluded that a slope of greater than 7° should be avoided.[11] A pearl to avoid excessive slope is to use an angel wing or similar type of device and place it in the cutting guide before the osteotomy is performed. The amount of bone resected anteriorly should be similar to that resected posteriorly (**Fig. 9–2**). If this occurs, then the slope is well within the 7° limit. The depth of the resection also needs to be precise to avoid the complication of a posterior plateau fracture. These fractures are multifactorial and certainly can be minimized

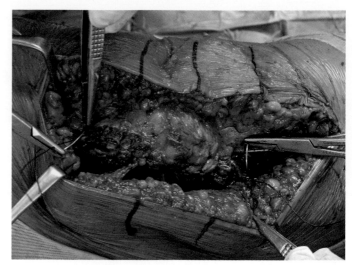

Figure 9-1 Use of a barbed suture (Quill Suture; Angiotech, Vancouver, British Columbia) to aid in watertight closure.

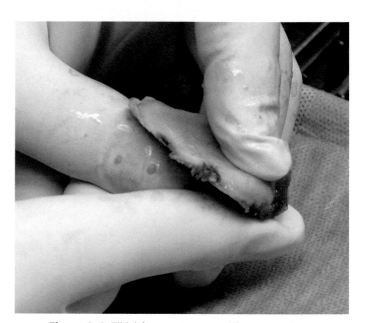

Figure 9-2 Tibial fragment assessed for proper slope.

with a more conservative initial cut (2–3 mm), with the ability to cut more bone if needed.

Limiting of guide fixation pins may also play a role, because the more pins utilized, the higher the risk of fracture. Seon et al. reported two occasions of shear fracture as a result of number of guide pins utilized.[12] Yang et al. showed similar results that appear to be associated with the technique related to the tibial osteotomy guide.[13] Van Loon et al. reviewed peripheral tibial plateau fractures and, once again, they appeared to be related to surgical technique. This complication can be avoided by limiting the number of fixation pins, achieving the proper cutting depth, exercising caution when utilizing the operative mallet, and ensuring proper component sizing.[14] Brumby et al. evaluated tibial stress fractures

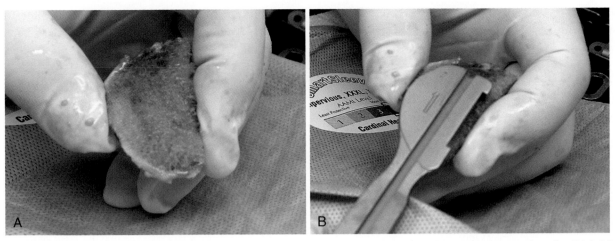

Figure 9-3 (A) Removing the tibial bone fragment whole for examination. **(B)** Use of the fragment as a template for tibial sizing.

and noted that the use of three or more fixation pins did increase their occurrence.[15] They felt that, if three or more pins were deemed necessary, the risk of stress fracture increases. Peripheral pins must not violate the medial cortex and should be avoided if at all possible.

One means to avoid damage to the anterior cortex of the tibia is using caution on removing the osteotomy fragment. We like to remove it in one piece because the osteotomy fragment can serve as a good template for the proper-size tibial component (**Fig. 9–3**). To remove it in one piece without damage to the anterior cortex, we often use a tibial guide and place an ostium on leveling off the tibial guide, not the anterior cortex. By pushing up from the anterior guide and pulling the tibial fragment forward, the piece can be removed intact to be used for sizing purposes and the anterior rim of the cortex is not damaged (**Fig. 9–4**).

Sagittal saw extension can be another source of error resulting in a reduction of the loading capacity of the tibia. When performing these cuts, the vertical cut should not penetrate greater than the total depth that is to be removed. Leaving in the same blade helps protect against undercutting the ACL insertion area.

Simpson et al. evaluated bone strain and found that a 40% increase is noted after implantation.[16] This increased stress reaction may be what contributes to the vague medial pain often seen in the initial 12 months following the unicompartmental procedure. Proper patient assurance is required if no fracture is found but medial pain exists. Unusually by the 12-month mark, these symptoms resolve as bone remodeling occurs.

CEMENT TECHNIQUE

Other surgical technical pearls to avoid complication are related to the cement technique. Retained cement leaves the surgeon with an unacceptable postoperative radiograph and

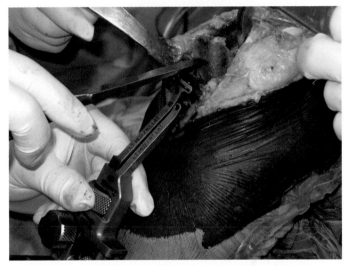

Figure 9-4 Use of an osteotome to wedge the tibial fragment without causing damage to the anterior tibial cortex.

may cause pain for the patient, requiring reoperation for removal of the retained cement. As with most things, prevention is the best treatment. This may involve the placement of a gauze posteriorly to allow for protection should posterior protrusion occur. The cement technique also can decrease the occurrence of retained cement. We like to wash, dry, and actually impact the cement off the plateau to allow for better bone penetration. Less cement is placed more posteriorly to help avoid protrusion, and the components are inserted in a posterior-to-anterior fashion to try to extrude the cement anteriorly around the posterior origin, where it is more difficult to see. Proper tools are also needed, such as curettes to remove any retained cement. In difficult cases an arthroscope can be placed and retained cement can be removed under direct visualization, but we find that with proper technique this is not often required.

Inserting the prosthetic component when the cement is in a less liquid form allows for easier removal of retained cement, although this is a bit of a gamble since no one wants the cement to harden before proper positioning has been achieved. To prevent loosening, more than proper cementing is required for a good cement-prosthesis interface. We have talked about pressurization of the bone cancellous surface but a cancellous surface needs to be prepped before the cement technique is performed. This includes washing as well as drying the tibial surface. Sclerotic bone can be drilled to allow better cement penetration and enhance tibial fixation. In all cases, cementing should include drilling, washing, drying, and then modern cement techniques as described with all retained cement removed.

FEMORAL COMPONENT

In regard to the femoral component, proper sizing is critical, and impingement needs to be avoided. Numerous systems allow for a linkage of the tibial cut to the femoral cut. The advantage here is that no intramedullary hole is placed, hence eliminating the blood loss that occurs from the intramedullary hole. The difficulty often encountered with the link system is that the distal cut is made in the extended position. One pearl is that the cut can be initiated in the extended position but completed with a flexed knee, which is more within most surgeons' comfort zones.

CONCLUSION

In closing, there are many ways in which unicompartmental arthroplasty provides long-term successful results. The above pearls and technical suggestions may help make the procedure a bit easier as well as help to avoid commonly seen complications.

REFERENCES

1. Engh GA, Ammeen D. Is an intact anterior cruciate ligament needed in order to have a well-functioning unicondylar knee replacement? Clin Orthop Relat Res 2004;(428):170-173.
2. Goodfellow J, O'Connor J. The anterior cruciate ligament in knee arthroplasty. A risk-factor with unconstrained meniscal prostheses. Clin Orthop Relat Res 1992;(276):245-252.
3. Cushner FD, La Rosa DF, Vigorita VJ, et al. A quantitative histologic comparison: ACL degeneration in the osteoarthritic knee. J Arthroplasty 2003;18:687-692.
4. Mullaji AB, Marawar SV, Luthra M. Tibial articular cartilage wear in varus osteoarthritic knees: correlation with anterior cruciate ligament integrity and severity of deformity. J Arthroplasty 2008;23:128-135.
5. Trompeter AJ, Gill K, Appleton MA, Palmer SH. Predicting anterior cruciate ligament integrity in patients with osteoarthritis. Knee Surg Sports Traumatol Arthrosc 2009;17:595-599.
6. Hamilton WG, Collier MB, Tarabee E, et al. Incidence and reasons for reoperation after minimally invasive uni-compartmental knee arthroplasty. J Arthroplasty 2006;21(6 Suppl 2):98-107.
7. Kim RH, Scuderi GR, Cushner FD, et al. Use of lidocaine with epinephrine injections to minimize blood loss in total knee replacement. Paper presented at the annual meeting of the Knee Society.
8. Pang HN, Lo NN, Yank KY, et al. Peri-articular steroid injection improved the outcome after uni-condylar knee replacement: a prospective, randomized controlled trial with a two-year follow-up. J Bone Joint Surg [Br] 2008;90:738-744.
9. Kissin YD, Cushner FD, Nett MP, Chadha P. Use of a novel suture to improve wound appearance and increase operating room efficiency. Paper presented at the annual meeting of the Eastern Orthopedic Association, Nassau, Bahamas, 2009.
10. Khanuja HS. Biomechanical comparison of medial parapatellar arthrotomy repair. Presentation at the annual AAOS Meeting, New Orleans, LA, 2009.
11. Hernigou P, Deschamps G. Posterior slope of the tibial implant and the outcome of uni-compartmental knee arthroplasty. J Bone Joint Surg [Am] 2004;86:506-511.
12. Seon JK, Song EK, Yoon TR, et al. Tibial plateau stress fracture after unicondylar knee arthroplasty using a navigation system: two case reports. Knee Surg Sports Traumatol Arthrosc 2007;15:67-70.
13. Yang KY, Yeo SJ, Lo NN. Stress fracture of the medial tibial plateau after minimally invasive uni-compartmental knee arthroplasty: a report of 2 cases. J Arthroplasty 2003;18:801-803.
14. Van Loon P, de Munnynck B, Bellemens J. Peri-prosthetic fracture of the tibial plateau after uni-compartmental knee arthroplasty. Acta Orthop Belg 2006;72:369-374.
15. Brumby SA, Carrinton R, Zayontz S, et al. Tibial plateau stress fracture: a complication of uni-compartmental knee arthroplasty using 4 guide pinholes. J Arthroplasty 2003;18:809-812.
16. Simpson DJ, Price AJ, Gulati A, et al. Elevated proximal tibial strains following uni-compartmental knee replacement—a possible cause of pain. Med Eng Phys 2009;31:752-757.

CHAPTER 10

Medial Unicompartmental Knee Arthroplasty: Fixed-Bearing Techniques

Jean-Noël Argenson and Sébastien Parratte

KEY POINTS

- Patient selection protocol and indications are essential.
- Implant and ancillaries selection should be adapted.
- Proper surgical technique is crucial in this "no-compromise" surgery.
- Ligament imbalance and bony deformities cannot be corrected with a UKA alone.
- Medial UKA should not be considered as a temporary procedure to wait for a TKA.

INTRODUCTION

The potential advantage of unicompartmental knee arthroplasty (UKA) over tricompartmental replacement is the preservation of the bone stock in the remaining compartment and the preservation of the ligaments. This concept requires an accurate and reproducible surgical technique. The most important evolution in UKA during the last decade is minimally invasive surgery, which can be defined as the ability to implant the components without an incision in the quadriceps tendon or the vastus medialis and without everting the patella.[1,2] When performing UKA, surgeons must bear in mind that proper implant positioning should not be compromised by using too small an incision.

Success of the procedure will be related not only to proper surgical technique but also to proper patient selection.[1–5] The indications for UKA are painful osteoarthritis or osteonecrosis limited to one compartment of the knee associated with significant loss of joint space on the radiographs on a stable knee.[5–9] Age and weight still represent debatable issues for the indication of UKA as the procedure is often presented as an alternative to either osteotomy or total knee arthroplasty (TKA).[5–9] Obesity itself is consequently not a contraindication. We do use the "SAW" concept (stability, alignment, and wear) to confirm the indication of UKA. Therefore, the knee should be stable and aligned and cartilage wear should be limited to one compartment of the knee. These criteria are checked preoperatively, and the physical examination should ensure that the knee is stable in the anteroposterior and sagittal planes and that the range of knee flexion is greater than 100° with a full knee extension. The patellofemoral joint should be clinically asymptomatic to confirm that wear is limited to one compartment.

To complete the physical examination, a systematic radiologic analysis should include anteroposterior and mediolateral views of the knee, full-length radiographs, stress radiographs,[10] and skyline views (**Fig. 10–1**). The radiographic analysis should ensure that there is no patellofemoral loss of joint space on skyline views at 30°, 60°, and 90° of flexion; the presence of full-thickness articular cartilage in the nonaffected compartment; and full correction of the deformity to neutral on stress radiographs performed with the patient supine using a dedicated knee stress system. The angle between the mechanical axis of the femur and the anatomic axis of the femur, as well as the mechanical axis of the lower limb, should be calculated on the full-length radiograph. A varus or valgus deformation of the lower limb greater than 15° may represent a contraindication for UKA as the correction of such deformation may require soft tissue release, which should not be performed when doing UKA.[11,12] When there is a question regarding the status of the anterior cruciate ligament (ACL) following the clinical examination, magnetic resonance imaging may be useful to confirm that the ACL is intact. This step, including patient selection and confirmation of the indication, represents probably the most important step and is really a basic warranty to the success of the procedure.

SETUP AND EQUIPMENT

The procedure can be performed under general or epidural anesthesia. We do use a tourniquet inflated at the proximal part of the thigh. We perform the procedure on a routine operating table using two leg holders, one below the foot and one against the thigh at the level of the tourniquet (**Fig. 10–2**). The leg holder below the foot should be positioned to maintain the knee flexed at 90° when the foot is resting on the leg

SYSTEMATIC PRE-OPERATIVE RADIOGRAPHIC EVALUATION

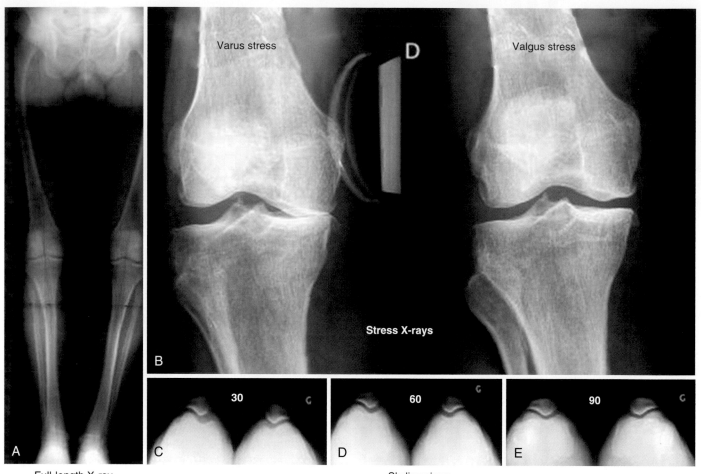

Full-length X-ray   Skyline views

Figure 10-1 To complete the physical examination, a systematic radiologic analysis should include anteroposterior and mediolateral views of the knee, full-length radiographs (**A**), stress radiographs (**B**), and skyline views (**C-E**). The radiographic analysis should ensure that there is no patellofemoral loss of joint space on skyline views at 30°, 60°, and 90° of flexion; the presence of full-thickness articular cartilage in the nonaffected compartment; and full correction of the deformity to neutral on stress radiographs performed with the patient supine using a dedicated knee stress system. The angle between the mechanical axis of the femur and the anatomic axis of the femur, as well as the mechanical axis of the lower limb, should be calculated on the full-length radiograph.

holder and the knee flexed at 110° when the foot is placed below the leg holder.

APPROACH

It is important to maintain proper visualization throughout the procedure to optimize implant positioning even when using a minimally invasive technique. Therefore, the length of the skin incision varies from 8 to 10 cm depending on skin elasticity and patient morphotype. Sufficient visualization is required throughout the procedure and can be achieved by frequent extension-flexion manipulations to preferentially visualize either the femoral side or the tibial side. The upper limit of the incision is the superior pole of the patella, and the incision extends distally either toward the medial side

of the tibial tuberosity for a medial UKA or toward the lateral side of the tibial tuberosity for a lateral UKA, ending 2 cm under the joint line previously located (**Fig. 10–3**). The proximal part of the incision is more essential for the procedure, and two thirds of the incision should be located above the joint line. For the medial UKA, a medial parapatellar approach is performed, extended proximally 1 or 2 cm in the quadriceps tendon. Once the synovial cavity is opened, the part of the fat pad in the way of the condyle is excised to properly visualize the condyle, the ACL and the corresponding tibial side of the tibial plateau. It is important to note that the principles of ligament balancing existing in TKA cannot be applied to UKA because the collateral ligaments should not be released in UKA. To protect the collateral ligament and safely perform the cuts, a dedicated curved, thin

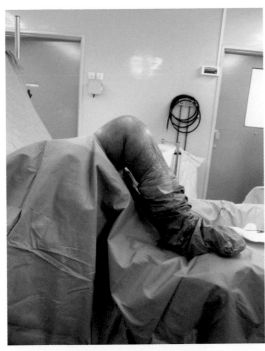

Figure 10-2 We perform the procedure on a routine operating table using two leg holders, one below the foot and one against the thigh at the level of the tourniquet. The leg holder below the foot should be positioned to maintain the knee flexed at 90° when the foot is resting on the leg holder and the knee flexed at 110° when the foot is placed below the leg holder.

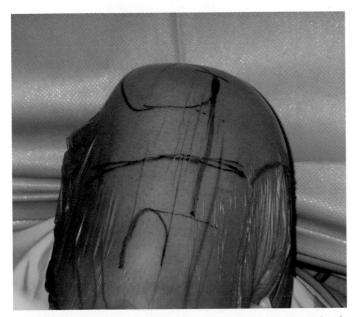

Figure 10-3 The upper limit of the incision is the superior pole of the patella, and the incision extends distally either toward the medial side of the tibial tuberosity for a medial UKA or toward the lateral side of the tibial tuberosity for a lateral UKA, ending 2 cm under the joint line previously located. The proximal part of the incision is more essential for the procedure, and two thirds of the incision should be located above the joint line.

Hohmann retractor is placed on the medial or lateral side of the incision.

Before proceeding to the bone cuts, the first step is to bring the knee to 60° of flexion to evaluate the joint by checking the resistance of the ACL with an appropriate hook and evaluating the state of both the opposite tibiofemoral joint and the patellofemoral joint (**Fig. 10–4**). The osteophytes are then removed on the medial femoral condyle, after which a relative lengthening of the medial collateral ligament and capsule is performed, allowing passive correction of the deformity. Then, osteophytes located in the intercondylar notch should also carefully be removed to avoid late impingement with the ACL on the notch (**Fig. 10–5**). This point is very important to preserve the ACL and avoid any so-called Marie-Antoinette effect related to the osteophytes developed in the intercondylar notch, which have a guillotine-like effect on the ACL.

TECHNICAL DESCRIPTION

It is important to bear in mind that in UKA the proper tension of the ligaments will be restored while filling the gap left by the worn cartilage with the unicompartmental components; therefore, UKA is a so-called surfacing procedure. The tibial cut is made using an extramedullary rod (**Fig. 10–6**). The guide is placed distally around the ankle with the axis of the guide lying slightly medial to the center of the ankle joint. The proximal part of the guide is resting on the anterior tibia pointing toward the axis of the tibial spines; with modern instrumentation, it is possible to have the cutting part of the guide resting only on the upper tibia (medial or lateral) to be resected. The diaphyseal part of the guide is parallel to the anterior tibial crest, and the anteroposterior position of the guide is adjusted distally to reproduce the natural upper tibial slope, usually between 5° and 7° of posterior slope. The amount of resection is decided after using a 4-mm probe located on the deepest part of the affected plateau, and particular care should be taken to properly define the level of the cut. A good anatomic landmark at this step is the deepest part of the deep layer of the medial collateral ligament. When the angel wing–shaped probe is inserted into the tibial guide, the tip of the probe should be at this level (**Fig. 10–7**). An insufficient cut on the tibia will lead to an overcorrection of the deformity, and cutting the tibia too low may lead to a tibial plateau fracture. To complete the tibial cut, the sagittal tibial cut can be done using one of the sagittal marks provided by the guide or made as a freehand cut. When the cut is made freehand, the cut should be aligned close to the tibial spine eminence, with the anterior starting point determined after checking the alignment of the edge of the femoral condyle on the tibial plateau when the knee is brought from flexion close to full extension (**Fig. 10–8**). At this step, once again, particular care should be taken to protect the ACL using a retractor or a pickle retractor.

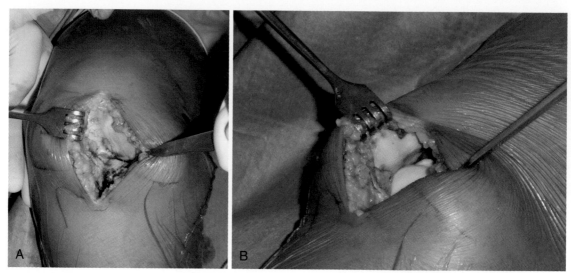

Figure 10-4 Before proceeding to the bone cuts, the first step is to bring the knee to 60° of flexion to evaluate the joint by checking the resistance of the ACL **(A)** and evaluating the state of both the opposite tibiofemoral joint and the patellofemoral joint **(B)**.

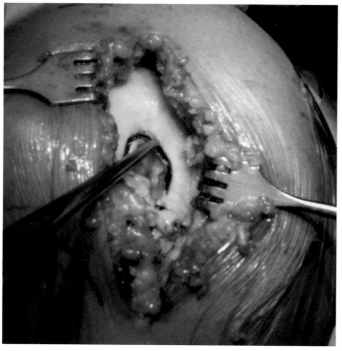

Figure 10-5 Osteophytes located in the intercondylar notch should carefully be removed to avoid late impingement with the ACL on the notch. This point is very important to preserve the ACL and avoid any so-called Marie-Antoinette effect related to the osteophytes developed in the intercondylar notch, which have a guillotine-like effect on the ACL.

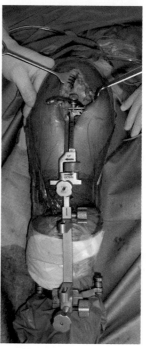

Figure 10-6 The tibial cut is made using an extramedullary rod. The guide is placed distally around the ankle with the axis of the guide lying slightly medial to the center of the ankle joint.

The drilling of the femoral medullary canal through a short incision often requires bringing the knee to 60° of flexion. In fact, in flexion, the tension from the patella on the intramedullary guide might induce incorrect alignment. Once the guide has been properly introduced, the distal femoral cut can be made by marking the angle between the anatomic and mechanical axis previously calculated on the full weight-bearing view. This angle is usually 4–6°. The amount of bone resected from the distal femur corresponds exactly, millimeter for millimeter, to the femoral prosthesis. The remainder of the femoral cuts (posterior cut and chamfers) will then be completed using the appropriate cutting block. The size of the femoral implant should be determined using the cutting block when this femoral finishing guide is positioned on the distal

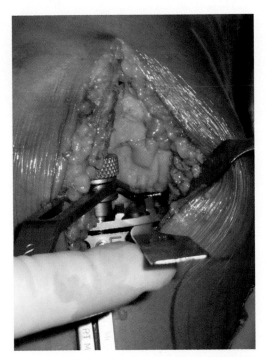

Figure 10-7 The amount of resection is decided after using a 4-mm probe located on the deepest part of the affected plateau, and particular care should be taken to properly define the level of the cut. A good anatomic landmark at this step is the deepest part of the deep layer of the medial collateral ligament. When the angel wing–shaped probe is inserted into the tibial guide, the tip of the probe should be at this level. An insufficient cut on the tibia will lead to an overcorrection of the deformity, and cutting the tibia too low may lead to a tibial plateau fracture.

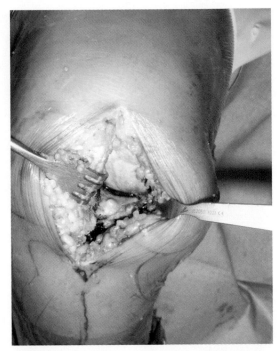

Figure 10-8 To complete the tibial cut, the sagittal tibial cut can be done using one of the sagittal marks provided by the guide or made as a freehand cut. When the cut is made freehand, the cut should be aligned close to the tibial spine eminence, with the anterior starting point determined after checking the alignment of the edge of the femoral condyle on the tibial plateau when the knee is brought from flexion close to full extension.

femoral cut, searching for the best compromise between an anatomically centered position on the femoral condyle and a long axis perpendicular to the resected tibial plateau (**Fig. 10–9**). The top of this finishing guide should be localized at least 1–2 mm above the deepest layer of the cartilage to avoid a potential notch between the femoral implant and the patella. To control the mediolateral position of the femoral cutting guide, which determines the position of the final implant, the use of tibial referencing based on the previously made tibial cut is probably the best landmark. Because the divergence of the medial condyle is different from one knee to another, checking the mediolateral position of the guide on the femoral condyle is also recommended. Once the posterior cut has been made and the cutting guide removed, removal of any posterior osteophytes is necessary using a curved osteotome to increase the range of flexion and avoid any posterior impingement with the polyethylene liner in high flexion (**Fig. 10–10**).

The size of the tibial tray should now be determined, managing the best compromise between maximal tibial coverage and overhang, which might induce pain. The anteroposterior size of the tibial plateau sometimes differs from the mediolateral one, especially for female knees, thus different sizing trials

are necessary to find the best compromise (**Fig. 10–11**). It is important to keep the depth of the tibial cut as conservative as possible to take advantage of the strength of the tibial cortex and the increased area of contact proximally. The knee is then brought into maximal flexion and externally rotated.

The final preparation of the tibia is completed with the appropriate guide, with the underlying keel impacted in the subchondral bone. Using a minimal incision, it is important to locate carefully the posterior margin of the tibial plateau to position the keel correctly in the anteroposterior direction. It is useful to precut the future location of the keel using a small osteotome. The flexion-extension gaps should be tested with the trial components in place and inserting a trial polyethylene liner (**Fig. 10–12**). Common causes of impingement are residual bone eminence, incorrect position of the tibial or femoral component, or an oblique tibial cut. Once this has been verified, it is important to check for 2 mm of protective laxity at close to full extension to avoid any overcorrection of the deformity, which could lead to progression of osteoarthritis in the unreplaced compartment. Important residual varus deformity should also be avoided, as recently reported, to minimize the risk of polyethylene wear when using flat polyethylene inserts. The ideal correction as measured on the postoperative full weight-bearing view will probably consist of a

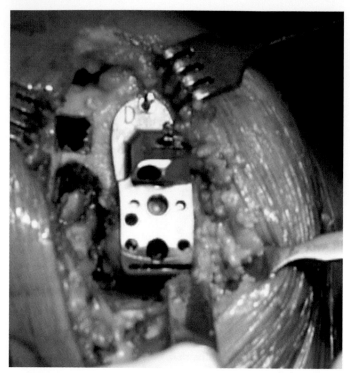

Figure 10-9 The size of the femoral implant should be determined using the cutting block when this femoral finishing guide is positioned on the distal femoral cut, searching for the best compromise between an anatomically centered position on the femoral condyle and a long axis perpendicular to the resected tibial plateau. The top of this finishing guide should be localized at least 1-2 mm above the deepest layer of the cartilage to avoid a potential notch between the femoral implant and the patella. To control the mediolateral position of the femoral cutting guide, which determines the position of the final implant, the use of tibial referencing based on the previously made tibial cut is probably the best landmark.

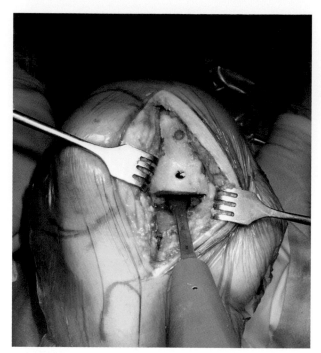

Figure 10-10 Once the posterior cut has been made and the cutting guide removed, removal of any posterior osteophytes is necessary using a curved osteotome to increase the range of flexion and avoid any posterior impingement with the polyethylene liner in high flexion.

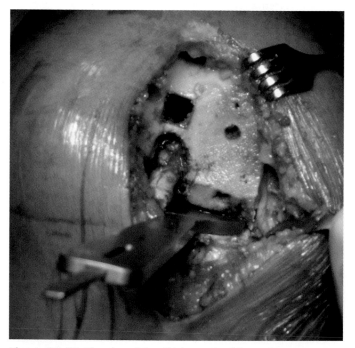

Figure 10-11 The size of the tibial tray should now be determined, managing the best compromise between maximal tibial coverage and overhang, which might induce pain. The anteroposterior size of the tibial plateau sometimes differs from the mediolateral one, especially for female knees, thus different sizing trials are necessary to find the best compromise.

tibiofemoral axis crossing the knee between the tibial spines and the lateral third of the tibial plateau for a medial UKA, as outlined by Kennedy et al. in their classification.[10]

We cement all components for better fixation because long-term results suggest loosening is not a common mode of failure with modern cemented fixed-bearing, metal-backed components. When cementing the components, it is important to avoid leaving any cement at the posterior aspect of the knee, and a 90° curved probe is useful to remove any posterior cement when using a minimal incision. Once the femoral implant has been cemented, bringing the knee close to extension helps remove any posterior cement, with the polyethylene liner inserted last. While the cement is curing, the knee should be maintained at 20° of flexion and not in full extension to avoid lift-off of the posterior aspect of the tibial plateau during this step (**Fig. 10–13**). Patellar tracking should be checked before closing; the absence of patellar eversion during the procedure is helpful for that step. The tourniquet is released

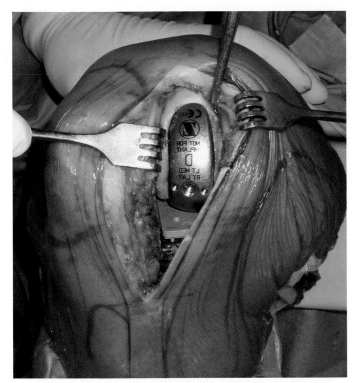

Figure 10-12 The flexion-extension gaps should be tested with the trial components in place and inserting a trial polyethylene liner. Common causes of impingement are residual bone eminence, incorrect position of the tibial or femoral component, or an oblique tibial cut. Once this has been verified, it is important to check for 2 mm of protective laxity at close to full extension to avoid any overcorrection of the deformity, which could lead to progression of osteoarthritis in the unreplaced compartment.

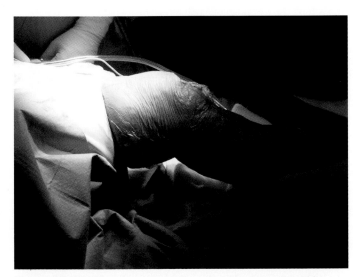

Figure 10-13 When the cement is curing, the knee should be maintained at 20° of flexion and not in full extension to avoid lift-off of the posterior aspect of the tibial plateau during this step.

before closure to adequately perform hemostasis. In our practice, one intra-articular drain is left for 36 hours.[12]

SPECIAL CONSIDERATIONS

Fixed-Bearing Lateral UKA[13]

In our practice, lateral UKA corresponds to 10% of the indications for UKA, and our published long-term results confirm previously published findings that lateral osteoarthritis can be treated successfully by unicondylar replacement. Some special technical considerations should be emphasized concerning lateral UKA. Using a minimal approach to the lateral compartment, the skin incision needs to be lateral, especially at the distal portion, owing to the frequent divergence of the lateral femoral condyle. When the lateral arthrotomy is performed, visualization of the joint is often easier than on the medial side due to the natural mobility of the lateral tibiofemoral joint. When performing a lateral UKA, it is recommended to not remove the osteophytes in order to optimize the femoral implant positioning considering the femoral divergence of the condyle. The tibial resection should stay minimal, because the disease is more often on the femoral side, and to respect the anatomy of the lateral tibial plateau, the cut should be performed without posterior slope. In cases of femoral dysplasia, it is often necessary to use a more "proximal-distal" femoral cut, and a dedicated femoral cutting guide can increase the thickness of the femoral cut. The alignment of the femoral cutting guide on the tibial cut is crucial due to the natural shape of the lateral femoral condyle. It is frequently necessary to mark the correct alignment in extension rather than in flexion to avoid any medial edge loading and impingement between the femoral implant and the tibial spines. The polyethylene insert is often thicker than for the medial side in cases of femoral dysplasia, even if the principle of undercorrection of the deformity for all cases of lateral UKA remains the basis for successful long-term results.

Fixed-Bearing UKA for Avascular Osteonecrosis of the Knee[14]

In our experience, the outcomes of UKA performed for osteonecrosis were comparable with the average reported results of TKA for osteonecrosis, with a revision rate of 3%. The special considerations related to UKA for osteonecrosis are related to patient selection and surgical technique. Patient preoperative analysis should ensure that the disease is limited to one compartment of the knee. The second consideration is the systematic use of cement to fix the UKA components in our series; this was previously emphasized in TKA for osteonecrosis of the knee, with reported improvement in patient outcomes by implementing the use of cement with all components. Finally, the use of a bone-cutting device combined with a femoral component including pegs most often permitted a resection of the entire osteonecrotic lesion and secured the implant fixation in healthy bone.

POSTSURGICAL FOLLOW-UP

Postoperatively, immediate weight bearing is recommended after the removal of the femoral nerve block catheter (left 12 hours postoperatively), protected by two crutches for 1 or 2 weeks. We recommend manual range-of-motion physiotherapy starting the day after surgery. Deep vein thrombosis prevention is managed using mechanical devices and low-molecular-weight heparin for 3 weeks postoperatively.[12] At 2 months, clinical and radiologic evaluation of the patient is performed. Pain-free full range of motion is usually acquired between 2 and 6 months, and during this period, we ask the patient to walk, swim, or ride a bike as often and as much as he or she can. Patients are allowed to go back to their previous sports activities at 6 months when they are performing low-impact activities and after 1 year when they are performing high-impact activities. Patients are followed yearly for 5 years and every 2 years after 5 years.[15] As polyethylene wear remains one of the first causes of failure after fixed-bearing UKA, this follow-up is particularly important. In fact, isolated polyethylene exchange can be successfully performed when the metal back has not been torn by the femoral compartment, and a regular patient follow-up may help to detect early polyethylene wear that may require a polyethylene exchange.[12]

TIPS AND PEARLS

- Check the proper indications: the SAW concept (stability alignment, wear).
- Do not perform too small an incision.
- Preserve the ACL and prevent the Marie-Antoinette effect by resecting the osteophytes in the intercondylar notch.
- Control the level of the tibial cut: "not too high, not too low."
- Do not oversize the femur: the anterior aspect of the femoral component should be 2 mm below the limit of the articular cartilage of the trochlea.
- Perform a four-points check at the time of the trialing: (1) the middle of the femoral component in the middle of the tibial plateau in flexion and in extension, (2) maintain a 2-mm laxity in valgus stress, (3) check for the absence of translation in constrained extension, and (4) check for the absence of impingement between the femoral component and the patella.
- Control the cementing technique: remove the cement at the posterior aspect of the tibial tray in extension using a 90° curved probe before the insertion of the polyethylene insert, and maintain the knee at 30° of flexion during the curing of the cement.

REFERENCES

1. Argenson JN, Parratte S, Flecher X, Aubaniac JM. Unicompartmental knee arthroplasty: technique through a mini-incision. Clin Orthop Relat Res 2007;(464):32-36.
2. Repicci JA, Hartman JF. Minimally invasive unicondylar knee arthroplasty for the treatment of unicompartmental osteoarthritis: an outpatient arthritic bypass procedure. Orthop Clin North Am 2004;35:201-216.
3. Argenson JN, Chevrol-Benkeddache Y, Aubaniac JM. Modern unicompartmental knee arthroplasty with cement: a three to ten-year follow-up study. J Bone Joint Surg [Am] 2002;84:2235-2239.
4. Argenson JN, Parratte S. The unicompartmental knee: design and technical considerations in minimizing wear. Clin Orthop Relat Res 2006;(452):137-142.
5. Berger RA, Meneghini RM, Jacobs JJ, et al. Results of unicompartmental knee arthroplasty at a minimum of ten years of follow-up. J Bone Joint Surg [Am] 2005;87:999-1006.
6. Cartier P, Cheaib S. Unicondylar knee arthroplasty: 2-10 years of follow-up evaluation. J Arthroplasty 1987;2:157-162.
7. Goodfellow J, O'Connor J, Murray DW. The Oxford meniscal unicompartmental knee. J Knee Surg 2002;15:240-246.
8. Insall J, Walker P. Unicondylar knee replacement. Clin Orthop Relat Res 1976;(120):83-85.
9. Gibson PH, Goodfellow JW. Stress radiography in degenerative arthritis of the knee. J Bone Joint Surg [Br] 1986;68:608-609.
10. Kennedy WR, White RP. Unicompartmental arthroplasty of the knee: postoperative alignment and its influence on overall results. Clin Orthop Relat Res 1987;(221):278-285.
11. Price AJ, O'Connor JJ, Murray DW, et al. A history of Oxford unicompartmental knee arthroplasty. Orthopedics 2007;30(5 Suppl): 7-10.
12. Argenson JN, Parratte S, Bertani A, et al. Long-term results with a lateral unicondylar replacement. Clin Orthop Relat Res 2008; (466):2686-2693.
13. Parratte S, Argenson JN, Dumas J, Aubaniac JM. Unicompartmental knee arthroplasty for avascular osteonecrosis. Clin Orthop Relat Res 2007;(464):37-42.
14. Parratte S, Argenson JN, Pearce O, et al. Medial unicompartmental knee replacement in the under-50s. J Bone Joint Surg [Br] 2009; 91:351-356.
15. Scott RD, Cobb AG, McQueary FG, Thornhill TS. Unicompartmental knee arthroplasty: eight- to 12-year follow-up evaluation with survivorship analysis. Clin Orthop Relat Res 1991;(271):96-100.

CHAPTER **11**

Unicompartmental Knee Arthroplasty: Mobile-Bearing Techniques

Michael J. Morris

KEY POINTS

- The Oxford mobile-bearing unicompartmental knee arthroplasty is indicated for anteromedial osteoarthritis with an intact anterior cruciate ligament.
- Long-term outcomes demonstrate greater than 92% survivorship at 20 years.
- Exceptionally low wear rates of 0.01 mm/yr have been noted.
- There is quicker recovery from surgery utilizing rapid recovery protocols compared to TKA.

INTRODUCTION

Anteromedial arthritis of the knee with an intact anterior cruciate ligament, as described by White et al., is a distinct pattern of osteoarthritis that is appropriately treated with unicompartmental arthroplasty when conservative measures fail.[1] Unicompartmental knee arthroplasty for anteromedial osteoarthritis with a functional anterior cruciate ligament utilizing a mobile meniscal polyethylene bearing (Oxford Unicompartmental Knee Arthroplasty, Oxford, UK) has demonstrated 92.3% survivorship at 20 years.[2] Clinical results have been good or excellent in 91% of patients at minimum 10-year follow-up utilizing Hospital for Special Surgery Knee Scores.[3] Wear rates of the polyethylene have been reported as 0.01 mm/year when the device is functionally normally without intra-articular or extra-articular impingement.[4] Rapid recovery protocol utilization has resulted in faster functional return than with total knee arthroplasty.[5] There remains concern regarding the increased difficulty in performing this operation, and early failures are often due to technical errors. New instrumentation has been developed (Oxford Microplasty Instrumentation; Biomet, Warsaw, IN) that allows more predictable execution of the procedure while minimizing technical errors. The enhanced performance of the operation should further improve the previously reported excellent clinical and survivorship successes of this mobile-bearing unicompartmental knee arthroplasty.

SETUP AND EQUIPMENT

A tourniquet should be placed on the proximal thigh of the operative limb. A hanging leg holder is utilized to have the operative extremity flexed 30° at the hip with enough abduction to allow at least 135° of knee flexion without impingement on the operative table (**Fig. 11–1**). The contralateral leg is placed in a well-padded foam leg holder. The foot of the bed is dropped perpendicular to the floor. A stiff, narrow reciprocating saw, a 12-mm-wide oscillating saw, and a double-armed vertical toothbrush saw are utilized during the operation (**Fig. 11–2**) (Oxford Knee Resection Procedure Three Pack; Synvasive Technologies Inc., El Dorado Hills, CA). A Woodson-style curette is an excellent cement removal tool. Standard knee retractors and instruments are used. Radiographs are reviewed for anteromedial arthritis and appropriate restoration of the knee with valgus stress radiograph (**Fig. 11–3A-D**). Preoperative templating of the femoral component size is performed using the lateral radiograph (**Fig. 11–3E**).

APPROACH

The operative extremity is exsanguinated and the tourniquet is insufflated to 350 mm Hg. The knee is allowed to flex 90° with gravity in the hanging leg holder. A slightly oblique skin incision is made from the superomedial edge of the patella to a point 3 cm inferior to the joint line, medial to the tibial tubercle (**Fig. 11–4A**). An arthrotomy is performed with proximal extension of 1–2 cm into the vastus medialis at the level of the superomedial pole of the patella (**Fig. 11–4B**). Electrocautery is used to expose the anteromedial aspect of the tibia to allow for later positioning and visualization of the tibial resection guide. None of the medial collateral ligament is released. The anterior horn of the medial meniscus is excised. A small portion of the retropatellar fat pad is excised to allow visualization of the anterior cruciate ligament and the lateral

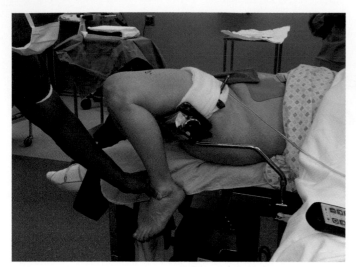

Figure 11-1 Patient positioning in the hanging leg holder. A tourniquet is placed on the upper thigh. The hip is flexed approximately 30° and abducted to allow at least 135° of knee flexion without impingement on the operative table.

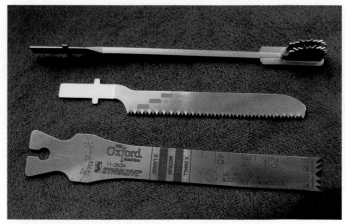

Figure 11-2 The three saws used during the procedure include a double-armed vertical toothbrush saw, a stiff narrow reciprocating saw, and a 12-mm-wide oscillating saw.

compartment of the knee (**Fig. 11–5**). If the anterior cruciate ligament is nonfunctional or there is full-thickness lateral compartment osteoarthritis upon inspection, conversion to a total knee arthroplasty is undertaken.

Assuming the anterior cruciate ligament and the lateral compartment are normal, the unicompartmental arthroplasty continues. Osteophytes are removed with an osteotome from the medial and lateral aspects of the intercondylar notch as well as from the medial margin of the medial femoral condyle. A small rongeur is used to remove the anvil osteophyte anterior to the anterior cruciate ligament insertion on the tibia. The anteromedial osteophyte on the tibia is removed and the blush of bleeding bone from its removal serves as a guide for depth of resection for the tibial osteotomy (**Fig. 11–6**).

TECHNICAL DESCRIPTION

The Oxford Microplasty femoral spoon of preselected size based on the preoperative templating is inserted into the medial compartment, capturing the medial femoral condyle in the sagittal plane. Appropriate tension and restoration of the joint space are achieved with the aid of sequential 1-mm spoons (range 1–3 mm) (**Fig. 11–7**). The proximal tibial resection guide is then placed and coupled to the spoon with the G clamp (**Fig. 11–8**). The G clamp comes in 3-mm and 4-mm options corresponding to the expected thickness of the polyethylene bearing at the completion of the procedure. Tension is removed from the Gelpi retractor prior to coupling to prevent inaccurate elevation of the planned resection level. A double check is performed confirming that the shaft of the tibial saw guide is parallel to the long axis of the tibia in the

coronal and sagittal planes. This will provide 7° of posterior slope utilizing the horizontal tibial resection guide. The tibial guide is secured in place utilizing one pin in the most lateral hole or two pins with one each medial and lateral. A curved Z retractor is placed medially to protect the medial collateral ligament.

The vertical cut is performed first with the stiff narrow reciprocating saw at the lateral edge of the medial femoral condyle and medial edge of the anterior cruciate ligament insertion on the tibia (**Fig. 11–9**). The blade should be directed at the head of the femur and along the flexion-extension plane. Care must be taken to avoid raising the blade during resection and damaging the posterior tibial cortex below the desired resection depth. The narrow saw blade is used to perform the horizontal osteotomy on the tibia. The blade must pass through the posterior cortex. The osteotomized bone is levered up with an osteotome and removed. The excised bone should demonstrate the classic findings of anteromedial arthritis with preservation of the posterior cartilage (**Fig. 11–10**). The remaining meniscus can now be removed.

The intramedullary rod with the distal coupling feature is placed retrograde up the femoral canal from a starting point 1 cm anterior to the anteromedial corner of the intercondylar notch, after drilling and opening the hole with an awl while the knee is in 45° of flexion. The Oxford Microplasty femoral alignment guide, which is set at the corresponding thickness of the flexion space measured by the plastic feeler gauges without the tension of retractors on the medial collateral ligament, is placed into the medial compartment. The linkage bar is used to couple the intramedullary rod to the Oxford Microplasty femoral alignment guide (**Fig. 11–11**). The 4-mm and 6-mm pilot holes are then drilled sequentially in the distal femoral condyle. The posterior femoral resection guide

Text continued on page 78

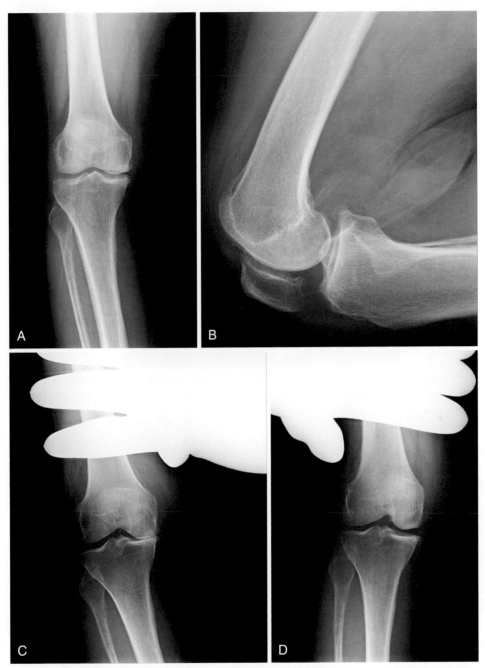

Figure 11-3 **(A)** Anteroposterior radiograph demonstrating varus deformity from medial osteoarthritis of the right knee. **(B)** Lateral radiograph demonstrating medial tibial erosion with maintenance of the posterior medial cartilage. This pattern is consistent with anteromedial arthritis with an intact anterior cruciate ligament. **(C)** Anteroposterior varus stress radiograph demonstrating complete collapse of the medial compartment. **(D)** Anteroposterior valgus stress radiograph demonstrating restoration of the limb alignment and maintenance of the lateral compartment of the knee.

Continued

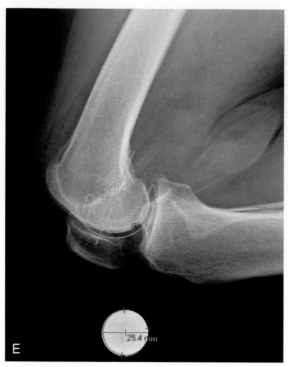

Figure 11-3, cont'd (E) Template of a size small femoral component. The central peg should parallel the shaft of the femoral axis. The prosthesis should lie about 3 mm distal and posterior to the bone on the template, which allows for the thickness of the articular cartilage.

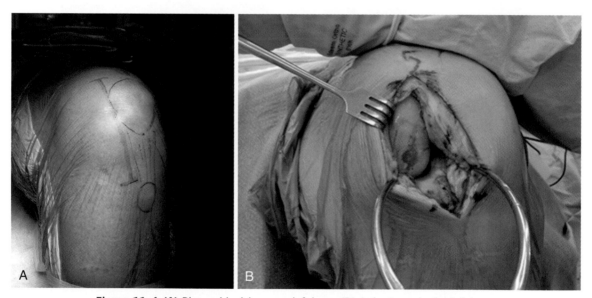

Figure 11-4 (A) Planned incision on a left knee. **(B)** Arthrotomy in the left knee.

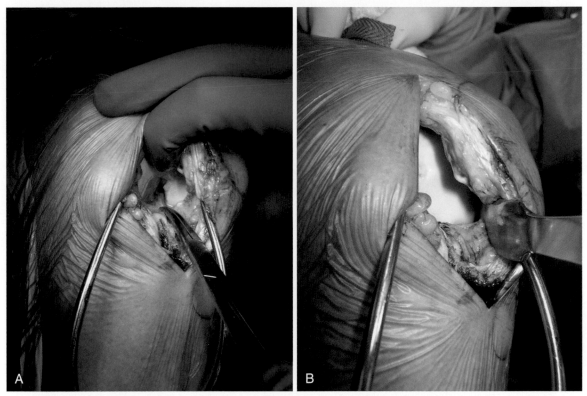

Figure 11-5 Intraoperative photographs demonstrating an intact anterior cruciate ligament **(A)** and the normal lateral compartment of the knee **(B)** during intraoperative inspection.

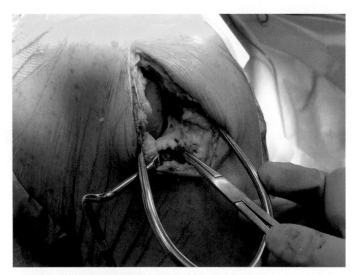

Figure 11-6 Intraoperative photograph of the anterior tibial osteophyte. Removal of the osteophyte leaves a blush of cancellous bone that is a good marker for transverse osteotomy level on the tibia.

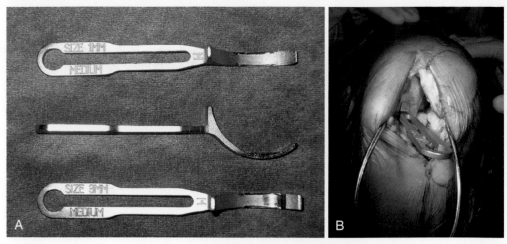

Figure 11-7 (A) Oxford Microplasty spoons ranging from 1 to 3 mm. **(B)** Intraoperative photograph of the Oxford Microplasty spoon tensioning the medial compartment to normal tension in flexion.

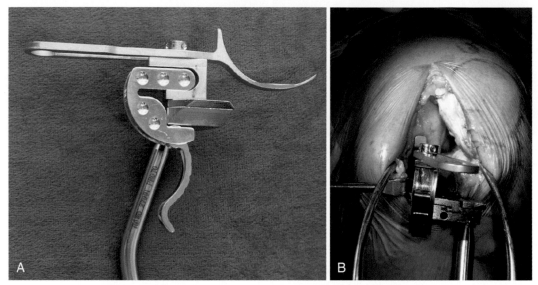

Figure 11-8 (A) Oxford Microplasty spoon and tibial resection guide linked by the G clamp. **(B)** Intraoperative photograph of G clamp–linked Oxford Microplasty spoon and tibial resection guide.

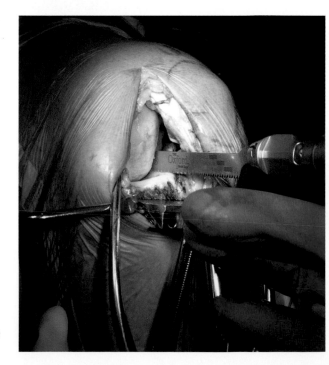

Figure 11-9 Intraoperative photograph demonstrating the vertical saw cut on the tibia. The saw should be aimed at the ipsilateral femoral head, and should be adjacent to the lateral aspect of the medial femoral condyle and medial edge of the anterior cruciate insertion on the tibia.

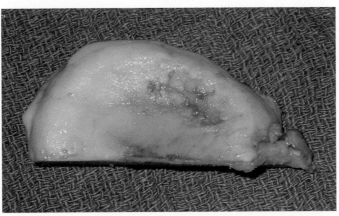

Figure 11-10 Excised tibial bone from a right knee demonstrating classic anteromedial arthritis with preservation of the posterior cartilage.

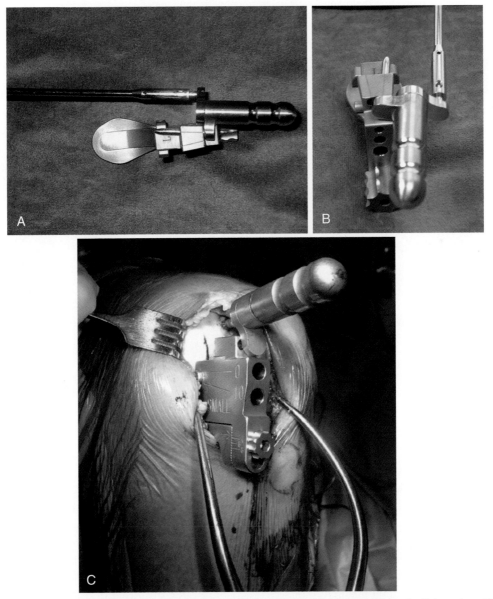

Figure 11-11 (A and **B)** Oxford Microplasty Flexion Gap Spacer coupled to the intramedullary rod by the linkage bar. **(C)** Intraoperative photograph demonstrating the Oxford Microplasty Flexion Gap Spacer coupled to the intramedullary rod by the linkage bar.

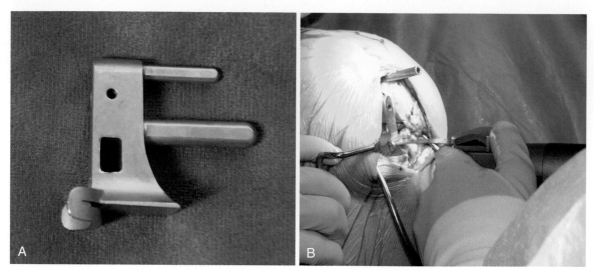

Figure 11-12 (A) Posterior femoral condylar resection guide. **(B)** Intraoperative photograph demonstrating the performance of the posterior femoral resection while protecting the medial collateral ligament with a retractor.

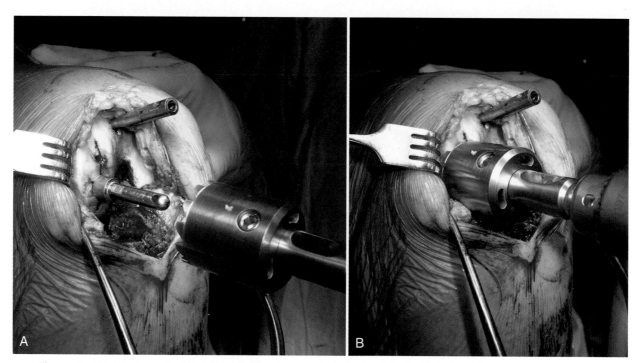

Figure 11-13 (A) Zero spigot inserted into the 6-mm pilot hole. **(B)** Spherical cutter used to mill the distal femur.

(**Fig. 11–12A**) is placed and then the posterior condyle is cut with the narrow saw while protecting the medial collateral ligament with the Z retractor (**Fig. 11–12B**). Milling is then performed on the distal femoral condyle starting with the zero spigot (**Fig. 11–13**). The tibial and femoral trials are placed and the feeler gauges are used to balance the flexion space (**Fig. 11–14A**). All retractors should be removed during trialing to prevent tension on the medial collateral ligament. The feeler gauge is removed and the knee is brought to 10–20° flexion.

Metal feeler gauges are then inserted to determine the balanced gap (**Fig. 11–14B**). The size of the flexion feeler gauge minus the size of the extension feeler gauge equals the spigot number that will be utilized to mill the remaining distal femur to balance the flexion-extension gaps. Trials are then replaced and gaps assessed. Further milling can be performed if necessary to balance the gaps. The Oxford Microplasty 2-in-1 anterior mill and the posterior osteophyte resection tool are placed (**Fig. 11–15**). The mill is used to remove the anterior femoral

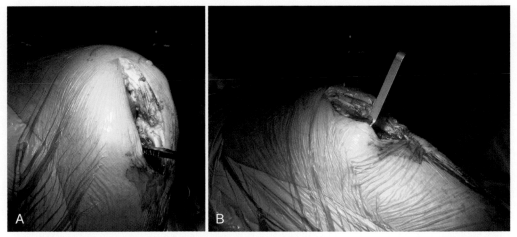

Figure 11-14 (A) Trial components with plastic feeler gauge balancing the flexion space. **(B)** Trial components in place with metal shim balancing the extension space at approximately 20° of flexion.

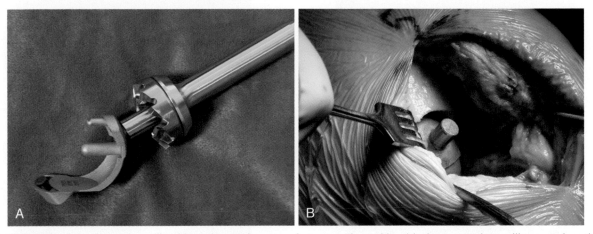

Figure 11-15 (A) The 2-in-1 anterior mill guide and posterior osteophyte resection guide with the appropriate mill engaged on the resection peg. **(B)** The guide seated on the medial femoral condyle prior to anterior milling.

condylar bone, which could be a source of impingement in extension. The angled osteotome is used through the capture mechanism to remove the posterior osteophytes that can cause impingement in high flexion.

Attention is given to the completion of the tibial preparation. The tibial base plate should cover the plateau adequately, and up to 2 mm of medial overhang is acceptable. It is critical to have the posterior margin of the component flush with the posterior cortex. This is accomplished by placing the universal removal hook into the posterior recess of the knee, pulling it forward to engage the posterior cortex, and then sliding the tibial component posteriorly until contacting the hook. It is common to have 1–2 mm of uncoverage anteriorly on the plateau. The tibial template nail is impacted through the tibial component. The toothbrush saw is utilized to prepare the keel and the bone is removed with the tibial groove gauge (**Fig. 11–16**). The trial tibial component is impacted gently into

position and then trialing is performed with the anatomic trial bearing. The bearing should restore the ligaments to normal tension, and range of motion should be smooth without impingement or instability.

The femoral and tibial bone is prepared to enhance cement interdigitation by drilling multiple small holes with the cement key drill (**Fig. 11–17**). The soft tissues of the knee are injected with a combination of ketorolac, ropivacaine, and epinephrine as part of our multimodal pain management protocol. The surfaces are copiously irrigated with pulse lavage and then dried. The tibial component is cemented first and impacted from posterior to anterior to force excess cement forward to allow ease of removal. The Woodson-style curette, with both the 45° and 90° arms, is an excellent tool to remove the excess cement. The suction is placed on the 4-mm anterior drill hole in the femur while finger impaction of the cement is performed on the femur. This negative-pressure

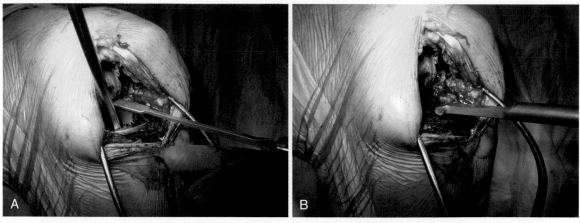

Figure 11-16 (A) After stabilizing the tibial base plate template with the tibial nail, the toothbrush saw is used to prepare the keel slot. **(B)** A tibial groove gauge is used to remove the bone in the keel slot.

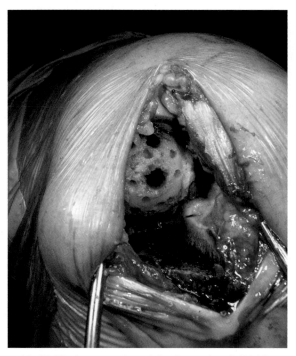

Figure 11-17 Final preparation of the femoral and tibial bone surfaces with the cement key drill.

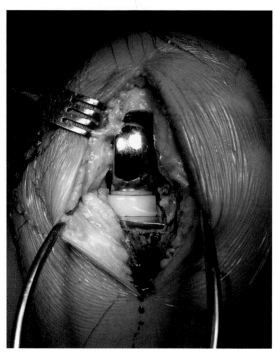

Figure 11-18 Final cemented components.

effect allows for excellent cement interdigitation. The femoral component is then impacted into position and excess cement is removed. The spacer bearing of appropriate thickness is inserted and then the leg is placed in 45° of flexion while the cement cures (**Fig. 11–18**). The bearing should be re-trialed after the cement cures. The appropriate size of polyethylene bearing is then inserted into the knee. A final check of range of motion ensures a smooth arc of motion with no impingement or instability of the bearing. Routine closure then ensues. Insertion of a drain is left to the discretion of the surgeon.

POSTSURGICAL FOLLOW-UP

The majority of patients spend 1 night in the hospital. The drain, if utilized, is removed on postoperative day 1. Lombardi et al. reported an average length of stay of 1.4 days (range 0–9) in the first 1000 unicompartmental knee arthroplasties performed in a two-surgeon series.[5] The patient returns at 6 weeks postoperatively for a clinical examination and radiographic evaluation (**Fig. 11–19**). The manipulation rate is 0.7% as reported by Berend in a series of 1000 consecutive unicompartmental knee arthroplasties (Berend KR, personal communication). Barring postoperative variances related to

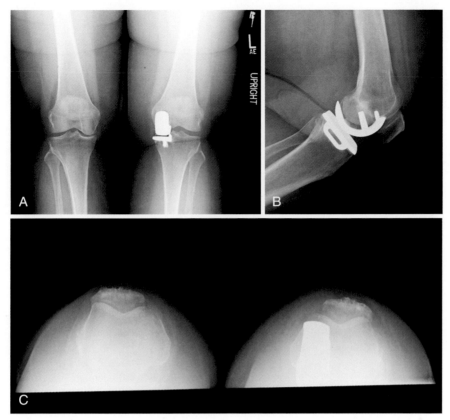

Figure 11-19 Postoperative anteroposterior **(A)**, lateral, **(B)** and Merchant's view **(C)** radiographs.

the arthroplasty, follow-up thereafter is annually with anteroposterior, lateral, and Merchant's view radiographs of the knee. No restrictions are placed on the patients, but high-impact repetitive exercise is discouraged.

TIPS AND PEARLS

- There is a tendency to place the bearing in too tight. However, it is recommended to leave the bearing relatively loose. If in between bearing sizes, choose the smaller thickness.
- Tibial plateau fractures are a rare but devastating complication. Protecting the integrity of the bone is paramount. Care when performing the vertical tibial osteotomy is critical. The saw blade should not cut the posterior cortex below the desired resection level. Prevention is best achieved by avoiding raising your hand during this resection. We also recommend drilling only one hole to secure the tibial resection guide to prevent weakening of the medial plateau below the resection level. Also, gentle impaction blows during insertion of the tibial component should be performed.
- The medial collateral ligament should be protected and never released during the operation. Retractors should be in place protecting the medial collateral ligament during all bone resections. Transection of the medial collateral ligament should be treated intraoperatively by converting to a total knee arthroplasty with appropriate constraint. In addition, all retractors should be removed during trialing to prevent false tensioning of the ligaments.
- Natural tibial slope should be reconstructed. The goal is 7° of posterior slope in the sagittal plane. Excessive slope is a known cause of posterior collapse and failure and should be avoided.

REFERENCES

1. White SH, Ludkowski PF, Goodfellow JW. Anteromedial osteoarthritis of the knee. J Bone Joint Surg [Br] 1991;73:582-586.
2. Price AJ, Murray DW, Goodfellow JW, et al. 20-year survival and 10-year clinical results of the Oxford uni knee arthroplasty [paper 046]. Presented at the 73rd Annual Meeting of the American Academy of Orthopaedic Surgeons, Chicago, IL, March 2006.
3. Price AJ, Waite JC, Svard U. Long-term clinical results of the medial Oxford unicompartmental knee arthroplasty. Clin Orthop Relat Res 2005;(435):171-180.
4. Kendrick BJL, Longino D, Pandit H, et al. Polyethylene wear in Oxford unicompartmental knee replacement: a retrieval study of 47 bearings. J Bone Joint Surg [Br] 2009;92:367-373.
5. Lombardi AV Jr, Berend KR, Walter CA, et al. Is recovery faster for mobile-bearing unicompartmental than total knee arthroplasty? Clin Orthop Relat Res 2009;(467):1450-1457.

CHAPTER 12
Medial Unicompartmental Knee Replacement: Cementless Options

Benjamin Kendrick, Nicholas Bottomley, Hemant Pandit, Andrew Price, Christopher Dodd, and David Murray

KEY POINTS

- Cementless fixation in unicompartmental knee replacement has the theoretical potential of very long-term biologic fixation.
- The indications for cementless UKR are identical to those in cemented UKR.
- Initial fixation is of paramount importance; implant design should allow an initial stable construct to allow effective osseointegration to occur.
- The incidence of radiolucency beneath the tibial component is reduced with cementless fixation compared with cemented fixation, and the clinical outcome is the same.

INTRODUCTION

Cementless fixation in unicompartmental knee replacement (UKR) is a developing field with advances in implant design and fixation surfaces. Although cementless options in unicompartmental replacement have been available for nearly 20 years, the operation has not become widespread. Cemented fixation is used in the majority of UKR procedures, with good clinical results. However, there is a concern over the suitability of cemented fixation in the younger, high-demand patient. Cementing in UKR is difficult and cementing errors, such as cement loose bodies, are common and may cause failure. In addition, the slow development and general acceptance of cementless UKR may be in part due to poor results from early designs. The use of cementless fixation in UKR is likely to increase with the aim for long-term biologic fixation being a realistic goal.

RATIONALE

The development of cementless UKR has mirrored that of total knee replacement (TKR), with the use of porous coatings, with and without hydroxyapatite, and, in some designs, the addition of cancellous screw augmentation. All designs have utilized a keel on the tibial component, although the shape, size, and direction have shown considerable variation (**Figs. 12–1 and 12–2**). The femoral component has usually mirrored the cemented equivalent for each design, although those femoral designs with a single peg had a second peg added for rotational stability.

One of the first advocates of cementless UKR was Jean-Alain Epinette,[1] who designed and developed a hydroxyapatite-coated tibial component. This component differed from most designs by employing a horizontal keel that slotted beneath the tibial spines, thus maintaining bone stock beneath the tibial tray. In addition, there were cancellous screws to augment the initial fixation. Kaiser and Whiteside further highlighted the importance of initial stability in 1990, with a cadaveric in vitro study demonstrating the additional stability provided by cancellous screws in a unicompartmental tibial component, compared with a posteriorly angled peg.[2]

Cementless fixation has many potential advantages over the more commonly used cemented fixation. In hip arthroplasty, cementless fixation has become ever more popular, whereas cementless total knee arthroplasty has remained less popular, particularly with regard to the tibial component. This is probably due to the increased difficulty in obtaining good initial fixation with a mostly flat tibial component resting on a flat tibial plateau. Although cementation provides an adequate fixation method in most cases, the use of cement results in several consequences that encourage perseverance with the development of cementless fixation. The disadvantages of cement use include possible thermal damage to the bony surfaces, an increased operative time, and the risk of cementing errors such as cement loose bodies or incorrect cement loose bodies, incorrect seating or impingement on cement. Cementless fixation avoids these problems and has the advantage of preserving tibial bone, as well as the theoretical potential of very long-term biologic fixation. However, cementless fixation in total knee arthroplasty has struggled to gain widespread acceptance due to some poor results, with a particular risk of failure of ingrowth.

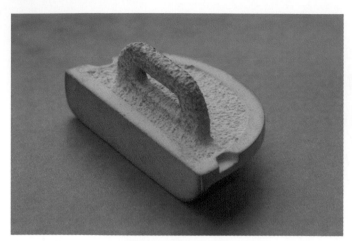

Figure 12-1 A cementless Oxford tibial component demonstrating a porous titanium layer with a hydroxyapatite coating.

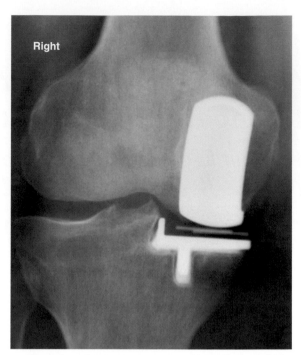

Figure 12-3 A physiologic radiolucency beneath a cemented Oxford tibial component.

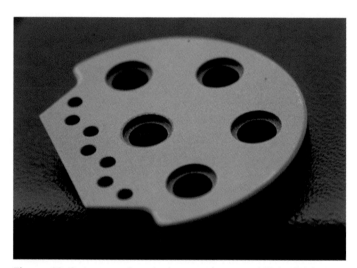

Figure 12-2 A cementless, hydroxyapatite-coated Unix tibial component with a horizontal keel and screw holes for additional fixation. (Photograph courtesy of Jean-Alain Epinette.)

Cementless fixation in UKR has mainly been used in the few centers that are strong advocates of unicompartmental surgery. The latest reports from the Australian and New Zealand joint registries show that cementless UKR accounts for 11% and 6% of all UKR procedures, respectively.[3,4] The Swedish register reported that all the UKRs performed in 2009 had both components cemented.[5] Neither the National Joint Registry of England and Wales nor the Canadian registry gives information regarding fixation method for UKR.[6,7]

Although the presence of thin, nonprogressive, radiolucent lines (**Fig. 12–3**) has long been recognized in knee arthroplasty, with no associated increase in failure rate, the exact cause and effect of these lines is still unknown. There is, however, a perception that a radiolucent line is indicative of

suboptimal fixation. The incidence of radiolucency differs beneath different implants, suggesting that the mechanical environment is important in their development. Forsythe et al.[8] reported an incidence of over 50% with the cementless Whiteside Ortholoc II UKR, whereas Pandit et al.[9] reported just 7% of cementless Oxford tibial components had a partial radiolucency, with none with a full radiolucency. There is also a reported increase in incidence of radiolucent lines with cemented Oxford components compared to the cementless version.[9] There is no clear consensus on the role or importance of thin ($\leq$1 mm), stable, so-called physiologic radiolucent lines, although there is evidence that they are not associated with either loosening or a decrease in clinical outcome scores. However, the greatly reduced incidence in cementless UKR is encouraging and suggests good bony fixation (**Fig. 12–4**). The Oxford UKR is particularly suited to cementless fixation because of the fully mobile bearing. The bearing movement causes a marked reduction in shear forces being transmitted through the tibial tray, and therefore the tray is mostly subjected to compression. This is an almost ideal mechanical environment for cementless fixation. Radiostereometric analysis studies of cementless fixation in TKR have shown a consistent pattern of migration, which differs from cemented fixation. Cemented components usually demonstrate continuous early migration, but the magnitude is small and stability is achieved by 2 years. In contrast, cementless components usually migrate a larger amount in the first few months before stabilizing. Onsten and Carlsson have

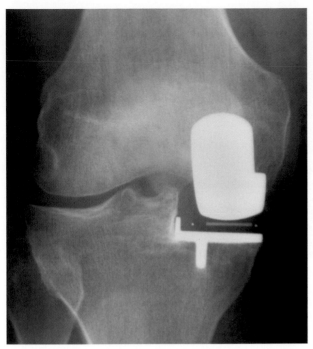

Figure 12-4 A well-seated cementless Oxford tibial component demonstrating no radiolucency at 5 years.

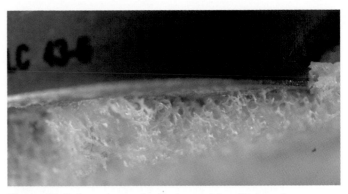

Figure 12-5 A specimen obtained at revision (for lateral compartment progression) 7 years after initial implantation, demonstrating bony apposition to the hydroxyapatite-coated undersurface of a Unix tibial component. (Photograph courtesy of Jean-Alain Epinette.)

demonstrated a reduction in the movement between 1 and 2 years postoperatively with the addition of a layer of hydroxyapatite to a porous-coated PFC tibial component.[10,11] Likewise, Regner et al. demonstrated the reduction in maximum total point movement at 5 years in the Freeman-Samuelson TKR tibial component with the addition of hydroxyapatite to the undersurface.[12]

INDICATIONS

The indications for UKR are controversial and vary according to the surgeon's philosophy. At Oxford, our view is that there should be full-thickness cartilage loss on both the medial tibial plateau and femoral condyle (bone-on-bone osteoarthritis), any intra-articular varus deformity should be correctable, and the anterior cruciate ligament (ACL) should be intact. Patellofemoral joint damage is ignored unless there is severe damage laterally. Cartilage damage on the lateral femoral condyle is permissible provided there is full-thickness cartilage present on a valgus stress radiograph and there is no full-thickness loss centrally. Full-thickness damage on the medial side of the lateral femoral condyle is not a contraindication.[13] We do not consider age, gender, activity level, or Body Mass Index to be contraindications. These indications are our routine for both cemented and cementless UKR. Bontemps also noted that the indications for cemented and cementless UKR are the same; however, due to cost saving, he favors cemented fixation in the elderly.[14] The suitability of cementless UKR in cases of

osteonecrosis or areas of bone loss is less easily described. The consensus in our group is that, if the knee is suitable for cemented UKR once the bony surfaces are prepared, then cementless UKR is also indicated. Our rationale for this is based on evidence that one does not require total bony ingrowth to maintain implant stability and therefore, if the bony surface can support the implant, then either fixation method is acceptable. Epinette's group demonstrated implant stability in cementless UKR when the amount of bony contact between tibia and component was between 38% and 52%[1] (**Fig. 12-5**).

SETUP AND EQUIPMENT

As with all arthroplasty surgery, the patient setup is of paramount importance. The patient should be set up as for routine medial unicompartmental knee arthroplasty. We recommend the use of a secure leg support, placed at midthigh, to allow the leg to hang and flex fully during surgery and to avoid pressure on the popliteal structures when fully flexed (**Fig. 12-6**). The Oxford cementless UKR uses the standard equipment trays in addition to the cementless tray. The specialist cementless tray includes instruments and trials specific for the cementless procedure. It contains cementless femoral trials, tibial templates with narrower keel slots, a narrower keel slot pick, and a cementless tibial component introducer. It is essential to use a narrower keel slot saw blade (Synvasive, Reno, NV). The keel slot width is of paramount importance, and therefore particular care needs to be taken when cutting the slot. The narrow keel slot pick also allows clearance of the keel slot without widening it unnecessarily. While the femoral component does not require any special equipment, implantation of the tibial component requires a specific introducer (**Fig. 12-7**). The introducer for implanting the Oxford tibial tray allows accurate placement of the tray,

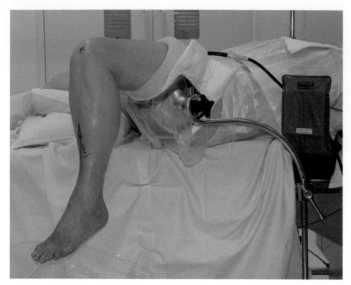

Figure 12-6 The correct setup for cementless Oxford UKR. The leg is able to hang vertically and can be flexed easily during surgery. The thigh support is midthigh so popliteal fossa compression does not occur.

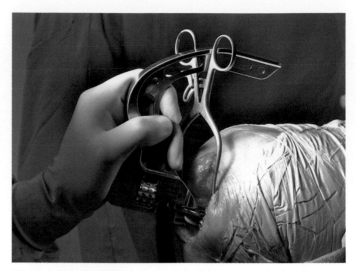

Figure 12-7 The Oxford cementless tibial tray attached to the specially designed introducer. The component can be accurately positioned and partially impacted before removal of the introducer to allow clearance of soft tissue beneath the tray and final impaction.

ensuring it is placed far enough back on the plateau before release and subsequent final seating. This facilitates firm seating on the posterior cortex and prevents anterior overhang.

APPROACH

Initially the Oxford UKR was implanted through a long midline incision as used for TKR. The Phase 3 instrumentation was introduced to allow the use of a short medial incision. Clinical studies have demonstrated that patients make a quicker recovery postoperatively and have equal outcome scores.[15–18] Therefore, the Oxford cementless UKR utilizes a short medial incision, from the medial pole of the patella to the tibial tubercle, as per the standard approach for cemented arthroplasty. Although there are advantages to a shorter incision, adequate exposure is important and the incision must be long enough to allow adequate inspection of the other compartments, retraction of the patella, and excision of osteophytes. The anteromedial corner of the tibia should be exposed to allow seating of the tibial cutting jig and exposure, and subsequent removal, of any osteophytes. Ligaments are never released, and care is taken to protect the medial collateral ligament (MCL). A specific retractor has been designed to help protect the MCL. The patella should not be inverted but can be retracted laterally. Introduction of a femoral intramedullary rod is helpful for alignment of the femoral component, as well as acting as an effective patellar retractor. Once the decision to proceed with UKR has been made, all osteophytes around the medial femoral condyle,

intracondylar notch, and anterior aspect of the medial tibial plateau should be removed. There is often an osteophyte anterior to the insertion of the ACL.

TECHNICAL DESCRIPTION

Careful and accurate preparation of the bony surfaces is of great importance as good initial fixation is reliant on a tight press-fit interface between both the femoral and tibial components and host bone. Different implant designs require different techniques. The following is a summary of the Oxford technique. An extramedullary tibial guide is used for tibial preparation. It should be positioned so the horizontal cut is just beneath the tibial defect unless this is very deep. The vertical tibial saw cut is made using a reciprocating saw (Synvasive, Reno, NV) placed just medial to the apex of the medial tibial spine and should be directed toward the hip joint or anterior superior iliac spine. The saw should be parallel to the tibial guide and should stop about 1 mm above the guide so as not to damage the bone supporting the implant. The horizontal cut is made with a 7° slope, taking care not to damage the MCL. Following removal of posteromedial femoral osteophytes, the size of the flexion gap should be checked to ensure that it is large enough for the minimum tibial component and bearing. If not large enough, more bone should be removed from the tibia. The position of the femoral component is determined using a femoral drill guide. Ideally the component should be flush with the original joint surface posteriorly and central on the femoral condyle. Bone is removed progressively from the distal femur until the flexion and extension gaps are balanced. The extension gap should be assessed in 20° of flexion so that the posterior capsule is lax. A meniscectomy is performed. Ideally, a small rim should be preserved medially to protect the MCL from the implant. Bone and cartilage are removed anterior and posterior to the implant to prevent impingement. A slot for the tibial keel is fashioned. A trial reduction is undertaken with the definitive trial components to ensure they seat fully, do not impinge, and function satisfactorily. The definitive implants are then impacted until secure.

POSTSURGICAL FOLLOW-UP

We use our standard postoperative rehabilitation regimen for both cemented and cementless UKR. Patients are allowed to weight-bear once comfortable. The patient is discharged once he or she is mobile on crutches and can safely negotiate stairs. In our institution, there is no difference in time to discharge between cemented and cementless UKR. Patients are advised to mobilize as comfort allows and are warned that it may take many months for the soreness, stiffness, and swelling to settle.

Before discharge, patients have routine radiographs with the anteroposterior view taken parallel to the tibial tray, allowing assessment of the component-bone interface. The lateral view is perpendicular to the femoral component, allowing assessment of bony contact around each peg. Using carefully screened radiographs enables proper evaluation of the interfaces and allows comparison with subsequent radiographs. The accuracy of detecting radiolucent lines, and hence assessment of whether they are progressive, is dependent on the reproducible acquisition of radiographs. The incidence of radiolucent lines beneath the cemented tibial component in Oxford UKR is approximately 62%.[19] However, the incidence in cementless Oxford UKR is markedly reduced at 1 year, with only 7% having a partial radiolucency and none having a complete radiolucency.[9] Radiographs taken in the first few days after surgery sometimes demonstrate a thin radiolucent line beneath the tibial tray (**Fig. 12–8A**). This is indicative of the tray not being fully seated at the time of surgery. However, with normal postoperative rehabilitation the radiolucent line disappears and the tray becomes securely seated on the tibial plateau (**Fig. 12–8B**).

CLINICAL RESULTS

Clinical results of cementless UKR are not commonly reported, and those reports evident in the literature are usually short series. A single randomized, controlled trial of cemented versus cementless UKR at Oxford has shown no difference in clinical outcome, and a reduced incidence of radiolucency with cementless fixation, at 2 years.[20] There have also been reports that contribute to the base of knowledge in UKR fixation, with lessons being learned and improvements made. A report from Keblish and Briard in 2004 regarding the LCS mobile-bearing UKR highlights the reasonable clinical results obtainable, but again shows that there are concerns regarding cementless fixation as all the failures of fixation in the study were in the cementless group.[21] The Porous Coated Anatomic

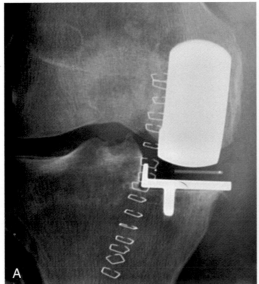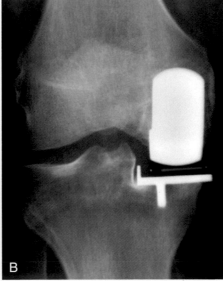

Figure 12-8 (A) A postoperative radiograph of a cementless Oxford UKR demonstrating a radiolucency beneath the tibial component. **(B)** A radiograph at 1 year of the same Oxford cementless UKR showing stabilization of the tibial component and no radiolucency. (Reproduced with permission and copyright © of the British Editorial Society of Bone and Joint Surgery from Pandit H, Jenkins C, Beard DJ, et al. Cementless Oxford unicompartmental knee replacement shows reduced radiolucency at one year. J Bone Joint Surg [Br] 2009;91:185-189. [Figures 3a and 3b].)

Table 12-1 Published Reports on Cementless Unicompartmental Knee Replacement

Authors (Implant, Year)	Number	Length of Follow-up	Failures due to Cementless Fixation	Failures due to Other Reasons	Success Rate	Comments
Bernasek et al.[22] (PCA, 1988)	28 (26 medial, 2 lateral)	Minimum 2 yr	4	2 (1 lateral progression, 1 patellar impingement)	22/28	
Magnussen and Bartlett[26] (PCA, 1990)	51 (42 medial, 9 lateral)	Minimum 2 yr	0	1 (lateral progression)	50/51	
Forsythe et al.[8] (Ortholoc, 2000)	57 (all medial)	1–8 yr (mean 3.3)	1	0	56/57	5 had loose beads with significant radiolucencies
Keblish and Briard[21] (LCS, 2004)	127 (additional 50 cemented included in paper)	5–19 yr	6	Not available as paper includes cemented UKR	Not available as paper includes cemented UKR	27 of 177 total UKR (cemented included) revised for bearing wear
Lecuire et al.[27] (Alpina, 2008)	120 (108 medial, 12 lateral)	Mean 6.5 yr	2	8 (3 lateral progression, 4 bearing fracture, 1 bearing wear)	110/120	Cementless failures revised early at 6 and 7 mo
Epinette and Manley[25] (Unix, 2008)	125 (111 medial, 14 lateral)	5–13 yr	0	2 (1 ACL deficiency, 1 lateral progression)	123/125	2/125 had peri-screw osteolysis, but no component loosening
Pandit et al.[9] (Oxford, 2009)	30 (all medial)	Minimum 1 yr	0	0	30/30	Reduced radiolucencies compared to cemented Oxford UKR (RCT)

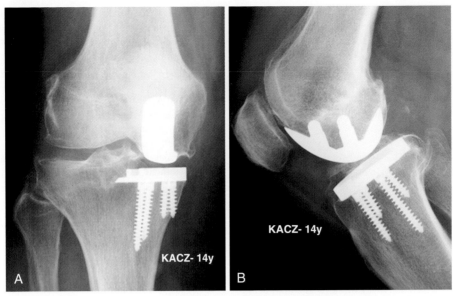

Figure 12-9 Anteroposterior **(A)** and lateral **(B)** radiographs taken 14 years postoperatively in a female patient who had a medial UKR for osteoarthritis at the age of 72. Note the absence of radiolucency either beneath the tibial component or around the screws. (Radiograph courtesy of Jean-Alain Epinette.)

UKR had initial success, using both cemented and cementless fixation methods. However, Bernasek et al. described an increased number of failures due to fixation in the early postoperative period, with fibrous tissue forming at the implant-bone interface[22] in the cementless components. Lindstrand and Stenstrom reported good results initially with the same implant, but then showed a deterioration between 4 and 8 years postoperatively.[23,24] Although the failures described in the midterm were mostly related to extreme polyethylene wear, this demonstrates the difficulty in obtaining long-term follow-up on UKR fixed without cement. Epinette and Manley have provided perhaps the best mid- to long-term follow-up of a cementless UKR.[25] At a minimum follow-up of 5 years, with a maximum of 13 years, there were no failures of fixation from 125 hydroxyapatite-coated Unix knee replacements. Radiographs obtained 14 years after surgery show that excellent fixation without the development of radiolucencies can be achieved (**Fig. 12–9**). The results of the available published reports are summarized in **Table 12–1**. The data presented demonstrate the need for further studies with longer follow-up in addition to focus on particular patient groups, such as the young with high demand.

SUMMARY

At present, cementless UKR is still an unproven long-term treatment for single-compartment osteoarthritis. However, the majority of reported failures are due to either inherent problems with design or progression in another compartment, rather than the fixation method. The important factors for success in cementless UKR surgery are the same as for any arthroplasty surgery: adherence to appropriate surgical indications, use of a well-designed implant, and meticulous surgical technique. Although due regard for the short- to midterm follow-up must be made, recent results show an encouraging future for cementless UKR.

REFERENCES

1. Bauer TW, Jiang M, Epinette JA. Hydroxyapatite-coated unicompartmental knee arthroplasty: histologic analysis of retrieved implants. *In* Cartier P, Epinette JA, Deschamps G, Hernigou P (eds). Unicompartmental Knee Arthroplasty. Paris: Expansion Scientifique Francaise, 1996, pp 43-50.
2. Kaiser AD, Whiteside LA. The effect of screws and pegs on the initial fixation stability of an uncemented unicondylar knee replacement. Clin Orthop Relat Res 1990;(259):169-178.
3. Australian Orthopaedic Association National Joint Replacement Registry. Annual Report. Adelaide: Australian Orthopaedic Association, 2009.
4. New Zealand Orthopaedic Association. The New Zealand Joint Registry: Annual Report. Wellington: New Zealand Orthopaedic Association, 2009.
5. Swedish Knee Arthroplasty Register. Annual Report. Lund: Swedish Knee Arthroplasty Register, 2009.

6. Canadian Institute for Health Information. Hip and Knee Replacements in Canada—Canadian Joint Replacement Registry. 2008–2009 Annual Report. Ottawa, Ontario: Canadian Institute for Health Information, 2009.

7. National Joint Registry of England and Wales. 6th Annual Report. Hemel Hempstead, UK: National Joint Registry of England and Wales, 2009.

8. Forsythe ME, Englund RE, Leighton RK. Unicondylar knee arthroplasty: a cementless perspective. Can J Surg 2000;43:417-424.

9. Pandit H, Jenkins C, Beard DJ, et al. Cementless Oxford unicompartmental knee replacement shows reduced radiolucency at one year. J Bone Joint Surg [Br] 2009;91:185-189.

10. Carlsson A, Bjorkman A, Besjakov J, Onsten I. Cemented tibial component fixation performs better than cementless fixation: a randomized radiostereometric study comparing porous-coated, hydroxyapatite-coated and cemented tibial components over 5 years. Acta Orthop 2005;76:362-369.

11. Onsten I, Nordqvist A, Carlsson AS, et al. Hydroxyapatite augmentation of the porous coating improves fixation of tibial components: a randomised RSA study in 116 patients. J Bone Joint Surg [Br] 1998;80:417-425.

12. Regner L, Carlsson L, Karrholm J, Herberts P. Tibial component fixation in porous- and hydroxyapatite-coated total knee arthroplasty: a radiostereometric evaluation of migration and inducible displacement after 5 years. J Arthroplasty 2000;15:681-689.

13. Kendrick BJ, Rout R, Bottomley NJ, et al. The implications of damage to the lateral femoral condyle on medial unicompartmental knee replacement. J Bone Joint Surg [Br] 2010;92:374-379.

14. Bontemps G, Brust K. Medial compartment knee replacement: cemented vs. uncemented. Combined Bristol and Oxford Unicompartmental Arthritis Symposium, Nuffield Orthopaedic Centre, November 18th 2009.

15. Price AJ, Webb J, Topf H, et al. Rapid recovery after Oxford unicompartmental arthroplasty through a short incision. J Arthroplasty 2001;16:970-976.

16. Rees JL, Price AJ, Beard DJ, et al. Minimally invasive Oxford unicompartmental knee arthroplasty: functional results at 1 year and the effect of surgical inexperience. Knee 2004;11:363-367.

17. Carlsson LV, Albrektsson BE, Regner LR. Minimally invasive surgery vs conventional exposure using the Miller-Galante unicompartmental knee arthroplasty: a randomized radiostereometric study. J Arthroplasty 2006;21:151-156.

18. Romanowski MR, Repicci JA. Minimally invasive unicondylar arthroplasty: eight-year follow-up. J Knee Surg 2002;15:17-22.

19. Gulati A, Chau R, Pandit HG, et al. The incidence of physiological radiolucency following Oxford unicompartmental knee replacement and its relationship to outcome. J Bone Joint Surg [Br] 2009;91:896-902.

20. Kendrick BJL, Pandit H, Jenkins C, et al. Cementless fixation of unicompartmental knee replacement decreases radiolucency at two years. Paper presented at the Annual Meeting of the British Association for Surgery of the Knee, Oxford, 2010.

21. Keblish PA, Briard JL. Mobile-bearing unicompartmental knee arthroplasty: a 2-center study with an 11-year (mean) follow-up. J Arthroplasty 2004;19(7 Suppl 2):87-94.

22. Bernasek TL, Rand JA, Bryan RS. Unicompartmental porous coated anatomic total knee arthroplasty. Clin Orthop Relat Res 1988;(236):52-59.

23. Lindstrand A, Stenstrom A. Polyethylene wear of the PCA unicompartmental knee: prospective 5 (4–8) year study of 120 arthrosis knees. Acta Orthop Scand 1992;63:260-262.

24. Lindstrand A, Stenstrom A, Egund N. The PCA unicompartmental knee: a 1–4-year comparison of fixation with or without cement. Acta Orthop Scand 1988;59:695-700.

25. Epinette JA, Manley MT. Is hydroxyapatite a reliable fixation option in unicompartmental knee arthroplasty? A 5- to 13-year experience with the hydroxyapatite-coated unix prosthesis. J Knee Surg 2008;21:299-306.

26. Magnussen PA, Bartlett RJ. Cementless PCA unicompartmental joint arthroplasty for osteoarthritis of the knee: a prospective study of 51 cases. J Arthroplasty 1990;5:151-158.

27. Lecuire F, Fayard JP, Simottel JC, et al. Mid-term results of a new cementless hydroxyapatite coated anatomic unicompartmental knee arthroplasty. Eur J Orthop Surg Traumatol 2008;18:279-285.

CHAPTER 13
Lateral Unicompartmental Knee Arthroplasty

Creighton C. Tubb, Karim Elsharkawy, and Wael K. Barsoum

KEY POINTS

- Isolated lateral compartment, noninflammatory arthritis in a ligamentously stable knee with less than 10° of valgus and more than 90° of flexion is uncommon.
- Fixed-bearing lateral UKA in properly selected patients can provide reliably good results.
- Surgical technique should focus on restoring appropriate soft tissue tension without overcorrecting the knee.
- Account for the "screw-home" mechanism by checking the tibial resection in flexion and extension.

INTRODUCTION

Degenerative joint disease is a common diagnosis among adults, with an estimated prevalence of knee osteoarthritis ranging from 4.9% to 16.7%.[1,2] Though difficult to pinpoint exactly, there has been an increase in the prevalence of osteoarthritis among adults in the United States.[1] Patients often present with degeneration of multiple knee compartments, although the process can involve a single compartment. Laskin[3] reported that less than 12% of patients in his practice had single-compartment disease and were candidates for unicompartmental knee arthroplasty (UKA). Moreover, isolated lateral compartment arthritis is quite uncommon and has received little attention in the orthopaedic literature. Scott[4] reported that lateral UKAs constitute less than 1% of all knee arthroplasties. Despite its low prevalence, the aging and increasingly active population ensures that orthopaedic surgeons will manage patients with isolated lateral knee compartment arthritis. For some of these, lateral UKA is a predictable solution.

The cause of lateral compartment knee arthritis is likely multifactorial. Valgus knee deformity, genetic factors, traumatic events, and meniscal pathology may all play a role.

The opinions and assertions contained herein are the private views of the authors, and are not to be construed as official or reflecting the views of the Department of the Army or Department of Defense.

Patients present with pain and often mechanical symptoms confined to the lateral aspect of the knee. The physical examination proceeds the same as for any patient with a degenerative knee process. Tenderness along the lateral distal femoral condyle and joint line are often noted. With advanced disease, the valgus deformity becomes more pronounced. Care should be taken to fully examine the knee to ensure the degenerative process does not involve the patellofemoral articulation or medial compartment. Likewise, ligament stability and the ability to passively correct a valgus deformity should be documented. Radiographic evaluation includes a weight-bearing anteroposterior film of both knees, a 45° flexed weight-bearing posteroanterior view, a lateral view, and a sunrise or comparable view of the patellofemoral articulation.

INDICATIONS

Orthopaedic surgeons entertain a host of management options for lateral knee compartment arthritis depending on patient characteristics and requirements. These options include nonsurgical modalities, osteotomies, total knee arthroplasty (TKA), or UKA. Our indications for lateral UKA are isolated lateral compartment degenerative changes and symptoms with intact knee ligaments and a passively correctable valgus deformity.

CONTRAINDICATIONS

Contraindications include advanced degenerative changes of the medial or patellofemoral compartments, inflammatory arthritic conditions, anterior cruciate or other ligament insufficiency, fixed valgus deformity or deformity greater than 10°, less than 90° of knee flexion, flexion contracture of greater than 10°, or a patient incapable of adhering to a postarthroplasty lifestyle.[5,6]

DISCUSSION

The potential benefits of UKA over TKA are faster recovery with shorter hospitalization and decreased morbidity, improved range of motion, better gait patterns, and bone conservation making future conversion to TKA easier should it be necessary.[7-10] Reports in the literature on medial unicompartmental arthroplasty have shown promising results.[11-14] Extrapolations of these data to the lateral compartment, however, may not be appropriate as it is quite different in terms of anatomic and biomechanical characteristics. There are limited studies that focus on the outcomes of lateral UKA.[5,10,15-18] Marmor[15] was the first to discuss unicompartmental arthroplasty for lateral compartment disease. He reported excellent results in 11 of 14 cases. Ohdera et al.[16] reported good results in 16 of 18 patients with greater than 5 years' follow-up. Ashraf et al.[17] reported on 88 patients with an average of 9 years' follow-up and felt that the results of lateral UKA were comparable to those found with medial UKA. Pennington et al.[5] reported on 29 knees among which there were markedly improved Hospital for Special Surgery knee scores and no revisions at greater than 12 years after lateral UKA. Early and midterm data suggest current-design lateral UKA offers reliable results.[5,10,16,17] As with any operative procedure, careful patient selection and adherence to proper indications and sound surgical technique influence these results. The remainder of this chapter reviews the preparation, surgical approach, technical factors, and postoperative management of lateral UKA.

SETUP AND EQUIPMENT

We utilize the same operating room setup as for a total knee replacement. The patient is positioned supine. A padded bump under the operative hip can be utilized at the surgeon's discretion. A footrest or sandbag secured to the bed allows the knee to be flexed to 90° and beyond. Others drop the foot of the bed to use a suspended leg technique that allows hyperflexion of the knee.[19-21] A well-padded tourniquet is positioned high on the thigh, with the lower extremity prepared and draped in a manner to allow the surgeon control of the extremity. The procedure is performed under tourniquet for modern cement technique and to improve visualization. Equipment will vary depending on the chosen implant. It is important to have a total knee system available in the event that intraoperative inspection reveals advanced degenerative changes affecting the medial or patellofemoral compartments. Likewise, preoperative counseling should include a discussion of the possibility for total knee arthroplasty. Other considerations include specialized retractors. We like to use a retractor in the notch that extends over the trochlea to protect the patellofemoral compartment. The need for these instruments is dependent on the chosen approach.

SURGICAL APPROACH (SEE VIDEO 13-1)

The lateral compartment can be easily accessed through a slightly lateralized oblique, extensile, paralateral incision running along the lateral border of the tibial tubercle and the patellar tendon (**Fig. 13–1**). A modified lateral parapatellar arthrotomy is then performed. There is some concern that this adds complexity in the event that conversion to a TKA is required or that future revision surgery will be more of a challenge. Sah and Scott[6,18] reported this concern and described their technique for lateral UKA through a medial parapatellar approach. To provide another perspective, the lateral parapatellar approach has been quite successful in the senior author's experience and has not posed problems intraoperatively or in the event of further surgery. The approach we describe provides excellent visualization of the surgical structures and minimizes soft tissue stripping.

The skin incision is from the superior pole of the patella to just lateral to the tibial tubercle. The length of the incision is adjusted to allow for adequate visualization as needed. Skin flaps are full thickness but not excessively undermined. Once through the skin and subcutaneous fat, the arthrotomy proceeds through the retinaculum, staying lateral to the patellar tendon (**Fig. 13–2**). A moderate amount of fat is excised under the patellar tendon to allow for adequate visualization in determining tibial rotation. The lateral edge of the tibial plateau is exposed for visualization and to allow proper retractor placement by elevating a small portion of the iliotibial band off of Gerdy's tubercle. The knee can be flexed and extended to allow visualization of the other compartments through this mobile soft tissue window. Final confirmation of isolated lateral disease is made prior to proceeding. Lateral femoral and tibial osteophytes should be removed. A patellar retractor is carefully placed after inspection of the anterior cruciate ligament to confirm its competence. A lateral Z retractor protects the iliotibial band and the lateral ligamentous and capsular structures after the visible portion of the lateral meniscus is excised.

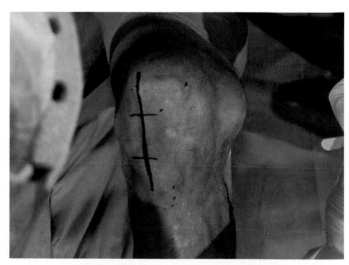

Figure 13-1 Paralateral skin incision.

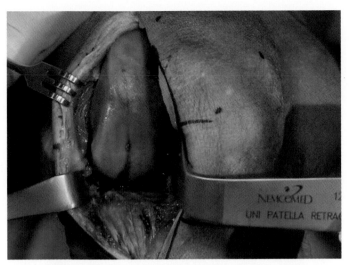

Figure 13-2 Lateral parapatellar arthrotomy offering excellent exposure of the lateral compartment.

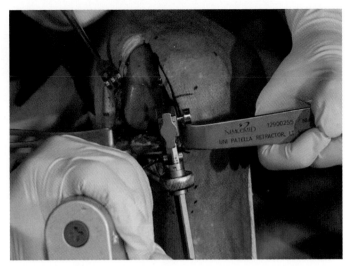

Figure 13-3 Extramedullary alignment rod and cutting jig for the tibial resection.

TECHNICAL DESCRIPTION

The exact steps of the procedure will vary depending on the chosen implant system, yet the principles are the same. We avoid mobile-bearing designs in the lateral compartment due to the risk of polyethylene dislocation.[22] Ultimately, the goal is a measured resection of the distal femur and proximal tibia to allow for implantation of components with correction of the valgus deformity. Care must be taken not to overcorrect the knee and place undue stress on the medial compartment and lateral ligamentous structures as this may lead to accelerated wear of the medial compartment. Beginning with a "tibia-first" approach, an extramedullary alignment rod is utilized to perform a tibial resection adequate enough to accept the tibial component bearing surface. The flexion gap is usually a bit larger than that for a medial UKA due to the greater mobility of the lateral compartment. Coronal alignment should match the mechanical axis of the tibia and sagittal alignment should reproduce the natural posterior slope for each knee. A sagittal saw blade is utilized to make the initial cut vertical to the cutting block. This cut is in line with the medial border of the lateral femoral condyle and slightly internally rotated to account for the rotational relationship between the femur and tibia in full extension as a result of the "screw-home" mechanism. Care must be taken to avoid injury to the tibial insertion of the anterior cruciate ligament. The sagittal saw blade can be left in place to prevent undermining the anterior cruciate ligament tibial insertion while a standard saw blade is used to complete the tibial resection using the cutting block (**Fig. 13–3**). The resected tibial surface can assist in determining the appropriate tibial implant size. It is frequently shorter and wider than the resected tibia in a medial UKA due to the configuration of the lateral tibial plateau.

Distal femoral resection is accomplished by implant-specific techniques but is performed to result in equal flexion and extension gaps. It is important to note that balancing the flexion and extension gaps is accomplished on the femoral side, most notably on the distal femoral cut as the posterior cut is usually a measured resection specific to the implant. After measuring the flexion gap, the extension gap is cut in a manner to allow for the same-size spacer block to fit as comfortably as that used in flexion. In comparison with a medial UKA, this feel is slightly looser. Our preferred system utilizes the cut tibial surface to assist in alignment with the knee in extension. After the distal femoral resection is complete, a 2-in-1 cutting block is utilized to perform the posterior condylar and posterior chamfer cuts. Posterior femoral osteophytes are then removed, and the remaining meniscal tissue is excised. A femoral trial implant is selected to ensure adequate surface coverage without extending too anteriorly, which risks inappropriate articulation of the component with the patella. The cut tibial surface is likewise measured and a trial placed. The knee should move naturally through a range of motion without increased laxity or limitations to flexion and extension (**Fig. 13–4**). Stability is checked in full extension, 30° of flexion, midflexion, and finally full flexion (**Fig. 13–5**). Sagittal plane stability should also be confirmed. It is important to check motion and stability with retractors removed to allow for a true representation of ligament tension.

Once satisfied with the construct, peg holes or keels can be prepared as per manufacturer recommendations, leaving the bone surfaces fully prepared for implantation (**Fig. 13–6**). The knee should be copiously irrigated with pulsatile lavage after areas of sclerotic subchondral bone are drilled with a small-diameter bit to improve cement interdigitation. A moistened

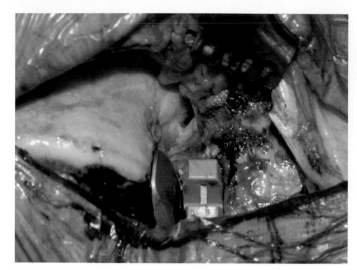

Figure 13-4 Trial components in knee extension (note proper component articulation).

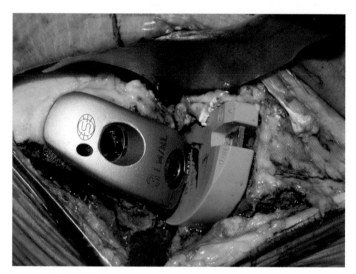

Figure 13-5 Trial components in knee flexion (note proper component articulation).

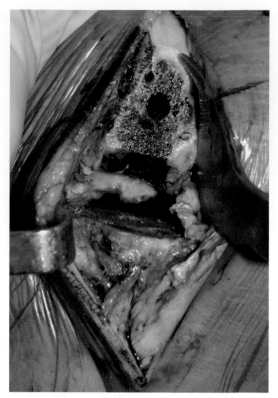

Figure 13-6 Prepared bone surfaces.

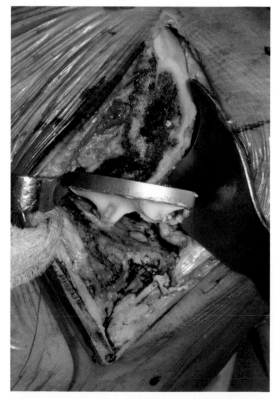

Figure 13-7 Implanting the tibial component from posterior to anterior, with surgical sponge placed to assist in excess cement removal.

surgical sponge placed with a tonsil forceps peripheral to the cut tibial surface aids in preventing retained lateral or posterior excess cement. With retractors positioned, the tibial implant is placed first. Cement technique is critical at this juncture as extruded posterior cement is difficult to retrieve with implants in place. It helps to place the posterior portion of the implant in first, then compressing it anteriorly so as to force the cement into the tibia and out anteriorly (**Fig. 13–7**). Extruded tibial cement is removed, as is the sponge. The femoral component is placed with a plastic tongue depressor sitting over the tibial baseplate to protect the femur from scratching (**Fig. 13–8**). We prefer an implant with femoral lugs that allow compression of the posterior condylar cement. Again, excess cement is removed and the polyethylene liner

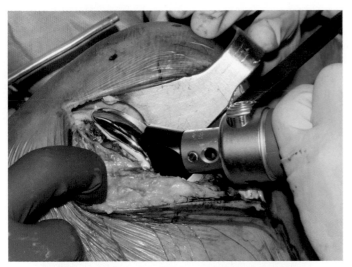

Figure 13-8 Implanting the femoral component.

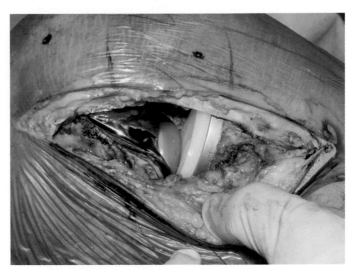

Figure 13-10 Final components in full flexion.

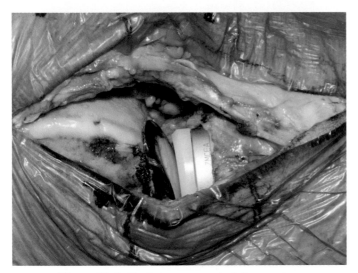

Figure 13-9 Final components in full extension.

impacted into the tibial tray if using a modular design. The knee should be held in extension to slight flexion until the cement is hardened to prevent the tibial component from lifting up anteriorly. Final inspection of the implant should ensure normal knee motion and stability without patellar impingement (**Figs. 13–9 and 13–10**).

Closure begins with deflation of the tourniquet and gaining hemostasis. The knee should be irrigated thoroughly as with any arthroplasty. The arthrotomy and skin are closed according to surgeon preference. A local injection of anesthetic and analgesic combination can assist with early mobility and postoperative pain management. A sterile dressing and lightly compressive wrap completes the case; surgical drains are not necessary.

SPECIAL CONSIDERATIONS

The unicompartmental arthroplasty of the lateral compartment is technically quite different than that of the medial compartment.[23] One of the more critical concepts unique to lateral UKA is the rotation of the tibial component. There is a tendency to introduce too much external rotation when preparing the tibia. The tibial resection is made with the knee flexed. As the knee extends, there is a relative external rotation of the tibia with respect to the femur. This screw-home mechanism results from the complex anatomy of the knee and the coupling of the cruciate ligaments.[24] Moglo and Shirazi-Adl[24] found the tibia to rotate internally 16.4° in 90° of knee flexion and externally 1.3° in knee hyperextension. If this tibial rotation is not taken into account during bone preparation, the tibial component will be externally rotated relative to the femoral component, causing edge loading of the polyethylene (**Fig. 13–11**). Pennington et al.[5] identified this unique aspect of lateral unicompartmental replacements and offer recommendations on how to avoid it. Essentially, the key is in the rotation of the tibial implant, which must be accounted for when performing the tibial resection.[5] By setting the tibial cutting guide in the appropriate alignment in flexion, the surgeon first ensures proper coronal plane alignment and reproduction of the posterior tibial slope. The vertical cut can be initiated after checking the orientation of this cut in full extension (**Fig. 13–12**). This will allow a better matching of the femoral condyle throughout the range of motion. If necessary, the femoral component can be lateralized slightly as well to improve articulation with the tibia.[6] However, if the articulation is significantly off in extension such that there is edge loading of the implants, the likely problem is the tibial rotation. Though unproven in the literature, abnormal implant articulation likely would diminish the survival of the implant.

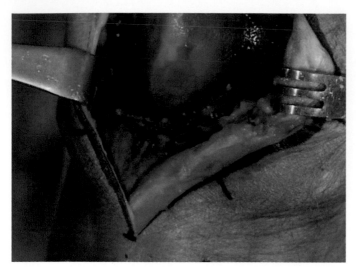

Figure 13-11 Initial tibial resection made in 90° of flexion and now visualized in full extension (note the improper rotation of the resected piece and the black ink mark indicating the proper rotational alignment of the tibial resection).

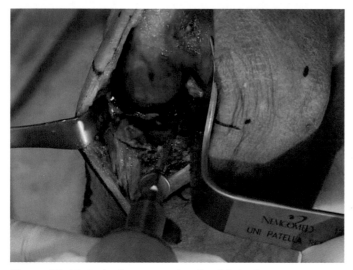

Figure 13-12 Sagittal saw resecting the tibia in the proper rotation.

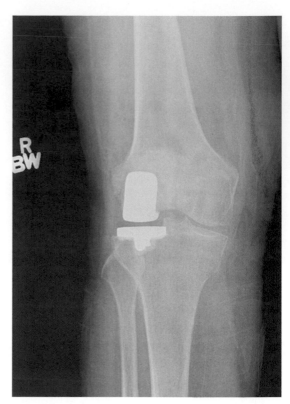

Figure 13-13 Postoperative anteroposterior view of a 75-year-old female with isolated lateral compartment arthritis.

Patients often remark how natural their knee feels after UKA. Preservation of the ligamentous structures of the knee, as well as the soft tissue, bone, and cartilage of the uninvolved compartments, likely provides proprioceptive feedback that account for this satisfaction. For the knee ligaments to function properly, it is critical to restore appropriate soft tissue tension without overcorrecting the deformity. If done correctly, ligamentous stability will be restored without overloading the uninvolved compartment. Trial components or spacer blocks are typically available with each system to assist in achieving the balance of a snug fit without requiring excessive force for insertion. Becoming familiar with the chosen implant system through training opportunities can reinforce the "feel" of properly balanced gaps for unicompartmental arthroplasty.

POSTSURGICAL MANAGEMENT

Interdisciplinary management from pain management services, physical and occupational therapy, and case management allows for rapid recovery. Patients are allowed immediate weight bearing under the supervision of physical therapy. Peripheral nerve catheters managed by anesthesia specialists are quite helpful in promoting adequate pain control to accommodate a rapid recovery protocol. Such protocols facilitate early mobility and decrease length of hospital stay.[25] Patients are hospitalized overnight and typically released home on the first or second postoperative day when deemed appropriate by the multidisciplinary team (**Figs. 13–13 and 13–14**). Prophylaxis against venous thromboembolic events includes early mobilization and sequential compression devices. Most patients also receive aspirin 325 mg twice daily for 4–6 weeks. High-risk individuals are discharged on enoxaparin rather than aspirin at the discretion of the surgeon. Assistive devices are used for ambulation as required. Outpatient physical therapy concentrates on gait training, strengthening, proprioception, and range of motion. Initial follow-up

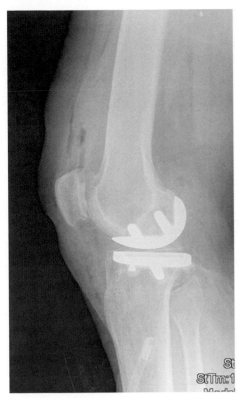

Figure 13-14 Postoperative lateral view of the same patient.

in the office occurs 2–4 weeks after surgery. The ability for a patient to return to work is dependent upon job description and demands but can be quite soon for many office-type jobs.

SUMMARY

The lateral UKA is a rewarding operation for appropriate patients with isolated lateral compartment arthrosis, even though this is not a particularly common diagnosis. The procedure is well supported by early and midterm data on the topic; we expect long-term studies to better define the expectations from this procedure. Proper indications and surgical technique are bedrock principles for orthopaedic surgeons regardless of the procedure. When these principles are applied to current-design lateral unicompartmental knee arthroplasties, surgeons can expect satisfying results while delivering patients an excellent solution to their knee pathology.

TIPS AND PEARLS

- Proper indications improve success rates.
- Do not damage or undercut the anterior cruciate ligament insertion.
- Tibial preparation should be initiated in flexion for coronal and sagittal alignment but then checked in extension to ensure proper rotational alignment. Avoid excessive external rotation.
- Ensure careful cement technique to provide good interdigitation without excess retained cement.
- Do not oversize the femoral side and err to lateralizing if need to prevent articulation with the patella.
- Do not overcorrect into varus.

REFERENCES

1. Lawrence RC, Felson DT, Helmick CG, et al. Estimates of the prevalence of arthritis and other rheumatic conditions in the United States. Part II. Arthritis Rheum 2008;58:26-35.
2. Grotle M, Hagen KB, Natvig B, et al. Prevalence and burden of osteoarthritis: results from a population survey in Norway. J Rheumatol 2008;35:677-684.
3. Laskin RS. Unicompartmental knee replacement: some unanswered questions. Clin Orthop Relat Res 2001;(392):267-271.
4. Scott RD. Lateral unicompartmental replacement: a road less traveled. Orthopedics 2005;28:983-984.
5. Pennington DW, Swienckowski JJ, Lutes WB, Drake GN. Lateral unicompartmental knee arthroplasty: survivorship and technical considerations at an average follow-up of 12.4 years. J Arthroplasty 2006;21:13-17.
6. Sah AP, Scott RD. Lateral unicompartmental knee arthroplasty through a medial approach: surgical technique. J Bone Joint Surg [Am] 2008;90(Suppl 2 Pt 2):195-205.
7. Laurencin CT, Zelicof SB, Scott RD, Ewald FC. Unicompartmental versus total knee arthroplasty in the same patient: a comparative study. Clin Orthop Relat Res 1991;(273):151-156.
8. Rougraff BT, Heck DA, Gibson AE. A comparison of tricompartmental and unicompartmental arthroplasty for the treatment of gonarthrosis. Clin Orthop Relat Res 1991;(273):157-164.
9. Chassin EP, Mikosz RP, Andriacchi TP, Rosenberg AG. Functional analysis of cemented medial unicompartmental knee arthroplasty. J Arthroplasty 1996;11:553-559.
10. Volpi P, Marinoni L, Bait C, et al. Lateral unicompartmental knee arthroplasty: indications, technique and short-medium term results. Knee Surg Sports Traumatol Arthrosc 2007;15:1028-1034.
11. Murray DW, Goodfellow JW, O'Connor JJ. The Oxford medial unicompartmental arthroplasty: a ten-year survival study. J Bone Joint Surg [Br] 1998;80:983-989.
12. Argenson JN, Chevrol-Benkeddache Y, Aubaniac JM. Modern unicompartmental knee arthroplasty with cement: a three to ten-year follow-up study. J Bone Joint Surg [Am] 2002;84:2235-2239.
13. Berger RA, Meneghini RM, Jacobs JJ, et al. Results of unicompartmental knee arthroplasty at a minimum of ten years of follow-up. J Bone Joint Surg [Am] 2005;87:999-1006.
14. Price AJ, Waite JC, Svard U. Long-term clinical results of the medial Oxford unicompartmental knee arthroplasty. Clin Orthop Relat Res 2005;(435):171-180.
15. Marmor L. Lateral compartment arthroplasty of the knee. Clin Orthop Relat Res 1984;(186):115-121.
16. Ohdera T, Tokunaga J, Kobayashi A. Unicompartmental knee arthroplasty for lateral gonarthrosis: midterm results. J Arthroplasty 2001;16:196-200.

17. Ashraf T, Newman JH, Evans RL, Ackroyd CE. Lateral unicompartmental knee replacement survivorship and clinical experience over 21 years. J Bone Joint Surg [Br] 2002;84:1126-1130.

18. Sah AP, Scott RD. Lateral unicompartmental knee arthroplasty through a medial approach: study with an average five-year follow-up. J Bone Joint Surg [Am] 2007;89:1948-1954.

19. Price AJ, Webb J, Topf H, et al. Rapid recovery after Oxford unicompartmental arthroplasty through a short incision. J Arthroplasty 2001;16:970-976.

20. Romanowski MR, Repicci JA. Minimally invasive unicondylar arthroplasty: eight-year follow-up. J Knee Surg 2002;15:17-22.

21. Bonutti PM, Neal DJ, Kester MA. Minimal incision total knee arthroplasty using the suspended leg technique. Orthopedics 2003; 26:899-903.

22. Robinson BJ, Rees JL, Price AJ, et al. Dislocation of the bearing of the Oxford lateral unicompartmental arthroplasty: a radiological assessment. J Bone Joint Surg [Br] 2002;84:653-657.

23. Romanowski MR, Repicci JA. Technical aspects of medial versus lateral minimally invasive unicondylar arthroplasty. Orthopedics 2003;26:289-293.

24. Moglo KE, Shirazi-Adl A. Cruciate coupling and screw-home mechanism in passive knee joint during extension–flexion. J Biomech 2005;38:1075-1083.

25. Klika AK, Gehrig M, Boukis L, et al. A rapid recovery program after total knee arthroplasty. Semin Arthroplasty 2009;20:40-44.

SELECTED READING

Laurencin CT, Zelicof SB, Scott RD, Ewald FC. Unicompartmental versus total knee arthroplasty in the same patient: a comparative study. Clin Orthop Relat Res 1991;(273):151-156.

Lawrence RC, Felson DT, Helmick CG, et al. Estimates of the prevalence of arthritis and other rheumatic conditions in the United States. Part II. Arthritis Rheum 2008;58:26-35.

Marmor L. Lateral compartment arthroplasty of the knee. Clin Orthop Relat Res 1984;(186):115-121.

Ohdera T, Tokunaga J, Kobayashi A. Unicompartmental knee arthroplasty for lateral gonarthrosis: midterm results. J Arthroplasty 2001;16:196-200.

Pennington DW, Swienckowski JJ, Lutes WB, Drake GN. Lateral unicompartmental knee arthroplasty: survivorship and technical considerations at an average follow-up of 12.4 years. J Arthroplasty 2006;21: 13-17.

Romanowski MR, Repicci JA. Technical aspects of medial versus lateral minimally invasive unicondylar arthroplasty. Orthopedics 2003;26: 289-293.

Rougraff BT, Heck DA, Gibson AE. A comparison of tricompartmental and unicompartmental arthroplasty for the treatment of gonarthrosis. Clin Orthop Relat Res 1991;(273):157-164.

Sah AP, Scott RD. Lateral unicompartmental knee arthroplasty through a medial approach: study with an average five-year follow-up. J Bone Joint Surg [Am] 2007;89:1948-1954.

Sah AP, Scott RD. Lateral unicompartmental knee arthroplasty through a medial approach: surgical technique. J Bone Joint Surg [Am] 2008;90(Suppl 2 Pt 2):195-205.

Volpi P, Marinoni L, Bait C, et al. Lateral unicompartmental knee arthroplasty: indications, technique and short-medium term results. Knee Surg Sports Traumatol Arthrosc 2007;15:1028-1034.

CHAPTER **14**

Computer-Guided Partial Knee Replacement

Thomas M. Coon and John H. Velyvis

KEY POINTS

- Make a perfect preoperative plan and execute it perfectly.
- Robotic limited cutting zones prevent injury.
- Minimally traumatic surgical technique allows rapid recovery.
- Robotically optimized implants allow efficient technique, and are based on traditional designs with a long successful track record.
- Multicompartment design allows resurfacing of only involved parts, and maintenance of normal ligaments.

INTRODUCTION

Over the past 10 years, partial knee replacement has risen in popularity. In large part this is due to the development of minimally invasive surgical techniques, which have become increasingly popular in all areas of surgical intervention. Minimally invasive techniques have promoted rapid recovery, lessened blood loss, and reduced postoperative pain.[1] In surgery of the knee, however, they have also increased the difficulty of arthroplasty surgery, particularly in the partial replacement environment, which utilizes even smaller incisions with the resultant constrictive soft tissue envelope. Such surgical constraints may lead to malalignment or malposition of implants by all but the most experienced of surgeons.[2,3] The same time period has seen rapid advancements in computer and electronic technology, and industry has utilized this technology to develop robotic machines that enhance the speed, efficiency, and accuracy of manufacturing far beyond the capabilities of human workers. Engineers and visionaries have long dreamed of the day such technologies could be applied to human surgical endeavors, and such a machine has been developed for the orthopaedic community by MAKO Surgical Corporation (Ft. Lauderdale, FL). The author first began use of this machine in June 2007, and has since performed approximately 300 robotic-assisted partial knee replacements with excellent results. This chapter outlines the theory, setup, performance, and early results of robotic-assisted partial knee arthroplasty.

The RIO (Robotic Arm Interactive Orthopaedic System) surgical system utilizes a mobile robotic arm that gives the surgeon tactile feedback of the cutting zone, so that bone cutting occurs only within the desired footprint area of the proposed implant, thus eliminating the risk of surgical bone-cutting error. The motorized burr is navigated by the computer, and if maneuvered out of the desired cutting area, simply shuts off. This is the first fully Food and Drug Administration–approved instrument widely available in the United States that enables surgical navigation of the cutting tool, thus taking computer navigation to the next level of sophistication.[4] To better exploit the capabilities of this novel cutting system, the engineers and surgeon consultants with MAKO Surgical Corporation have designed a complimentary robotically optimized implant system that uses the robot's unique ability to accurately sculpt bone into complex curves and shapes, thus creating a unique implant system of thin-section shape-matching implants that are ideally suited to partial knee replacement.[5] Because the implants measure approximately 3 mm in cross section, they are ideally suited to use in younger, more active patients who may in the future require revision surgery. The use of these thinner implants should ease revision issues of bone loss for the surgeons of tomorrow. This implant system (Restoris MCK; MAKO Surgical Corporation) is modular and multicompartmental in nature, consisting of tibial onlay or inlay components, femoral condylar components, trochlear components, and patellar components. The components can be mixed and matched based on computed tomography (CT) scan planning like jigsaw puzzle pieces, giving the patient a knee construct that is individualized for his or her unique anatomy, while still maintaining the efficiency of off-the-shelf manufactured components.[6] Like any partial knee replacement system, the ligamentous structures are retained, and the navigation component of the robotics allows nearly perfect dynamic gap balancing to allow excellent anterior cruciate ligament (ACL) and posterior cruciate ligament function of the partial knee construct.

PATIENT SELECTION

Patient selection remains one of the most important determinants of successful partial knee replacement. The arthritis should be confined to the individual compartment that is proposed to be resurfaced. One significant advantage of the multicompartment knee system is that one or two compartments can be resurfaced individually with the decision made at the time of the surgery, so absolute clinical accuracy is perhaps slightly less critical than it is with other systems.

Since the partial knee replacement relies on intact ligamentous structures for stability, it is important that all ligaments remain intact and generally normal range of motion (ROM) is desired. For medial compartment arthritis, it is generally considered optimal to have an intact ACL, although this is not an absolute requirement.[7] If the patient does not have symptomatic instability, a medial unicompartmental knee arthroplasty (UKA) can be performed with good success. ACL reconstruction can be performed at a later date if instability becomes a problem. For isolated patellofemoral (PF) arthroplasty, it is important that the remaining compartments of the knee have minimal pathology, as failure of these implants is usually caused by progression of disease in the other compartments. It is probably also ideal to avoid cases with severe patellar malalignment issues or excessive bony deficiency. Bicompartmental arthroplasty combines medial UKA with PF arthroplasty. The unique shape-matching ability of the Restoris MCK system allows computer matching of various sizes of implants to yield a perfect implant fit. It is still important to assure intact cartilage of the contralateral compartment and intact ligamentous structures to allow anatomic tracking of the construct.

PLANNING

The robotic technology is based on three-dimensional CT images of the patient's knee. Once a compatible CT scan is obtained, the scan segments are inputted into the robotic computer, and a process called segmentation is performed. In this process each CT image is outlined with a computer probe and the cortical bone shape thus inputted into the computer. The robot then utilizes this information to construct an accurate three-dimensional image of the knee. The Makoplasty technician then uses shape matching to align computer models of the implants to the cortical bone surface, planning for the implants to be approximately 1 mm proud of the bone to mimic the thickness of hyaline cartilage. The computer allows accurate positioning of the implants on the bone, and measures the alignment in relation to the mechanical axis of the extremity as determined from the CT scout views of hip, knee, and ankle.[8]

Implant placement of UKA components is based on fairly traditional alignment parameters that can be found in any

tome on unicompartmental arthroplasty. Once alignment of the trochlear component is begun, however, positioning parameters are less clear since this is a shape-matching component. The author has had good success with generally matching the cortical shape of the trochlear groove, taking care to deepen the groove slightly to avoid overstuffing the patellofemoral joint. It is very important to pay close attention to the medial and lateral transition zones to assure smooth transition of the patella from the trochlea onto the femoral condylar surface, and thus avoid a "speed bump" effect when the patella tracks through the range of motion (**Fig. 14–1**).

OPERATING ROOM AND PATIENT SETUP

The introduction of any complex technology into the operating room environment always adds its own special problems and difficulties.[9] In the case of robotics, there are issues of placement of the robot unit as well as the camera and console for the Makoplasty technician. These items must be placed in an appropriate position near enough to the patient to allow full effectiveness of the robotic arm while still allowing adequate line-of-sight visibility for the optical trackers, and leaving room for the surgeon and assistant to perform the technical aspects of the surgery (**Fig. 14–2**). The author finds it most effective to place the robot on the side of the table opposite the operated leg, thus bringing the robotic arm into the wound directly from the side of the extremity that carries the incision; for example, for a left medial UKA, the robot would be placed on the right side of the patient and the robotic burr delivered directly into the medial parapatellar incision. The camera and technician console are opposite the robot approximately 5 feet from the table to give the optimal camera view of the optical arrays. The arrays are placed

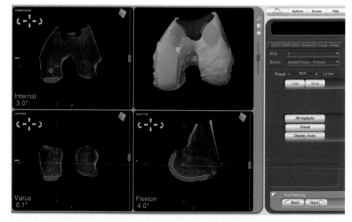

Figure 14-1 Computer-guided implant placement allows the surgeon to visualize precise implant position and interaction prior to cutting bone, thus easing preparation of the critical transition zone between the femoral and trochlear components.

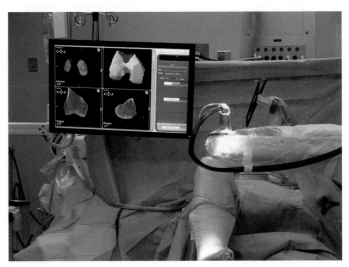

Figure 14-2 Placement of the robotic arm so that it enters the joint directly on the side of the incision eases access to deep recesses of the joint.

anterolateral so there is an unobstructed view of the camera. Alternative setups can be utilized but limit camera view or robotic access, or allow excess bone debris to be expelled onto the arrays (see Fig. 14–2).

SURGICAL APPROACH

For medial or patellofemoral arthritis, a medial parapatellar approach is utilized. The incision begins at the superior pole of the patella and extends to the midtibial tuberosity. A smaller incision may be utilized; however, this makes placement of the high-flex femoral component more difficult. The arthrotomy mimics the skin incision, with care taken to avoid cutting of the vastus medialis muscle. A medial retinacular T-shaped incision is made in the joint capsule midway between the vastus medialis and medial meniscus to allow increased access to the joint and also ease placement of and access to the femoral mechanical checkpoint, placed later in the procedure for reference of the robotic registration.[1] The deep fibers of the medial collateral ligament are then elevated, and the infrapatellar fat pad removed. Following this, a thorough examination of the joint should reveal an intact patellofemoral joint, lateral compartment, and ACL for a medial UKA, and isolated patellofemoral arthritis if a PF arthroplasty is the plan. The approach for a lateral UKA mirrors that of the medial, the main difference being that extra care must be taken to avoid retractor placement that puts pressure on the peroneal nerve, located posterior to the fibular head. Also, the surgeon should be extra mindful of landmarks, since the medial approach is more familiar, and when working from the lateral side one can easily become confused and misplace landmarks or malalign a component.

Registration

Registration is perhaps the most critical portion of the early preparation for robotic-assisted arthroplasty. It begins with placement and recording of the positions of the mechanical checkpoints. These are important reference points, and are frequently referred to as a double check during the bone preparation process. They should be firmly fixed to good-quality bone, and care should be taken to avoid displacing them throughout the procedure. Femoral and tibial registration occurs next, and follows a prescribed pattern set by the robotic software. Points should be collected accurately, and care taken to avoid perforating deep to the cortical surface, but soft tissue or cartilage should be penetrated to record only the bony surface. It also is helpful to collect the individual points in a linear pattern rather than a cluster, this giving the computer a larger picture of the cortical plane to match with the parent CT scan. Combined exposure and femoral and tibial registration typically takes the author approximately 10–15 minutes, and accurate results are the key to efficient use of the robot.

Dynamic Ligament Balancing

One of the most exciting features of the robotic software is that which allows dynamic ligament balancing of the completed procedure *prior* to cutting any bone. Once the bones are registered, the knee can be moved through a range of motion, and a series of data points captured while stressing the knee into "anatomic" or corrected alignment. This mimics the final corrected alignment of the knee as best determined by the experienced "feel" of the surgeon. Also, the alignment can be viewed on the computer screen and the limb alignment corrected to neutral, or more commonly slightly undercorrected for the UKA to avoid overloading the contralateral side of the joint; in other words, a varus knee is usually undercorrected to 1° of mechanical varus alignment.[7] Once this "ideal" alignment position is determined and recorded by the computer, the implant position can be microadjusted within these ligament parameters until the flexion and extension gaps are perfectly balanced, usually to within 0.1 mm. This ligament-balancing technique leads to excellent ACL function and tension, and very early and rapid return of ROM postoperatively (**Figs. 14–3 through 14–5**).

Bone Cutting

Cutting the footprints for the femoral and tibial components is probably the least familiar to the orthopaedic surgeon new to robotics, and is in fact the easiest portion of the operation. Since all the preparation work has already been done during the planning and registration stages, cutting the bone simply involves moving the burr through the haptic field created by the planning process. It is simply a matter of execution. The burr is placed into the haptic "room", and once inside cannot

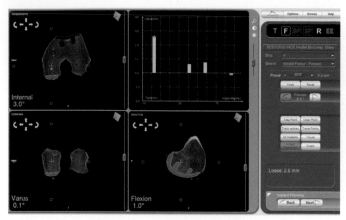

Figure 14-3 Dynamic ligament balancing allows microadjustment of implant position to fine-tune ligament balance prior to cutting bone. In this instance, the femoral component is too posterior, leading to tightness of the flexion gap (right side of graph below the line).

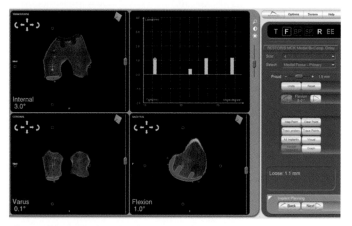

Figure 14-4 Moving the femoral component anteriorly loosens the flexion gap so that both flexion and extension gaps are equal (right and left bars are equal), thus promoting superior ligament balance.

come out until it is intentionally released. The surgeon simply moves the burr throughout the space until all of the "green" areas of bone (those inside the footprint of the implant) are removed. The haptic field does not allow the surgeon to "color outside the lines" (cut outside the desired area of bone resection). The zone guarantees placement of the implant to within 0.5 mm of the planned position. If the burr is accidentally or intentionally moved outside of this area, the burr stops cutting, thus virtually eliminating the chance of erroneous bone cuts or ligament or other soft tissue injury. The software guides the surgeon through the appropriate steps for preparing the bone surfaces, including drilling of anchoring holes and keels. The Restoris MCK implants have been designed to use this robotic technique, and all surfaces are manufactured with a 3-mm

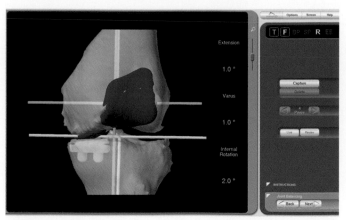

Figure 14-5 Appropriate microadjustment of implants leads to desired 1° undercorrection of varus and excellent ligament balance.

radius of curvature to be compatible with the 6-mm burr, so that no additional preparation is required. Minimal additional surgical preparation, including removal of the meniscus and any osteophytes or loose bodies, is required.

Implant Placement

After final bone and soft tissue preparation is completed, trial implants are used to determine the final polyethylene thickness required. Because of variability in surgeon ligament tensioning, occasionally it is necessary to use a thicker polyethylene spacer, and very rarely cutting of additional depth of the tibial component may be required. Final implant placement and cementing are done in the traditional fashion, with care taken to remove all excess cement and ensure complete seating of the tibial polyethylene component into the tibial baseplate.

RESULTS

The combination of minimally invasive surgical exposure, minimally traumatic bone removal, and outstanding ligament balance allows rapid postsurgical recovery and very early attainment of ROM goals, increasing patient satisfaction. Additionally, the robotically guided implant alignment leads to excellent postoperative radiographs, thus improving surgeon satisfaction and hopefully long-term implant survival as well (**Figs. 14–6 through 14–9**).[10] The author studied his first 67 robotic-assisted UKAs and compared them to his previous 67 consecutive manually instrumented UKAs. Because of the curved nature of the femoral component, measurements of tibial alignment were taken to test for accuracy of alignment. The root-mean-square (RMS) error of the tibial slope was 3.7° manually compared to 1.2° robotically. In addition, the variance using manual instruments was 9.8 times greater than the robotically guided implantations ($p < .0001$).

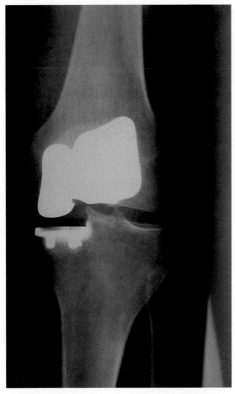

Figure 14-6 Postoperative anteroposterior radiograph of bicompartmental arthroplasty 1 year after surgery.

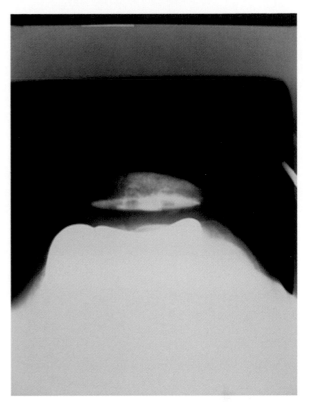

Figure 14-8 Postoperative Merchant's view of bicompartmental arthroplasty 1 year after surgery.

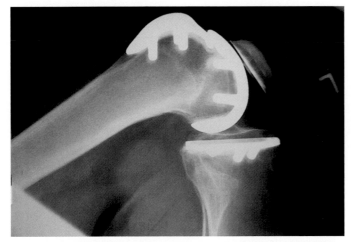

Figure 14-7 Postoperative lateral radiograph of bicompartmental arthroplasty 1 year after surgery.

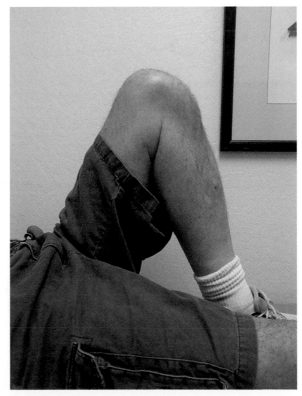

Figure 14-9 Excellent knee flexion and "normal" kinematics 1 year after surgery.

In the coronal plane, the average error was $3.0 \pm 2.2°$ more varus using manual instruments compared to $0.3 \pm 1.9°$ when implanted robotically ($p < .0001$), while the varus/valgus RMS error was 3.7° manually compared to 1.8° robotically. In terms of patient function, patents with either technique had equivalent ROM and Knee Society scores. There was no significant difference in terms of average Knee Society score, change in

Knee Society score, or Marmor rating between the two groups at any of the follow-ups. Furthermore, there were no significant differences in the measures that comprise these scores, such as ROM, pain, and use of assistive devices ($p > .05$), except for ROM at 3 weeks, which was significantly higher for the robotically assisted inlays (116 ± 12) compared to the manual onlays (110 ± 13; $p < .01$).[11,12]

Bicompartmental arthroplasty is a new addition to the robotic armamentarium. As of the time of this writing, the author has performed approximately 40 such procedures with satisfactory early results—it does remain a procedure under development at this time. Study of the first 15 procedures is ongoing; however, preliminary results at only 6 weeks' follow-up show patients recovered their preoperative ROM ($p = .20$). Knee Society Knee Scores significantly improved from a preoperative average of 61 ± 12 (range: 50–90) to a postoperative average at 6 weeks of 87 ± 15 (range: 50–96) ($p < .001$). Every patient was released after 1 day of hospital stay. Radiographically, there was no evidence of loosening, wear, or progression of osteoarthritis. There were also no perioperative complications.[13] Using computer simulation, the amount of bone removed using bicompartmental arthroplasty compared to traditional total knee arthroplasty (TKA) was predicted. Total bone removed on the femur and the tibia using a standard TKA implant is 3.5 times the bone removed using a bicompartmental onlay implant and 4 times the bone removed when using a bicompartmental inlay implant.[13]

SUMMARY

Novel technologies lead to novel solutions. The addition of computer guidance to implant planning and surgical execution has ushered in a new era of accuracy in implant placement and ligament balance, with resultant improvements in early patient function and satisfaction. Only time will tell if concurrent improvements in longevity are evident, but historically improved implant placement has generally led to improvements in survival rates. Further evolution of implant design to exploit the strengths of surgical robotics is likely to extend the range and complexity of robotic procedures and the breadth of pathology amenable to this groundbreaking technology.

REFERENCES

1. Tria AJ Jr. Advancements in minimally invasive total knee arthroplasty. Orthopedics 2003;26(8 Suppl):s859-s863.
2. Fisher DA, Watts M, Davis KE. Implant position in knee surgery: a comparison of minimally invasive, open unicompartmental, and total knee arthroplasty. J Arthroplasty 2003;18(7 Suppl 1):2-8.
3. Kort NP, van Raay JJ, Cheung J, et al. Analysis of Oxford medial unicompartmental knee replacement using the minimally invasive technique in patients aged 60 and above: an independent prospective series. Knee Surg Sports Traumatol Arthrosc 2007;15:1331-1334.
4. Lonner JH. Indications for unicompartmental knee arthroplasty and rationale for robotic arm-assisted technology. Am J Orthop 2009;38(2 Suppl):3-6.
5. Banks SA. Haptic robotics enable a systems approach to design of a minimally invasive modular knee arthroplasty. Am J Orthop 2009;38(2 Suppl):23-27.
6. Lonner JH. Modular bicompartmental knee arthroplasty with robotic arm assistance. Am J Orthop 2009;38(2 Suppl):28-31.
7. Berger RA, Nedeff DD, Barden RM, et al. Unicompartmental knee arthroplasty: clinical experience at 6–10 year followup. Clin Orthop Relat Res 1999;(367):50-60.
8. Roche MW, O'Loughlin PF, Musahi V, et al. Robot-assisted unicompartmental knee arthroplasty: preoperative planning and surgical technique. Am J Orthop 2009;38(2 Suppl):10-15.
9. Coon TM. Integrating robotic technology into the operating room. Am J Orthop 2009;38(2 Suppl):7-9.
10. Lonner JH, John TK, Conditt MA. Robotic arm-assisted UKA improves tibial component alignment: a pilot study. Clin Orthop Relat Res 2010;(468):141-146.
11. Coon TM, Driscoll MD, Horowitz S, et al. Robotic assisted UKA is more accurate than manually instrumented UKA. Podium presentation at the 21st Annual Congress of ISTA, October 1–4, 2008, Seoul, South Korea.
12. Coon TM, Driscoll MD, Conditt MA. Early clinical success of a novel tactile guided UKA technique. Podium presentation at the 21st Annual Congress of ISTA, October 1–4, 2008, Seoul, South Korea.
13. Coon TM, Kreutzer S, Horowitz S, et al. Robotically guided bicompartmental arthroplasty. Podium presentation at the International Society for Computer Assisted Orthopedic Surgery Annual Meeting, June 16–19, 2010, Paris, France.

CHAPTER 15

Individualized Unicompartmental Knee Arthroplasty

Wolfgang Fitz

KEY POINTS

- Individualized UKA addresses anatomic differences between medial and lateral condyles regarding width, anterior length, and different anterior radiuses, as well as geometric differences between medial and lateral tibial plateaus.
- Individualized UKA also addresses shortcomings in respect to larger AP and ML dimension seen in large males.
- For the first time, a lateral UKA is introduced to address the different anatomic variances of the lateral tibiofemoral joint.

INTRODUCTION

Forty years ago, knee arthroplasties were introduced with one or more femoral and tibial sizes. Gradually, left and right components as well as more sizes were added to better match smaller and larger knees in different patients. The components' shape and dimensions were optimized using anthropometric data, and asymmetric femoral and tibial components were introduced. However, to this day there is no specific implant for the lateral tibiofemoral joint, on the femoral and on the tibial side. Common practice is to use a left medial component for the right lateral and a right medial for the left lateral tibial plateau. One would imagine that, besides anteroposterior (AP) and mediolateral (ML) dimensions and their ratio, different shapes or different curvatures would have been introduced to optimize each patient's anatomy and to restore closer to normal knee kinematics. However, this is not the case. Shapes are determined by manufacturers and come in different magnifications of their geometries. This is done for both femoral and tibial components. On the femoral side, each manufacturer offers one specific J-curve with different magnifications, matching the condylar geometry to some degree. One manufacturer even offers a single-radius femoral component. The question remains whether a more anatomic reconstruction of the joint surfaces would further enhance

clinical outcome. More sophisticated measures are needed, such as measurement of proprioception, muscle function, and gait analysis to reflect the changing demographics of younger, more active patients considering knee replacement surgery.

The selection of a specific off-the-shelf implant is driven by a surgeon's familiarity with surgical technique and implants, quality of sales support, and ease of a surgical technique. Off-the-shelf implants lack the ability to best fit for an individual surface geometry. Pricing has and will play a more important role in the future. An implant should not be chosen for any other reason besides it being the best fit for a patient.

FEMORAL COMPONENTS

The overall goal of selecting a femoral component is optimal fit. The femoral component should not overhang, but it should be wide enough and match the geometry without impingement of the medial spine or the posterior cruciate ligament. The transition to the femoropatellar joint should be smooth, not prominent, and the femoral component should not be too long, specifically on the lateral side to avoid patellofemoral (PF) impingement. Hernigou and Deschamps[1] reported on 99 unicompartmental arthroplasties (UKAs) with a mean follow-up of 14 years. Of these, 29% were symptomatic due to patellar impingement through the femoral component. In this group, lower Knee Society scores were related to problems climbing stairs. They proposed two failure mechanisms; one may be related to an over-resection off the posterior condyle, which consequently moves the femoral component more anteriorly. They also hypothesized that poor intraoperative judgment of the linea terminalis, which describes the trochleocondylar junction, could lead to oversizing the femoral component. **Figure 15–1** shows the transition between the medial and lateral condyles to the trochlea. The linea terminalis is the result of the medial and lateral meniscal impression on the femur and can be seen on lateral radiographs. In Herningou and Deschamps's series, the trochleocondylar junction was an average of 3 mm anterior on the medial and 4 mm posterior on the lateral side relative to a line representing the slope of the intercondylar roof.[1] Berger et al.[2] reported

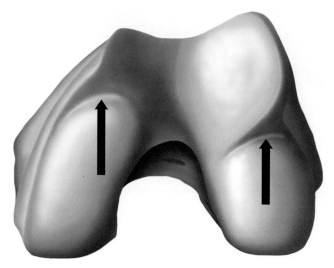

Figure 15-1 The linea terminalis is more anterior medially as compared to the lateral side.

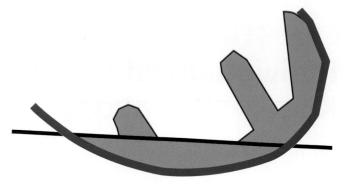

Figure 15-2 Only-femoral designs are prone to surgical errors. Too much flexion of the femoral component can lead to patellofemoral impingement.

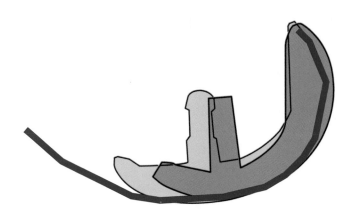

Figure 15-3 Only-femoral designed components rely on a distal femoral bone cut. The edge of the femoral component thins, but does not go below the subchondral bone.

the results of 59 UKAs with a follow-up of 11–15 years. The main failure mode was symptomatic patellofemoral osteoarthritis in 10%; this was observed despite a pristine PF joint preoperatively. In a group of 48 living patients who had an average radiographic follow-up of 17 years, Squire et al. reported evidence of PF osteoarthritis in 35 patients (87%).[3] A total of 14 knees were revised. Six patients were revised for disease progression, but it was not defined whether this was related to PF osteoarthritis.

The linea terminalis has to be respected to avoid PF impingement. Both surgical technique and femoral implant design play a role. The distal femoral cut in most systems is not based on an intramedullary rod, but solely on the tibial cut. It is difficult for the surgeon to judge the correct amount of flexion of the distal femoral cut. This step determines the amount of flexion in which femoral component is implanted. If the knee is hyperextended, the distal femoral cutting block cuts in more extension. If the knee is held in more flexion, the component results in a more flexed position. However, the tibial cut can vary depending on whether there is more or less slope, which additionally contributes to more or less flexion or extension. Individualized femoral jigs may help to resolve this source of surgical error. **Figure 15–2** shows a femoral component in too much flexion, resulting in PF impingement. All three studies cited above reported increasing PF osteoarthritis in the second decade. All studies used an only-femoral component (**Fig. 15–3**), which means that the anterior edge is not curved below the subchondral bone. This is in contrast to a recessed femoral component where the edge of the implant extends below the subchondral bone as shown in **Figure 15–4**. Using a recessed single-radius femoral component, progression of PF osteoarthritis was not seen in a series with a

follow-up between 10 and 20 years.[4] It remains unclear, since there is no reported 10- to 20-year follow-up series of a tapered J-curve design, whether this is related to the recesses design itself or to the single-radius design. The single-radius femoral implant restores the posterior condylar offset by balancing the flexion gap prior to the extension gap, so the surgical technique is very focused on restoring the posterior condyle. Additionally, its shorter design, replacing only the posterior condyle, may increase femoropatellar offset, which may result in decreasing PF stresses and thereby reducing the likelihood of PF osteoarthritis. However, since PF peak stresses are lowest in extension and increase during flexion,[5,6] J-curve femoral components reconstructing the posterior condyle should achieve the same offset compared to a single-radius design (see Fig. 15–4). Restoring the cylindrical posterior condyle,[7] therefore, should not result in significantly different PF stresses.

Only-femoral designs may be more susceptible to PF osteoarthritis as a failure mode in the second decade due to

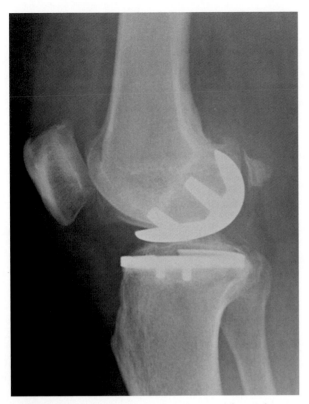

Figure 15-4 J-curve and single-radius designed femoral components are available where the edge of the component extends below the subchondral bone.

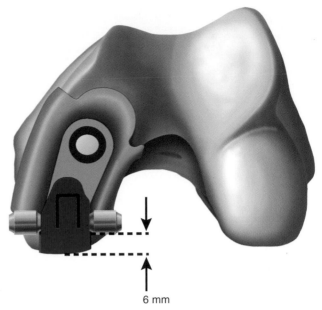

6 mm

Figure 15-5 A preoperative surgical plan provides detailed information on how much bone needs to be resected off the posterior condyle. A specific instrument (L-guide, in blue) facilitates appropriate posterior resection. The instrumentation is individualized and single use.

impingement between the patella and the edge of the femoral implant. This may be additionally enhanced with the decreasing of cartilage thicknesses as we get older. Individualized UKAs have several advantages compared to off-the-shelf implants: computed tomography (CT) data are utilized to identify the linea terminalis and the implant is designed with respect to the transition to the PF joint with short lateral and longer medial components. The length of the components is related to the restoration of the posterior condyle. A surgical plan provides detailed information on how much bone needs to be resected off the posterior condyle. An example of 6 mm of posterior condylar resection is shown in **Figure 15–5**. Therefore, an incidental too-anterior placement of the femoral component is addressed by preoperative planning, individualized femoral cutting blocks, and cross-checking through the correct amount of resected bone. In order to address the problem of PF impingement, the anterior edge is recessed below the subchondral bone. **Figure 15–6** shows a three-dimensional model demonstrating this design feature.

Width

The medial condyle appears narrower and the lateral condyle wider. Some authors, such as Yoshioka et al.,[8] could not find a difference. Others described a wider lateral condyle: Mensch

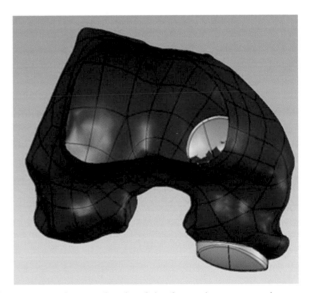

Figure 15-6 The anterior tip of the femoral component is designed to recess underneath the subchondral bone to address femoropatellar impingement.

and Amstutz[9] described an average width of 26.6 mm for the medial condyle and 26.9 mm for the lateral condyle in 30 cadaver knees. Erkman and Walker[10] studied 50 radiographed knees and found similar measurements, but values were 10% larger, suggesting magnification differences. We found an average medial condylar width of 26.1 mm (range, 21–32 mm)

Table 15-1 Minimum and Maximum Widths of Currently Available U.S. Femoral Components		
Implant	*Minimum Width (mm)*	*Maximum Width (mm)*
Stryker Triathlon	19.0	24.0
DePuy HP	18.0	25.0
Zimmer HF	21.0	26.0
Smith and Nephew Journey	18.0	25.0
Biomet Oxford	19.0	23.0
Wright Advance	19.0	22.0

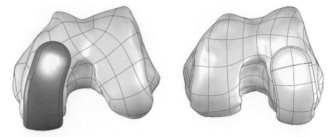

Figure 15-7 Medial and lateral individualized UKAs demonstrating more curvature on the medial side, and a shorter and wider lateral femoral condyle, optimizing condylar coverage.

and an average lateral condylar width of 28.5 mm (range, 22–36 mm) on 48 CT scans.[11] Our data are very similar to published data. Looking at off-the-shelf femoral components (**Table 15–1**), the width is narrower compared to the femoral condyles' dimensions. This is necessary to allow the surgeon to find the best implant placement and fit, since the bone is cut to fit the implant. The advantage of individualized femoral components are wider femoral components. However, whether this will be an advantage resulting in better long-term results with less femoral loosening still has to be proven. There may, however, be an advantage in heavier patients in that a wider femoral component reduces the overall stresses on implant and fixation.

Geometry

Medial and lateral condyles differ in form and appearance; the anterior edges of both menisci result in an indentation of the inferior surface of both condyles, which is more prominent on the lateral side and represents the anterior part of the J-curve.[12] In all implant designs, this anterior part of the J-curve is changed, removing the indentation to reflect the absence of the menisci. The posterior two parts represent two different radii with a constant ratio of 2 : 1.[12] Mensch and Amstutz[9] found similar values of 1.9 : 1. The first radius, which is larger laterally than medially, represents the weight-bearing surface between extension and 45° and the posterior radius between 45° and 120°. The anterior of the two radii of the lateral condyle averaged 5.9 mm more than the medial condyle (**Fig. 15–7**). The posterior radii are very similar.[9] Prosthetic replacement with equal radii diminishes the lateral and increases the medial condylar anterior radii and may affect knee kinematics.[9] Howell et al. compared the posterior radii of medial to those of lateral condyles, and found no significant difference between medial and lateral radii,[13] confirming the findings of Shinno and of Mensch and Amstutz for the posterior condyles of the two radii.[9,12] Eckhoff et al. observed the cylindrical geometry of the posterior condylar radius and found slightly larger medial condyles.[7] While both make arguments for a single-radius designed femoral component, the work of Shinno and of Mensch and Amstutz clearly

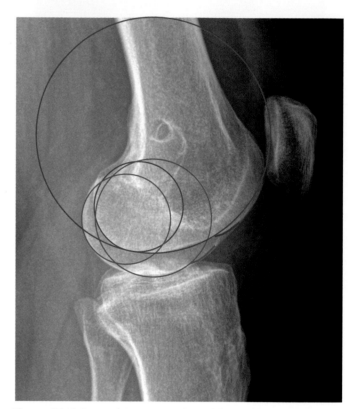

Figure 15-8 Femoral J-curve consists of three different parts. The posterior two parts are best described through two different radii with a fixed ratio and the anterior part is the result of meniscal indentation (medial red and lateral blue).

underlines the importance of describing all parts of the femoral J-curve. The posterior two arcs have different radii, and Eckhoff et al. and Howell et al. described only the very posterior part, which is important between 45° and 120°. A single-radius design does not match the J-curve, but only the posterior radius which is the smallest radius.[9,12] Since the ratio between the two radii is constant, there may be an argument for the off-the-shelf implant (**Fig. 15–8**). However, there is a difference between the more anterior two radii of the medial and lateral femoral condyles that warrants different medial and lateral femoral condylar designs. The lateral anterior radius is twice as large as the medial.

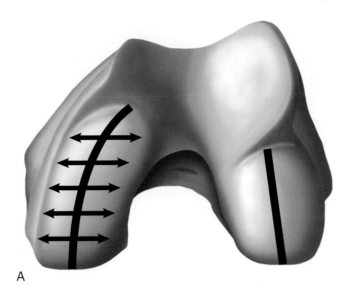

A

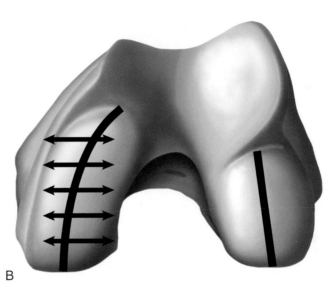

B

Figure 15-9 Front view of a left knee. The medial condyle is longer and slightly curved. The lateral condyle is shorter, wider, and less curved. Placement of a curved component on the left and a straight on the right would be preferable.

Individualized femoral components offer a solution to address these different condylar geometries, and therefore have the potential to improve knee kinematics and to restore a close-to-normal ligament tensioning. Just by looking at the medial and lateral condyle, there are two additional variations of the shape and geometry of both condyles to be observed. First, the medial condyle extends from the posterior condyle to the transition to the femoropatellar joint appearing not straight, but rather curved with the proximal part pointing more toward the notch. However, the lateral condyle appears less curved. Most available implants are asymmetric, and one could argue it would be preferable to use a more curved asymmetric femoral component to replace the medial condyle,

while using a less curved or almost straight component for the lateral side (**Fig. 15–9**). The only two remaining symmetric implants on the U.S. market are the Biomet Oxford and the Wright Advance. Biomet's Oxford is contraindicated for the lateral side, but could be used in combination with a fixed-bearing tibial tray. However, no manufacturer offers this option, and it is solely at the surgeon's discretion to choose implants for best fit between medial and lateral condyles. Individualized implants solve the different shape and geometry of the medial and lateral condyles. Another problem of off-the-shelf femoral components is the way femoral component sizes grow. We know the J-curve has three different elements with a defined ratio of the posterior two radii.[9,12] Most implant sizes

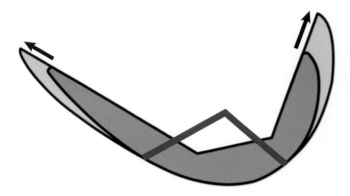

Figure 15-10 Smaller and larger sizes increase or decrease with shorter or longer anterior or posterior extensions, while the central portion of the J-curve remains unchanged.

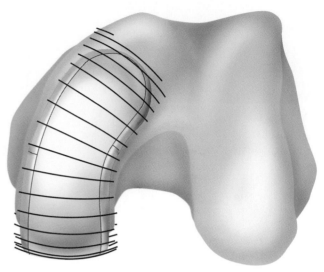

Figure 15-12 Individualized femoral component design follows the medial condylar curvature and the anterior twist of the surface toward the notch. The coronal surface is engineered to optimize contact area with the tibial component.

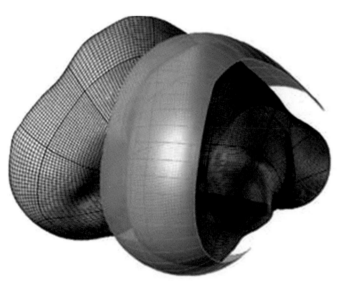

Figure 15-11 Individualized femoral component design is based on patient's specific J-curve. The implant is 3.5 mm offset from the subchondral bone with a prosthetic coronal curvature.

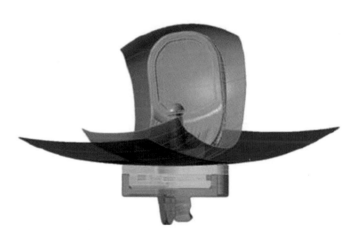

Figure 15-13 The surface radius of the prosthetic coronal curvature (orange) drives the tibial surface radius (blue) to optimize contact area.

are not a true magnification of the J-curve. **Figure 15–10** shows one example of how larger and smaller sizes are generated. The central third of the J-curve, which is specific to each manufacturer, does not change, and the posterior and anterior thirds are elongated evenly with larger sizes. This concept does not really respect the anatomic principle of the three parts of the J-curve and can result in incomplete coverage of the posterior condyle (see Fig. 15–10).

Individualized femoral components are based on the individual J-curve 3.5 mm above the subchondral bone (**Fig. 15–11**). This represents the necessary thickness for the femoral component for mechanical strength, but on the other side it restores the individual joint surface. Each individual J-curve receives an engineered coronal radius (**Fig. 15–12**) to optimize the tibial contact area (**Fig. 15–13**). The mean contact

area and the mean contact stress showed comparable values to off-the-shelf fixed-bearing implants during heel strike, toeoff, and midstance positions, with small standard deviations.[14] Steklov et al. concluded that a constant coronal curvature can be applied to individualized J-curves to combine unique benefits of individualized implants with proven concept for minimizing polyethylene wear.[14]

Tibial Plateau

Medial and lateral tibial joint surfaces are not similar in their geometry. This prompts the question whether the use of the same implant is justified. We presented CT data on 48 patients (24 females and 24 males) showing that the medial tibial

Table 15-2 **Tibial Implant Dimensions of UKAs Currently Available in the United States**						
Implant	_Size 1 (mm)_	_Size 2 (mm)_	_Size 3 (mm)_	_Size 4 (mm)_	_Size 5 (mm)_	_Size 6 (mm)_
Stryker Triathlon						
AP	41.0	44.0	47.0	50.0	53.0	56.0
ML	23.0	25.0	27.0	29.0	31.0	33.0
DePuy HP						
AP	42.0	45.0	48.0	51.0	54.0	57.0
ML	24.0	26.0	28.0	30.0	32.0	34.0
Zimmer HF						
AP	41.0	44.0	47.0	50.0	53.0	56.0
ML	23.0	25.0	27.0	29.0	31.0	33.0
Smith and Nephew Journey						
AP	38.0	42.0	46.0	49.0	52.0	55.0
ML	24.0	25.0	27.0	29.0	30.0	32.0
Biomet Oxford						
AP	38.0	41.0	44.0	47.0	50.0	53.0
ML	26.0	26.0	28.0	30.0	32.0	34.0
Wright Advance						
AP	40.0	44.0	49.0	54.0		
ML	24.0	26.0	29.0	33.0		

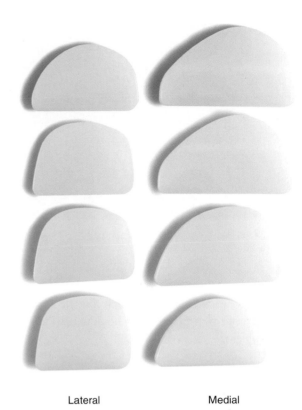

Lateral   Medial

Figure 15-14 Different geometries of medial and lateral tibial trays.

plateau measured 5 mm below the lowest point is different, with an ML/AP ratio of around 0.6 while that of the lateral tibial plateau is 0.7.[11] This means the medial tibial plateau is more oval and the lateral side is rounder. Servien et al.[15] found similar AP/ML ratios of 0.56 for the medial side and 0.63 for the lateral side. Their measurements are smaller compared to our data, but their series had five times more females than males, resulting in smaller values. Surendran et al.[16] studied CT scans of 100 (50 males and 50 females) cadavers and described the dimensions 6 mm below the lowest point of the medial tibia with a slope of 7°. They found reasonable coverage with off-the-shelf implants for the Korean population. There was only one male with an AP length of more than 58 mm. No Korean male had a tibial cut wider than 33 mm, which is different from our series, where 8 of 25 males had a medial tibia of more than 33 mm. They did not study the lateral tibial side at all. Comparing our measurements with the actual dimensions of tibial plateaus in commercial implants available in the United States (**Table 15–2**), we found for the medial tibial plateau that 13% of males have not enough AP coverage, and 25% of males and 4% of females have too much ML coverage. On the lateral side, 4% have not enough AP and 27% not enough ML coverage. Servien et al.[15] did not compare the actual tibial plateau measurements with implant dimension, but they concluded that optimal AP coverage may lead to medial overhang.

Besides looking at the actual dimensions, the shape of the tibial plateau varies too. We know the lateral tibial plateau is not as D-shaped as the medial—it is instead rounder. Fitzpatrick et al. observed the shape of the tibial cuts 5 mm below the

joint surface in 34 CT scans, and calculated how much cortical rim would be covered by a D- and/or a teardrop-shaped implant.[17] The D-shaped implant was better than the teardrop-shaped implant, with a maximum of 74% cortical coverage on the medial side and 60.5% on the lateral side. They used a theoretical model to calculate how much cortical coverage could be obtained with an optimized implant design and concluded that 76% could achieve cortical rim coverage and felt there was room for improvement in implant design. Individualized implants have the advantage of being able to reproduce each patient's geometry. **Figure 15–14** shows different geometries observed in my recent patients. Specifically, the rounder geometry of the lateral tibial plateau is quite obvious and explains the findings of poor cortical coverage more so on the lateral tibial plateau that Fitzpatrick et al. described. Shortcomings of off-the-shelf implants are reflected in variations of surgical techniques published in the past. There are two recommendations: one is to place the lateral tibial plateau more mesial (moving it closer to the lateral tibial spine) and leaving the very lateral aspect of the tibial condyle uncovered.[18] The second recommendation is to internally rotate the tibial component for better coverage.[19] **Figure 15–15** shows the effect on a sawbones of internally rotating the lateral tibial tray to improve lateral cortical coverage. However, this may lead to decreased coverage toward the posterior cruciate ligament

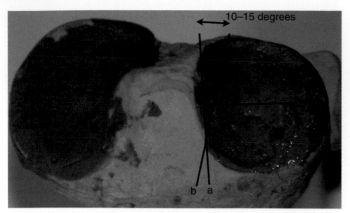

Figure 15-15 Rotating the lateral tibial plateau more internally decreases the coverage toward the PCL.

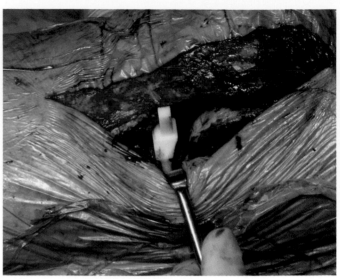

Figure 15-16 Individualized chips in incremental different thicknesses matching the tibial surface topography are inserted during the balancing step. A corresponding amount is resected off the tibia. Thicker chips result in less tibial resection.

(PCL) and may cause the lateral femoral condyle to roll backward with flexion toward the PCL. Individualized tibial trays solve this problem.

Ligament Balancing

The reconstruction of the geometry of femoral and tibial articulating surfaces may play a more important role in total knee arthroplasty and more so in UKA to restore more physiologic kinematics and ligament tensioning. Unicompartmental arthroplasties restore close-to-normal knee kinematics, whether they are mobile bearing[20] or fixed bearing.[21] The Oxford experience taught surgeons that the balancing of the medial collateral ligament has to be obtained within 1 mm to avoid meniscal bearing dislocation and to restore normal joint kinematics. This is a little less than the recommended 1–3 mm.[22] Exact numbers of how much play or laxity should be obtained after knee arthroplasty remain unclear. Recently, one implant introduced a tensiometer and early results demonstrated that women had 10–15N less tension compared to men.[23] However, this device resulted in 4.9% dislocation rate in mobile-bearing UKA within 2 years. One magnetic resonance imaging study showed that, in normal living knees, a lateral joint gap opened under the stress of 6.7 mm versus 2.1 mm medially. There was a tendency that female gaps had more laxity, but it did not reach statistical significance. The lateral side is 4.6 mm laxer in flexion, and authors questioned the concept of rectangular flexion gaps in total knee replacement.[24] However, this confirms that the balancing of medial and lateral UKAs in flexion should be different and looser laterally. In extension, the balancing under stress should be around 1–2 mm medially and 2–3 mm laterally.

After removing all osteophytes, it is important during the balancing step to avoid tightness. This would result in overcorrection and potentially lead to progressive osteoarthritis of the contralateral side. Most off-the-shelf implants use some type of spacer blocks to allow precise balancing. Individualized

UKAs introduce an individualized spacer-block concept. After the removal of osteophytes and residual articular cartilage, individual chips in various thicknesses designed to match the surface topography of the tibia are inserted. **Figure 15–16** shows an inserted navigation chip with a gap opening of about 2–3 mm. The chip can be exchanged to be thinner or thicker, depending on the surgeon's liking. The thicker the chip, the less bone is resected off the tibia, and vice versa.[25] The gap opening after the components are cemented equals the gap opening during the balancing step.

Alignment

Restoration of coronal alignment within 2.4–7.2° of valgus results in the lowest failure rate of 0.5% in total knee replacement.[26] Choong et al.[27] demonstrated, in a randomized prospective study comparing computer-assisted navigation to hand navigation in total knee replacement, that International Knee Society and Short Form-12 scores were significantly better at 6 weeks and 3, 6, and 12 months if coronal alignment within 3° of neutral was achieved. Better alignment correlates with better knee function and improved quality of life.[27] Improvement of coronal alignment using non–image-based navigation was demonstrated in a randomized prospective study of UKAs, resulting in 95% with an alignment with a range between 0° and 4°. However, no study has yet shown better alignment to improve clinical outcome in UKA. Individualized instruments, using the mechanical alignment of femur and tibia published recently, resulted in correction of the varus coronal alignment from 7° to 1° in 32 individualized UKAs. Also the medial proximal tibial angle was corrected from 87° to 89°, demonstrating the high accuracy of single-use, individualized, and prenavigated surgical instrumentation.[28]

CONCLUSIONS

The use of individualized instrumentation using long-axis mechanical information facilitates accurate component positioning along the mechanical axis. Individualized UKAs have several advantages compared to off-the-shelf implants: CT data are utilized to identify the linea terminalis and manufacture an implant respecting this important anatomic landmark for both the medial and lateral condyles and respecting their anatomic variances. The different lengths of medial and lateral condyles are respected, and the surgical technique incorporates the appropriate posterior condylar resection to avoid anterior placement (see Video 15-1). A surgical plan provides detailed information to the surgeon for each patient to optimize implant position. Width and geometry and the differences of the medial and lateral condyles are respected in individualized femoral implants. Deficiencies of tibial implant sizes for large males on the medial side as well as on the lateral side are addressed. Long-term results for lateral UKA are needed to demonstrate the superiority of this novel technology.

REFERENCES

1. Hernigou P, Deschamps G. Patellar impingement following unicompartmental arthroplasty. J Bone Joint Surg [Am] 2002;84:1132-1137.
2. Berger RA, Meneghini RM, Sheinkop MB, et al. The progression of patellofemoral arthrosis after medial unicompartmental replacement: results at 11 to 15 years. Clin Orthop Relat Res 2004;(428): 92-99.
3. Squire MW, Callaghan JJ, Goetz DD, et al. Unicompartmental knee replacement: a minimum 15 year followup study. Clin Orthop Relat Res 1999;(367):61-72.
4. Svard UC, Price AJ. Oxford medial unicompartmental knee arthroplasty: a survival analysis of an independent series. J Bone Joint Surg [Br] 2001;83:191-194.
5. Huberti HH, Hayes WC. Patellofemoral contact pressures: the influence of q-angle and tendofemoral contact. J Bone Joint Surg [Am] 1984;66:715-724.
6. Marder RA, Swanson TV, Sharkey NA, Duwelius PJ. Effects of partial patellectomy and reattachment of the patellar tendon on patellofemoral contact areas and pressures. J Bone Joint Surg [Am] 1993;75:35-45.
7. Eckhoff DG, Bach JM, Spitzer VM, et al. Three-dimensional mechanics, kinematics, and morphology of the knee viewed in virtual reality. J Bone Joint Surg [Am] 2005;87(Suppl 2):71-80.
8. Yoshioka Y, Siu D, Cooke TD. The anatomy and functional axes of the femur. J Bone Joint Surg [Am] 1987;69:873-880.
9. Mensch JS, Amstutz HC. Knee morphology as a guide to knee replacement. Clin Orthop Relat Res 1975;(112):231-241.
10. Erkman MJ, Walker PS. A study of knee geometry applied to the design of condylar prostheses. Biomed Eng 1974;9:14-17.
11. Fitz W, Losina E. Why we need individualized partial knee replacements. Presented at the 9th EFORT meeting, Vienna, Austria, 2009.
12. Shinno N. Statico-dynamic analysis of movement of the knee. I. Modus of movement of the knee. Tokushima J Exp Med 1961;8: 101-110.
13. Howell SM, Howell SJ, Hull ML. Assessment of the radii of the medial and lateral femoral condyles in varus and valgus knees with osteoarthritis. J Bone Joint Surg [Am] 2010;92:98-104.
14. Steklov N, Slamin J, Srivastav S, D'Lima D. Unicompartmental knee resurfacing: enlarged tibio-femoral contact area and reduced contact stress using novel patient-derived geometries. Open Biomed Eng J 2010;4:85-92.
15. Servien E, Saffarini M, Lustig S, et al. Lateral versus medial tibial plateau: morphometric analysis and adaptability with current tibial component design. Knee Surg Sports Traumatol Arthrosc 2008;16: 1141-1145.
16. Surendran S, Kwak DS, Lee UY, et al. Anthropometry of the medial tibial condyle to design the tibial component for unicondylar knee arthroplasty for the Korean population. Knee Surg Sports Traumatol Arthrosc 2007;15:436-442.
17. Fitzpatrick C, FitzPatrick D, Lee J, Auger D. Statistical design of unicompartmental tibial implants and comparison with current devices. Knee 2007;14:138-144.
18. Scott R. Total Knee Arthroplasty. Philadelphia: WB Saunders, 2005.
19. Pennington DW, Swienckowski JJ, Lutes WB, Drake GN. Lateral unicompartmental knee arthroplasty: survivorship and technical considerations at an average follow-up of 12.4 years. J Arthroplasty 2006;21:13-17.
20. Price AJ, Rees JL, Beard DJ, et al. Sagittal plane kinematics of a mobile-bearing unicompartmental knee arthroplasty at 10 years: a comparative in vivo fluoroscopic analysis. J Arthroplasty 2004; 19:590-597.
21. Patil S, Colwell CW Jr, Ezzet KA, D'Lima DD. Can normal knee kinematics be restored with unicompartmental knee replacement? J Bone Joint Surg [Am] 2005;87:332-338.
22. Whiteside LA. Making your next unicompartmental knee arthroplasty last: three keys to success. J Arthroplasty 2005;20(4 Suppl 2):2-3.
23. Hoffmann F, Campbell D, et al. Ligament balancing in unicondylar knee prothesis: early clinical results of a multicentre study on 175 cases. Presented at the 9th EFORT meeting, Vienna, Austria, 2009.
24. Tokuhara Y, Kadoya Y, Nakagawa S, et al. The flexion gap in normal knees: an MRI study. J Bone Joint Surg [Br] 2004;86: 1133-1136.
25. Fitz W. Unicompartmental knee arthroplasty with use of novel patient-specific resurfacing implants and personalized jigs. J Bone Joint Surg [Am] 2009;91(Suppl 1):69-76.
26. Fang DM, Ritter MA, Davis KE. Coronal alignment in total knee arthroplasty: just how important is it? J Arthroplasty 2009;24(6 Suppl):39-43.
27. Choong PF, Dowsey MM, Stoney JD. Does accurate anatomical alignment result in better function and quality of life? Comparing conventional and computer-assisted total knee arthroplasty. J Arthroplasty 2009;24:560-569.
28. Koeck FX, Beckmann J, Luring C, et al. Evaluation of implant position and knee alignment after patient-specific unicompartmental knee arthroplasty. Knee 2010;August 3. [Epub ahead of print]

CHAPTER 16
The Patella in Medial Unicompartmental Knee Arthroplasty

Keith R. Berend

KEY POINTS

- The premise behind Oxford criteria is that UKA is utilized to treat anteromedial osteoarthritis. When these criteria are present, other unnecessary contraindications such as age, weight, and the status of the patellofemoral articulation can be safely ignored without affecting the outcome of Oxford UKA.
- Correction of varus deformity with preservation of the anterior cruciate ligament has a protective effect on the patellofemoral joint, even if there is significant arthritic disease present.
- The author employs the surgical technique described and taught by the implant designers.
- Cementing technique is critical to prevent loosening, and the removal of impinging osteophytes is paramount to reduce the potential for dislocation and increased wear.
- Medial UKA is a conservative procedure that can accurately correct malalignment, and restore an arthritic knee to its predisease functional status with normal kinematics and tremendous pain relief.
- Mobile bearing, with its inset femoral component, may be more tolerant to patellofemoral disease than a polyradial/polycentric femoral component used in fixed-bearing UKA.

INTRODUCTION

Unicompartmental knee arthroplasty (UKA) or partial knee replacement represents the ultimate minimally invasive procedure for treating degenerative joint disease of the knee in the appropriately indicated patient. The conservative nature of the procedure stems from the bone conservation, the preservation and correction of normal ligamentous structures, and the restoration of normal knee kinematics. These outcomes cannot be achieved with any total knee arthroplasty (TKA). By incorporating a fully congruent, meniscal bearing,

the Oxford UKA (Biomet, Inc., Warsaw, IN) has demonstrated some of the lowest wear rates seen with any knee implant in both retrieval studies and RSA studies, averaging 0.02 mm per year in both.[1,2] Thus, wear does not appear to be a limiting factor in the indications for or contraindications against UKA using this device. The fully congruent articulation provides a larger contact area and reduces the contact stresses, leading to significantly decreased wear when compared to fixed bearing, noncongruent designs. Other design-specific differences, such as an inset, spherical femoral component, may specifically address the patellofemoral joint problems seen with many fixed-bearing UKA designs. The long-term outcomes that have been published using this device make it one of the most successful devices available today for the treatment of medial compartmental disease of the knee and therefore make this device the logical choice for UKA. Survivorship rates out to 15 years and 20 years have been 95% and 92%, respectively, in an independent series.[3]

The indications for UKA have been debated widely over the past several decades. Classical indications, when followed closely, have included only a very small percentage of degenerative knees. The Kozinn and Scott criteria limit the utilization of UKA to those patients older than 60 years, weighing less than 82 kg, and exclude active individuals. Additionally, these classical indications exclude cumulative deformity of more than 15°, any fixed flexion contracture of more than 5°, and more than minimal arthritic changes in the patellofemoral joint.[4] With these indications, only between 2% and 12% of arthritic knees would meet the criteria for UKA.[5,6] The so-called Oxford criteria are somewhat more liberal and encompass an anatomic and radiographic philosophy for inclusion or exclusion of patients. The premise behind these expanded criteria is that UKA is utilized to treat a specific disease entity: anteromedial osteoarthritis. Anteromedial disease is defined as the combination of full-thickness cartilage loss in the medial compartment, a correctible intra-articular varus deformity, and preserved lateral joint space seen with a valgus stress radiograph. By definition, these criteria are only present when the ligaments are functionally intact and the disease is confined to the anterior one third or

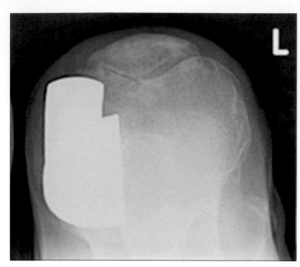

Figure 16-1 Skyline radiograph of left knee 2 years status post-Oxford Medial Mobile Bearing UKA. Full-thickness cartilage loss and grooving are present in the medial facet of the patellofemoral joint. The patient reports no pain and full range of motion (0–135°).

two thirds of the tibial plateau. When these criteria are present, other unnecessary contraindications such as age, weight, and the status of the patellofemoral articulation can be safely ignored without affecting the outcome of Oxford UKA.

In the United States, perhaps the biggest area of debate is the status of the patellofemoral joint. Concern over the status of this joint in an otherwise suitable candidate for UKA is also unwarranted. It is this author's opinion that the correction of varus deformity with preservation of the anterior cruciate ligament has a protective effect on the patellofemoral joint, even if there is significant arthritic disease present. Despite ignoring patellofemoral disease, the long-term results of Oxford UKA have not been affected by progression of patellofemoral disease or anterior knee pain (**Fig. 16–1**).

TECHNIQUE

The author employs the surgical technique described and taught by the implant designers. The operative leg is placed in a specialized leg holder to suspend the limb while allowing unrestricted flexion past 110°. After a minimally invasive exposure, the proximal medial tibial plateau is exposed. It is critical that no medial release be performed as the procedure is designed to correct the knee back to its predisease state, and any medial release will result in overcorrection. The proximal tibial resection is performed and the explanted plateau measured for tibial baseplate sizing. The flexion gap is then measured (this should be 4 mm or more). Using an intramedullary alignment guide, the femoral drill guide is positioned on the distal femur. Based upon preoperative templating, the

correct-size femoral instruments are selected. The femoral alignment guide places drill holes for the posterior resection and for use with balancing the flexion and extension gaps with the use of novel spigots and reamers. Once the posterior resection is made, the distal femur is reamed with a cylindrical reamer to convert the condyle from a polycentric shape to the spherical shape of the Oxford UKA implant. The flexion and extension gaps are then balanced to within less than 1 mm of each other, accuracy that is not currently achievable with TKA. This balancing is done through the use of spigots, which allow for reaming of the distal femur. After balancing the gaps, the final tibial preparation is done and trials are inserted. The final implant is a fully congruent spherical device that allows for considerably more malalignment than fixed-bearing designs. Additionally, the component is inset into the femur, and cannot articulate with the patellofemoral joint. Cementing technique is critical to prevent loosening, and the removal of impinging osteophytes is paramount to reduce the potential for dislocation and increased wear.

RESULTS

To date we have performed over 1500 medial Oxford UKAs. At 6 years, the cumulative survivorship is better than 98%. We reported on 318 medial compartmental UKAs in 268 patients using the aforementioned Oxford indications.[7] Isolated medial pain was present preoperatively in 211 knees (67%). Anterior knee pain was described in 20 knees (6%) and lateral pain described in 9 knees (3%). Posterior knee pain was described in 9 knees (3%), and in 65 knees (21%) the pain was described as global in nature. Follow-up averaged 8 months (range, 6 weeks to 28 months). There were six revisions in this group for an early survivorship of 98.1%. Survivorship in knees with preexisting radiographic signs of patellofemoral joint disease was no different than in those knees without patellofemoral disease. In fact, there was a trend toward a higher average Knee Society pain score in knees with preexisting patellofemoral joint disease ($p = .052$). The preoperative site of pain was not a significant predictor of survivorship or failure with the device, nor did preoperative location of pain influence postoperative knee scores.

DISCUSSION

Medial UKA is a conservative, truly minimally invasive procedure that can accurately correct malalignment, and restore an arthritic knee to its predisease functional status with normal kinematics and tremendous pain relief. An anatomic basis for establishing the indications and contraindications based upon the pathognomonic findings of anteromedial disease appears to provide reproducible good results in up to 30–35% of arthritic knees. The long-term published outcomes have been

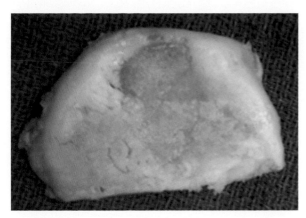

Figure 16-2 Clinical photograph of excised tibial bone. The pathognomonic findings of anteromedial osteoarthritis are demonstrated with eburnated bone in the anterior two thirds of the tibia. Note the intact bone and cartilage posteriorly. When these findings are present, the deformity is correctible and patellofemoral disease can safely be ignored.

good, with very little wear and, specifically, no failures from patellofemoral progression or anterior knee pain.

Kuipers et al. recently described factors associated with reduced early survivorship using the Oxford Phase 3 device.[8] They noted that young age (<60 years) was the only variable associated with early revision, but that preoperative patellofemoral arthritis was not associated with decreased implant survivorship and the status of the patellofemoral joint should not be considered as an indication or contraindication when using this device. Beard et al. studied a consecutive series of 100 Oxford UKAs, specifically evaluating the role of preoperative anterior knee pain and patellofemoral arthritis on the outcomes.[9] More than half the patients reported anterior knee pain preoperatively and yet no patients were revised at 2 years for patellofemoral pain or progression. Furthermore, 54% of

patients had degenerative changes in the patellofemoral joint and, again, no patient failed from progression. Similar to our findings, the preoperative status of the patellofemoral joint did not affect the outcomes, unless bone-on-bone lateral facet disease was present with grooving and subluxation. In these cases, Beard et al. reported lower knee scores in this subset of patients. This severe lateral patellofemoral disease, while not associated with failure, did have a negative effect on outcomes, and its presence should be seen as a relative contraindication to medial UKA.

It appears that the mobile bearing, with its inset femoral component, may be more tolerant to patellofemoral disease than a polyradial/polycentric femoral component used in fixed-bearing UKA. Berger et al. described a rapid increase in second-decade patellofemoral symptoms with a fixed-bearing UKA design. At 10 years only 1.6% of patients were thought to have anterior knee pain, and this rose to 10% at 15 years.[10] At 15 years, survivorship of this fixed-bearing design began to decline, predominantly due to patellofemoral progression, dropping from 98% at 10 years to 95.7% at 15 years.[10] This is remarkably different than the second-decade survivorship seen with the medial mobile-bearing device. The Oxford group followed 824 consecutive UKAs performed between 1998 and 2005. Full-thickness cartilage loss was observed in the trochlea in 13% of knees and full-thickness loss in any area of the patellofemoral joint was seen in 16%. The severity of patellofemoral disease did not influence outcome in this series.[11] It is hoped that the early success in the United States will mirror the excellent long-term results seen in other series. At 6 years, survivorship of better than 98%, despite ignoring the status of the patellofemoral joint, is being reported. The data clearly demonstrate that not only should anterior knee pain and patellofemoral disease be ignored, but that its presence preoperatively has no effect on outcome or failure (**Fig. 16–2**).

REFERENCES

1. Kendrick BJ, Longino D, Pandit H, et al. Polyethylene wear in Oxford unicompartmental knee replacement: a retrieval study of 47 bearings. J Bone Joint Surg [Br] 2010;92:367-373.
2. Price AJ, Short A, Kellett C, et al. Ten-year in vivo wear measurement of a fully congruent mobile bearing unicompartmental knee arthroplasty. J Bone Joint Surg [Br] 2005;87:1493-1497.
3. Price AJ, Waite JC, Svard U. Long-term clinical results of the medial Oxford unicompartmental knee arthroplasty. Clin Orthop Relat Res 2005;(435):171-180.
4. Kozinn SC, Scott R. Unicondylar knee arthroplasty. J Bone Joint Surg [Am] 1989;71:145-150.
5. Ritter MA, Faris PM, Thong AE, et al. Intra-operative findings of varus osteoarthritis of the knee: an analysis of pre-operative alignment in potential candidates for unicompartmental arthroplasty. J Bone Joint Surg [Am] 2004;86:43-47.
6. Laskin RS. Unicompartmental knee replacement: some unanswered questions. Clin Orthop Relat Res 2001;(392):267-271.
7. Berend KR, Lombardi AV Jr, Adams JB. Obesity, young age, patellofemoral disease, and anterior knee pain: identifying the

unicondylar arthroplasty patient in the United States. Orthopedics 2007;30(Suppl 5):19-23.
8. Kuipers BM, Kollen BJ, Bots PC, et al. Factors associated with reduced early survival in the Oxford phase III medial unicompartmental knee replacement. Knee 2010;17:48-52.
9. Beard DJ, Pandit H, Gill HS, et al. The influence of the presence and severity of pre-existing patellofemoral degenerative changes on the outcome of the Oxford medial unicompartmental knee replacement. J Bone Joint Surg [Br] 2007;89:1597-1601.
10. Berger RA, Meneghini RM, Sheinkop MB, et al. The progression of patellofemoral arthritis after medial unicompartmental replacement: results at 11 to 15 years. Clin Orthop Relat Res 2004;(428):92-99.
11. Beard DJ, Pandit H, Ostlere S, et al. Pre-operative clinical and radiological assessment of the patellofemoral joint in unicompartmental knee replacement and its influence on outcome. J Bone Joint Surg [Br] 2007;89:1602-1607.

CHAPTER 17

Minimally Invasive Surgery: Medial Fixed-Bearing Onlay Unicompartmental Knee Arthroplasty

William Macaulay and Amrit Goyal

KEY POINTS

- Select patients properly (carefully consider Kozinn and Scott criteria).
- Avoid overcorrection (resect enough tibial bone and use a thin tibial insert).
- Properly size and rotate both components.
- Do not undersize the tibia: the tibial component spans the tibial spine and medial cortex of the tibia (no overhang).
- Balance the flexion-extension gap.

INTRODUCTION

Unicompartmental knee arthroplasty (UKA) has gained popularity in the past decade. The concept of unicondylar knee replacement was introduced in the 1970s by Marmor. He reported pain relief in 86.6% of his patients at an average of 11 years of follow-up with this prosthesis.[1] However, Insall and Aglietti[2] and Laskin[3] reported high failure rates of 26% and 20%, respectively, especially with medial compartment arthroplasty. Most of the failures in subsequent reviews have been attributed to inappropriate patient selection, technical errors, and poor implant design.[1] O'Rourke et al.[4] recently reported a survivorship of 96% at 5 years and 84% at 20 years of follow-up with the Marmor prosthesis. Over the years, refinement in the surgical technique and improved implant designs and instrumentation have led to the resurgence of interest in UKA. The purported advantages of UKA over proximal tibial osteotomy are better pain relief, quicker return to function, fewer complications, and better long-term results. Furthermore, compared to a total knee arthroplasty (TKA), UKA has a more physiologic gait and better range of motion as the cruciate ligaments, contralateral menisci, and other structures are preserved.[5] Also, the recovery is faster[6] and it can be easily revised to a TKA with minimum morbidity if required for failure.

Since 2002, the senior author has been using a reproducible and accurate minimally invasive surgical technique (modified slightly from that described by Gesell and Tria[7]), with a cemented modular fixed-bearing Miller-Galante (MG) implant (Zimmer, Warsaw, IN), which is described in detail in this chapter. Naudie et al.[8] reported a 94% survivorship at 5 years and 90% at 10 years with the MG prosthesis. Argenson et al.[9] also found survivorship of 97% at 5.5 years of follow-up with the same implant. Berger et al.[10,11] reported Jorge Galante's MG survivorship of 98% at 10 years and 95.7% at 13 years of follow-up. Minimally invasive surgery (MIS) has evolved over the years from more traditional UKA with the use of better instrumentation and modified surgical technique. MIS philosophy does not mean a small skin incision but aims at bone-sparing technique and preservation of all possible soft tissues. Also, during arthrotomy and surgery the quadriceps tendon is not incised and the patella is not averted, thereby preserving the integrity of the quadriceps mechanism.[12] MIS allows for a faster, less painful recovery, shorter hospital stay, and better cosmesis. Attempts to perform MIS surgery with a careless surgical technique can lead to component malposition, malalignment, and significant soft tissue damage. Coon[12] found that short-term results of MIS UKA were comparable to that of traditional UKA. Pandit et al.[6] also found survival rates of 97.3% at 7 years with MIS technique. Since failures if they occur are more common early on, Pandit et al. believed that results of MIS should be comparable to the traditional UKA in the long term.

PREOPERATIVE EVALUATION

One of the most important requirements for a successful outcome of UKA is patient selection. Kozinn and Scott[13] summarized their patient selection criteria in their UKA review paper from 1989. Those that we consider most important are as follows.

The ideal candidate for unicondylar knee arthroplasty is a low-demand, thin patient (>55 years of age) with isolated medial unicompartmental disease. The range of motion of the knee joint should be greater than 90° and a flexion contracture, if present, should be 5° or less. The valgus deformity should be less than 15°, and varus less than 10° should be passively correctable to neutral. There should be no rest pain or evidence of inflammatory arthropathy. There should not be diffuse pain or significant involvement of other knee compartments. The lateral compartment should have full-thickness joint space on the anteroposterior radiograph and also well-preserved meniscus and articular cartilage. Patellofemoral pain is a relative contraindication. The knee should be stable without any insufficiency of the cruciate or collateral ligaments. Medial or lateral subluxation or posterior tibial bone loss is suggestive of crucial ligament insufficiency. Patients with osteonecrosis of a single femoral condyle should not have extensive metaphyseal-diaphyseal involvement. Ideally the patient should be able to pinpoint the medial compartment as the source of pain, which worsens significantly with weight bearing (the so-called one-finger test).[14]

A thorough history, physical examination, and radiographic examination are done for all patients. Radiographic examination is of the utmost importance for medial UKA planning. The patient should have anteroposterior standing weight-bearing radiographs of the knee in extension and 45° of flexion (the so-called tunnel view) on a large film to judge the mechanical alignment. There should be no tibiofemoral subluxation or translocation, which denotes involvement of the contralateral compartment. A skyline view should be done to assess the patellofemoral compartment. The lateral view is helpful to determine the posterior tibial slope, look for any posterior femoral osteophyte that might impinge in deep flexion, and determine if the tibial wear pattern is excessively posteromedial (which could connote anterior cruciate ligament [ACL] insufficiency). A notch view or tunnel view (anteroposterior view with flexed knee) also helps in evaluation of cartilage thinning, which is much more impressive in flexion. Magnetic resonance imaging is required in some cases of osteonecrosis to evaluate the extent of involvement. It may also help in evaluating the other compartments' and the cartilage thickness.

SURGICAL TECHNIQUE FOR MEDIAL FIXED-BEARING ONLAY UKA

Positioning and Draping

We prefer that UKA patients undergo regional anesthesia unless contraindicated. The anesthesia team should be aware of the fact that the patient will be required to walk and start with the physical therapy soon after completion of surgery. Care is taken not to give drugs that might overly sedate patients for many hours. Patient preparation is done as per standard protocols. The patient is positioned supine on the operating table. The tourniquet is placed high up on the thigh so flexion contracture can be more easily seen, and an impervious drape is applied to prevent wetness below the tourniquet that could damage the skin. The patient operative site shaving is done just before prepping with a safety razor. A prescrub with chlorhexidine soap and water is done and the skin is prepped with tinted chlorhexidine solution. The skin of the extremity is draped with iodine-impregnated plastic draping to make the operative field impervious and decrease skin flora. Also, the MIS approach requires continuous repositioning of the knee to different degrees of flexion to optimize visualization, so care is taken to drape the extremity free with slackness in the drapes. We prefer a bump positioned at 90° of flexion, but a leg holder can be equally effective.

Approach

The skin incision (**Fig. 17–1**) is slightly medial to the midline, extending from the superior edge of the patella to the medial aspect of the tibial tubercle. The incision is approximately 10 cm long depending on patient size and adipose tissue, and can be extended to avoid applying too much tension to skin during retraction. A "mobile window" is created by releasing adipose tissue from the retinaculum approximately 2 cm circumferentially around the incision. A medial parapatellar arthrotomy (**Fig. 17–2**) is performed from a level 1 fingerbreadth above the superior pole of patella to a point approximately 15 mm distally to the tibial joint line. The arthrotomy does not damage the vastus medialis muscle. Also, the technique does not require eversion or dislocation of the patella, thus preserving the suprapatellar pouch. This may reduce postoperative pain and allow faster quadriceps control, since disruption of the extensor mechanism is minimal.

The medial compartment is exposed by excising a small portion of the fat pad in the area just medial and posterior to

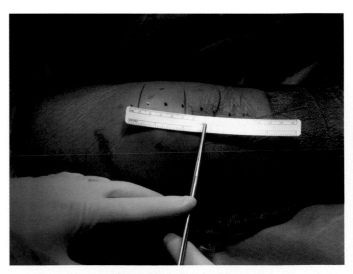

Figure 17-1 Skin incision.

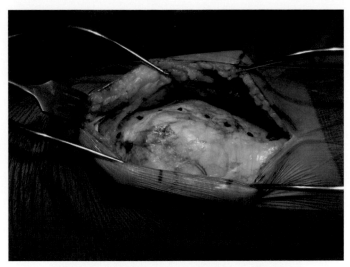

Figure 17-2 Medial parapatellar arthrotomy.

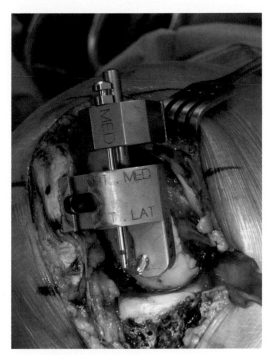

Figure 17-3 The distal femoral intramedullary valgus cutting guide.

the patellar tendon. All the lateral compartment structures and the cruciate ligaments are protected during the exposure. The patellofemoral compartment (easily visible), the lateral compartment (obstructed view), and the ACL are inspected. If significant arthritis is seen, conversion to TKA should be done, which should always be ready as a backup plan. The medial release is limited to a minimal medial subperiosteal release (enough to perform the tibial resection only). In varus knees that are not 100% correctable to neutral by a gentle valgus stress applied at 20° of flexion, the deep medial collateral ligament may be released if required to correct the alignment slightly (no more than 5°). Avoiding overcorrection of the knee alignment is essential to prevent loading of the opposite compartment, and therefore we prefer to undercorrect to about 2°. Any osteophytes from the intercondylar notch are removed to prevent impingement on the ACL.

Femoral Preparation

We use the intramedullary technique for femoral preparation. The site for inserting the intramedullary guide is 1 cm anterior to the origin of the posterior cruciate ligament and just anterior to the femoral intercondylar notch. With the knee flexed approximately 30°, a starting point is made with the punch. An 8-mm drill is used to make the path for the femoral intramedullary guide. The femoral canal is suctioned to remove the fat to decrease the chances of fat embolism. A fringe benefit of this hole is that it can be used for a patellar retractor later and for the entire case. The medial distal femoral resection guide (**Fig. 17–3**), which is attached to an intramedullary rod, is placed according to the side being operated. A shorter rod is used if the patient has altered femoral anatomy or a long-stemmed hip prosthesis. The guide is placed flush with the femoral condyle (which helps in making sure that

proper thickness of bone is resected) and fixed in place if needed. The guide is stabilized with holding pins and the distal cutting adjustable valgus guide placed. The valgus angle is determined by evaluating the mechanical on preoperative standing radiographs. This usually corresponds to a 4° valgus cut on the distal femur. The distal femoral resection is deep enough only to match the depth of the femoral prosthesis. Medial osteophytes can be removed at this stage. Also, the surface may be rasped to remove any bony prominences to make it completely flat, which is important for subsequent jig placement.

Next, the intramedullary patellar retractor (**Fig. 17–4**) is inserted (upon removal of the medial distal femoral resection guide), which allows for better exposure and prevention of patellar damage during the procedure. The femoral finishing guide (**Fig. 17–5**) is applied next to the distal femoral cut surface. Sizing and correct placement of this guide is one of the most crucial steps of the surgery. The size of the femoral component should be such that it leaves 1–2 mm of exposed subchondral bone on the anteromedial edge of the cut surface. The implant should be big enough to cover almost all of the condyle, but small enough to prevent patellar impingement. The guide rests on the posterior condyle and should be flush against the bone, or the accuracy of the cuts and subsequent component placement may be compromised. The femoral guide, properly rotated, is stabilized with holding pins and the anterior and posterior femoral posts are drilled and then

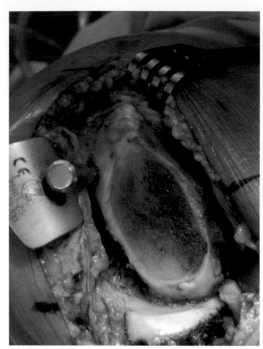

Figure 17-4 Intramedullary patellar retractor is a key retractor for exposure.

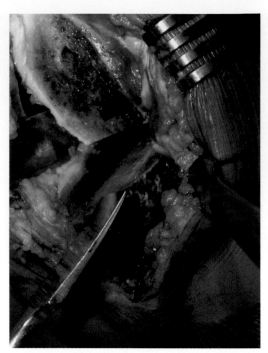

Figure 17-6 Curved osteotome used to remove any posterior femoral osteophytes.

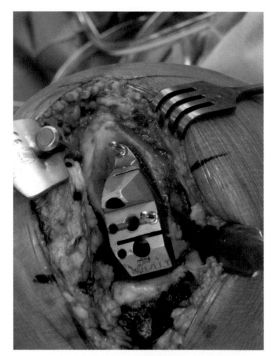

Figure 17-5 Sizing and correct placement of the femoral finishing guide.

surfaces must be smoothed out of any bony irregularities. The femoral guide should be placed parallel to the long axis of the tibia at 90° of flexion and full extension. It is important to align the femoral component so as to later avoid edge loading on the polyethylene insert. The femoral component is generally smaller than the femoral condyle and, if in between sizes, the smaller of the two should be chosen. Attention is now paid to the tibial side.

Tibial Preparation

The tibial preparation is done using an extramedullary guide. Intramedullary instrumentation requires patellar eversion and wider exposure, which is difficult with MIS technique. The distal portion of the tibial alignment rod is positioned at the center of the ankle mortise (over the anterior tibial tendon) and held with the spring. The longitudinal axis of the rod is aligned parallel to the long axis of the tibia. Proximally the guide is fixed with the rod centered at the tibial spine. Care should be taken while draping to avoid heavy drapes around the ankle to help in alignment for the tibial cut. The posterior slope of the tibial cut is set to match the patient's posterior tibial slope.[15] A 2-mm depth gauge is used to take the tibial cut from the deepest defect in the tibia. By applying it a little loose (with regard to knob tightness), a 3- or 4-mm resection can be taken to avoid overstuffing the medial compartment. The tibial resection guide (**Fig. 17–7**) is fixed with guide pins and all of the knobs are tightened once the position has been confirmed. A retractor is placed medially to protect the medial

chamfer and posterior condylar cuts made. An anterior femoral holding peg may be used to stabilize the guide while drilling the posterior post. After the cuts are made, posterior osteophytes are removed with a curved osteotome (**Fig. 17–6**) and curette to prevent impingement in deep flexion. The

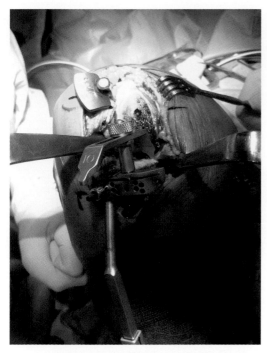

Figure 17-7 MIS tibial cutting jig.

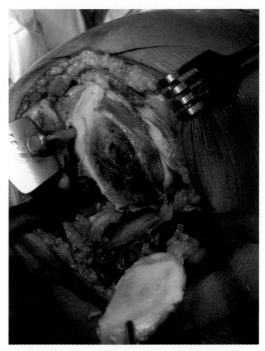

Figure 17-8 Minimal tibial resection and the cut tibial surface.

collateral ligament and another in the intercondylar notch to protect the lateral structures. The front-to-back conservative vertical cut into the tibial spine is made with a reciprocating saw (preserving the attachment of the ACL) on the tibial surface. At the same time the cut is made as close to the ACL attachment as possible to get a broad tibial cortical support for the tibial baseplate. Also, care is taken to make the cut in proper rotation without damaging the posterior cruciate ligament. It is also critically important to avoid any anterior or posterior tibial bony cortical extension of the vertical cut and to avoid undercutting of the tibial spine.

After the cut, the tibial resected surface (shaped like a "half-lollipop") is removed (**Fig. 17–8**). Any irregularities of the tibia are smoothened with a rasp (**Fig. 17–9**). The osteophytes tenting the medial collateral ligament are removed, and removal of the medial meniscus may be easiest at this stage. The tibia sizer is used to determine the best tibial size for covering the tibial surface in both anteroposterior and mediolateral dimensions (**Fig. 17–10**). Also, the resected tibial surface can be used for estimating the size of the tibial baseplate. The largest possible tibial size is chosen, making sure that there is minimal to no overhang and the implant rests on strong cortical bone. An undersized tibial component has higher chances of subsidence, especially if the tibial resection is deeper than anticipated. A quarter-inch osteotome is used to make a starting slot for the central fin of the tibial baseplate (**Fig. 17–11**). The trial tray is then impacted into place and secured. The tibial post holes are prepared with the tibial peg drill to complete the tibial preparation.

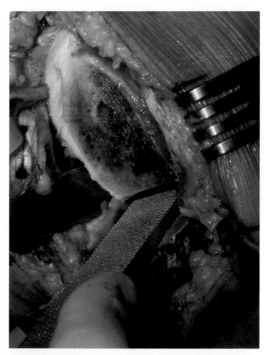

Figure 17-9 Rasping the cut surface to remove any bony irregularities.

Trial Reduction

The provisional femoral component is put in with the help of a T-handle inserter with the leg in deep flexion and patellar retractor in place. Trial reduction is performed with the tibial provisional insert that will get the patient to about 2–3° of

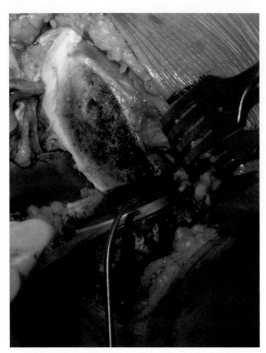

Figure 17-10 Sizing of the tibial tray with help of a curved rake on the posterior border of the tibia.

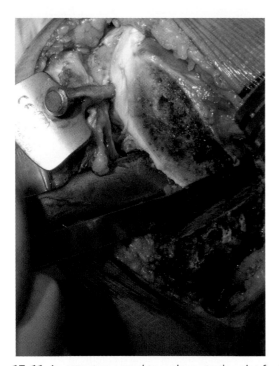

Figure 17-11 An osteotome used to make a starting slot for the central fin of the tibial baseplate.

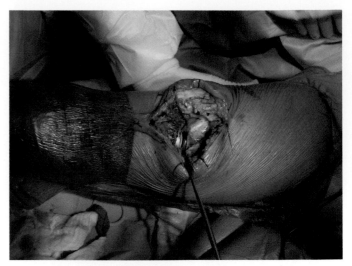

Figure 17-12 Trial components in extension to check alignment and balance.

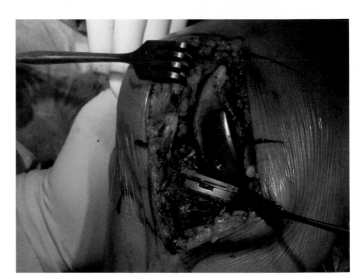

Figure 17-13 Trial components in flexion to check the flexion gap.

varus (usually an 8-mm insert when a small tibial resection has been made), and the knee is checked for the range of motion and ligament balance through the range of motion (**Figs. 17–12 and 17–13**). This can be checked with a plastic tongue depressor that is 2 mm thick on one side and 3 mm thick on the other. The 2-mm end should fit between the femoral component and tibial insert easily at 0° and 90° of flexion, while the 3-mm side is very tight. Ideally there should be 2 mm of laxity in 90° of flexion and in full extension. The femoral component should be centered over the tibial component in flexion and extension and does not follow the anatomic femoral condyle orientation. If required, it should be reoriented.

Determination of alignment in UKA differs from that of TKA. In UKA, thickness of the polyethylene insert controls alignment, whereas in TKA alignment is determined by cuts. For a tight flexion and extension gap, decreasing the size of the polyethylene insert or lowering the tibial cut can help in balancing the knee. For a tight extension gap and normal flexion balance, the tibial cut may be redone by decreasing the posterior slope slightly. This has the effect of increasing the extension gap while not changing the flexion gap so the two will balance. Therefore, any correction of flexion contractures or a tight extension gap should be corrected by modifying the tibial side. Similarly, excessive flexion gap tightness causes the tibial prosthesis to lift up anteriorly as the femoral component rolls posteriorly. It can limit postoperative flexion and also subject the polyethylene articular insert to excessive loading. This can be corrected either by using a smaller polyethylene articular insert or slightly increasing the posterior slope of the tibial resection. The patellar tracking should be checked, making sure that the femoral component does not encroach anywhere close to the patella.

Final Components and Cementing

The trial components are removed and the knee joint is irrigated with pulse lavage to remove all the bony debris and blood clots. The raw bony surfaces are dried with sponges. If required, drill holes are made in the sclerotic tibial or femoral surface to achieve a better cement-bone bonding. The tibial component is cemented first. We prefer a type of cement that is viscous and workable immediately upon mixing. The cement is applied more on the anterior surface than the posterior, and the posterior portion of the tibial component is placed to engage the tibia prior to the anterior portion of the tibial component contacting the tibia so as to encourage cement to leave the interface anteriorly. A sterile gauze sponge can be placed behind the tibia to aid in removal of any posterior excess cement, but care must be taken not to incarcerate the gauze within the interface. The tibial baseplate is then impacted with the help of a tibial impactor to fully seat the implant on the tibial cut surface. The posteriorly placed gauze is removed at this point and a curved nerve root retractor is used to remove cement from the posterior aspect of the tibia if there is any. The femoral component is then inserted in deep flexion with the patella retractor in place. The leg is then brought into slight midflexion to clear the patella and then repositioned again in deep flexion to complete the femoral component insertion. A trial polyethylene insert is put in and the leg straightened, allowing the cement to harden. The alignment is checked again to verify that it is not overcorrected. At the end of the cementing, the trial insert is removed and all the extra cement is meticulously removed from the joint despite the limited exposure afforded by this technique. The original polyethylene articular insert is finally put in (**Figs. 17–14 and 17–15**). The joint is thoroughly lavaged to remove any bony debris and loose bodies. The incision is closed in three layers (**Figs. 17–16 and 17–17**). A sterile dressing is applied and the limb bandaged loosely with an Ace bandage as the tourniquet is taken down.

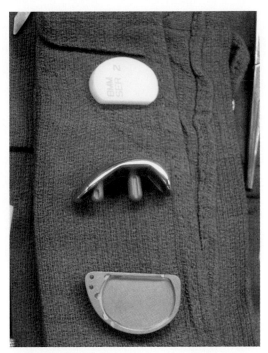

Figure 17-14 The final components ready for implantation.

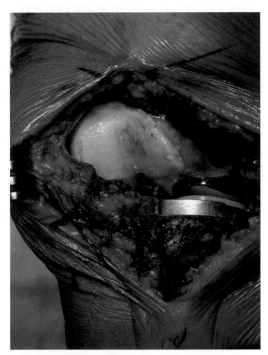

Figure 17-15 Cemented final components.

POSTSURGICAL CARE AND FOLLOW-UP

The patient is transported to the recovery room, where the spinal anesthetic wears off, but a femoral block, if employed, is useful in avoiding more than half of the pain. The patient is given adequate preemptive analgesia so that the pain does not rise to a level that will prevent mobilization. The patient

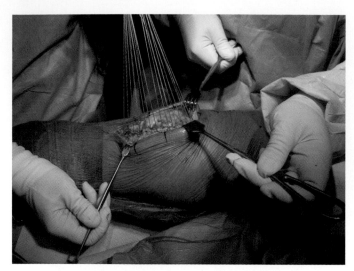

Figure 17-16 Closure of arthrotomy.

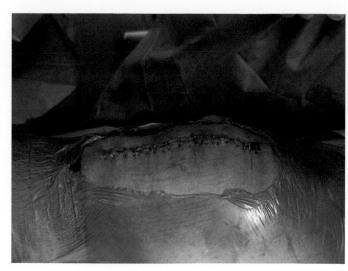

Figure 17-17 Skin closed with staples.

generally undergoes a multimodal regimen including aspirin and pneumatic compression for venous thromboembolic prophylaxis. The patients may be discharged the same day or admitted for a day or two until the time they are comfortable with walking and balance. The recovery observed is much faster compared to that with a total knee replacement. Also, the subjective feeling of the patient is more like that of a normal knee. A physical therapist at home helps the patients with range-of-motion and strengthening exercises. The patient is seen at 4 weeks and 3 months in the office and evaluated clinically and radiographically.

SUMMARY

Minimally invasive medial unicondylar knee arthroplasty with this technique preserves bone stock and allows accurate component positioning. Proper preoperative selection of patients, meticulous surgical execution, and attention to detail make the operation reproducible and are necessary for a successful clinical outcome.

REFERENCES

1. Marmor L. Unicompartmental knee arthroplasty: ten- to 13-year follow-up study. Clin Orthop Relat Res 1988;(226):14-20.
2. Insall JN, Aglietti P. A five to seven-year follow-up of unicondylar arthroplasty. J Bone Joint Surg [Am] 1980;62:1329-1337.
3. Laskin RS. Unicompartmental tibiofemoral resurfacing arthroplasty. J Bone Joint Surg [Am] 1978;60:182-185.
4. O'Rourke MR, Gardner JJ, Callaghan JJ, et al. The John Insall Award. Unicompartmental knee replacement: a minimum twenty-one-year follow-up, end-result study. Clin Orthop Relat Res 2005;(440):27-37.
5. Andriacchi TP, Galante JO, Fermier RW. The influence of total knee replacement design on walking and stair-climbing. J Bone Joint Surg [Am] 1982;64:1328-1335.
6. Pandit H, Jenkins C, Barker K, et al. The Oxford medial unicompartmental knee replacement using a minimally-invasive approach. J Bone Joint Surg [Br] 2006;88:54-60.
7. Gesell MW, Tria AJ Jr. MIS unicondylar knee arthroplasty: surgical approach and early results. Clin Orthop Relat Res 2004;(428):53-60.
8. Naudie D, Guerin J, Parker DA, et al. Medial unicompartmental knee arthroplasty with the Miller-Galante prosthesis. J Bone Joint Surg [Am] 2004;86:1931-1935.
9. Argenson JA, Chevrol-Benkeddache Y, Aubaniac JM. Modern unicompartmental knee arthroplasty with cement: a three to ten year follow-up study. J Bone Joint Surg [Am] 2002;84:2235-2239.
10. Berger RA, Nedeff DD, Barden RM, et al. Unicompartmental knee arthroplasty: clinical experience at 6- to 10-year followup. Clin Orthop Relat Res 1999;(367):50-60.
11. Berger RA, Meneghini RM, Jacobs JJ, et al. Results of unicompartmental knee arthroplasty at a minimum of ten years of follow-up. J Bone Joint Surg [Am] 2005;87:999-1006.
12. Coon TM. Minimally invasive unicompartmental knee arthroplasty using the quad-sparing instrumentation. Operative Techniques Orthop 2006;16:195-206.
13. Kozinn SC, Scott R. Unicondylar knee arthroplasty. J Bone Joint Surg [Am] 1989;71:145-150.
14. Bert JM. Unicompartmental knee replacement. Orthop Clin North Am 2005;36:513-522.
15. Hernigou P, Deschamps G. Posterior slope of the tibial implant and the outcome of unicompartmental knee arthroplasty. J Bone Joint Surg [Am] 2004;86:506-511.

SECTION 4
Outcomes

CHAPTER **18**

Mobile-Bearing Uni: Long-Term Outcomes

Nicholas Bottomley, Benjamin Kendrick, Hemant Pandit, Christopher Dodd, David Murray, and Andrew Price

KEY POINTS

- The fully mobile meniscal bearing is a design against wear.
- Indications for surgery, implantation technique, and surgical expertise are all relevant to both midterm and long-term outcome.
- Outcome studies show survivorship of up to 92% at 20 years.
- Relatively few failures occur in the second decade.

INTRODUCTION: PROSTHESIS DESIGN

The mobile-bearing unicondylar knee arthroplasty design comprises a spherical metal component and a flat tibial baseplate with a fully congruent mobile polyethylene bearing. The aim of the device when first conceived in 1976 was to protect against polyethylene wear and component failure while retaining a high range of motion. The principles of the design were to provide an implant constrained only by the restored natural tensions of the ligaments and muscles. A fully congruent bearing allowing maximal contact area between the prosthesis and bearing reduces polyethylene wear and, to enable this congruity without constraining the prosthesis, the bearing is fully mobile. The upper surface of the mobile meniscal polyethylene bearing is spherically concave, matching the spherical surface of the prosthetic femur. The undersurface of the meniscal bearing is flat, lying on the tibial baseplate. This configuration of a spherical femur, flat tibia, and fully unconstrained and mobile meniscal bearing enables physiologic tension to be maintained in the retained anterior cruciate and medial collateral ligaments over the entire range of knee flexion. The meniscal bearing allows sliding and rolling with mainly a compressive stress applied to the underlying bone, decreasing shear stress at the implant-bone interface, which is an important factor in component loosening.

The implant most commonly used is the Oxford unicompartmental knee replacement.[1] This design was originally used

as a bicompartmental device but was first used as a unicompartmental device in 1982 (Phase 1). Since then two further design phases have been introduced, retaining the design features while improving the instrumentation and the method of implantation. In Phase 1 the femoral surface was prepared with cutting blocks to remove angular cuts of bone to fit the nonarticular surface of the femoral component. However, this did not allow accurate balance of the flexion-extension gap at implantation, and the Phase 2 prosthesis was introduced in 1987 and sought to improve this. The femoral component was changed to a spherically concave inner surface and the femoral bone surface was prepared with a mill rotating around a spigot. Incremental 1-mm milling of the distal femoral surface allows careful balancing of the knee ligaments throughout flexion (**Fig. 18–1**). The Phase 3 design, introduced in 1998, provided new instruments and an increased range of components to facilitate the implantation through a short incision. The aim was to gain the short-term advantages associated with this less invasive incision[2] while maintaining the longer term survival, by maintaining the original design features of the fully congruent articulation (**Fig. 18–2**). Although the Oxford mobile-bearing unicompartmental knee was the first of its kind, there are several other mobile-bearing knees based on a similar philosophy. The AMC knee (Uniglide) utilizes a fully mobile bearing restoring the natural tension within the knee; however, there is a difference in the shape of the femoral component. The radius of the femoral component is constant up to 45° of flexion but decreases toward the posterior portion of the condyle.

We have reviewed the long-term results of the prostheses mentioned above. There is substantial literature regarding the Oxford Knee and more limited literature about the other prosthesis. Long-term outcome is an important factor since impressive early results of an implant may dramatically change with longer term follow-up. For example, in the PCA fixed-bearing unicompartmental prosthesis, 90% of patients were reported as having a satisfactory functional result at 2 years,[3] yet the cumulative survival at 3.7 years was only 77%.[4] Our aim is to review the long-term results, at 10 years and greater, of mobile-bearing unicompartmental replacements.

MEASURING OUTCOME: EXPLANATION OF STUDY TYPES

Assessing Survivorship

The measurement of success in arthroplasty surgery is important to provide information not only for the surgeon selecting the type of surgery and individual prosthesis to use but also when counseling patients regarding expected outcome from an intervention. The most commonly used measure of success is the survival of the implant (time to revision), but it is also

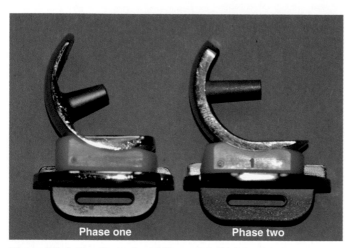

Figure 18-1 The Phase 1 and Phase 2 Oxford Partial Knee Replacement, showing the progression from distal femoral cuts in the Phase 1 to spherical distal femoral surface in Phase 2.

important to assess the functional outcome of the arthroplasty in surviving patients, since this provides more complete information regarding the success of the patients' treatment than pure survival analysis.[5] Modern survival analysis will define a failure end point and provide an assessment of how many patients failed and how long after the operation this failure occurred. It is therefore important to understand the exact nature of the defined end point in each study as some authors use removal of the implants as the failure end point, whereas others use further surgery of any type. The difference between the two end points may affect the reported survival. Survival analysis may be performed using the life table method or Kaplan-Meier method. Whichever is employed, there are a number of features that must be understood about the reported data. Survival figures are cumulative, which allows a prediction of the expected failure rate in the long term, reducing the need for large numbers of prostheses to have reached the long-term follow-up point. However, the number at risk at each time point must be known since, if this number reduces to less than 15, it becomes difficult to interpret the data. Loss to follow-up is also important, and studies should present worst- and best-case scenarios.

Study Types

Results on mobile-bearing unicompartmental replacements are available from three main sources. The first of these are cohort studies, second prospective trials, and third from the results of arthroplasty registers.

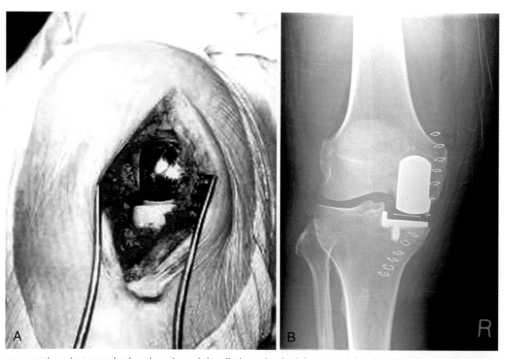

Figure 18-2 (A) Intraoperative photograph showing the minimally invasive incision possible with the Phase 3 Oxford Partial Knee Replacement. **(B)** Postoperative radiograph of the Phase 3 Oxford Partial Knee Replacement. Note the skin clips in place to show the incision.

Cohort Studies

Cohort studies are usually based around the observed results of cases treated by a single or small group of surgeons. Their advantage is that the groups of patients are followed in detail and with often near-complete follow-up. However, the total number of patients is often small from noncontinuous series with exclusions, and results may be significantly affected by individual preoperative indications, intraoperative technique, and postoperative indications for revision. Additionally, these studies are open to bias as they are often reported by the designer or enthusiasts, which may not be representative of the implant in general orthopaedic practice. Despite this, they do offer important information as to the success or failure of the intervention.

Prospective Trials

Prospective randomized controlled trials of a prosthesis or surgical technique allow many of the flaws of cohort studies outlined above to be overcome. They are, however, much less common, which is a reflection of the cost and complexity of organization and execution of such studies. When available, they provide better quality data than cohort studies. Some studies of this type are available for interpretation, although there is no published cumulative revision rate at 10 years from a randomized controlled trial.

Joint Registers

The prime function of registers is to assess the success of treatment in large, often nationwide, population-based cohorts. They provide data that represent clinical practice without the inherent bias in cohort studies and can be used to compare outcome of implant designs. For this reason, registers have always taken "revision" as the marker of failure and the "cumulative revision rate" as the comparator between implants. While revision is an event that will invariably bring a patient back into contact with a surgeon and is therefore easily measured, there are some difficulties with the interpretation of the revision rates. Unfortunately, arthroplasty registers collect few data and exert no control over patient selection, surgical expertise, and indication for revision. The term *surgical routine* was defined by Robertsson et al.[6] in 2001 to describe these factors, and it was shown that the revision rate in centers that performed fewer than 23 unicompartmental knee arthroplasties (UKAs) annually had a risk of revision 1.63 times higher than centers with higher volumes of work. Over the last 10 years, the New Zealand Joint Registry has introduced patient-reported outcome data (PROMS) into the joint register. This allows additional information to be gained regarding true clinical outcome and patients' functional score at the time of revision surgery, which offers an improved assessment of the true success of arthroplasty. Analysis of these data shows that, in every category of clinical outcome, a UKA is between four and six times as likely to be revised as a total knee arthroplasty (TKA). This highlights the problem of using registry data to compare between UKA and TKA, whereas a comparison between UKA designs is more relevant.

What Is Long-Term Outcome?

Ideally long-term outcome would reflect the results and outcome of all patients for their entire lifespan—in other words, when the patient is either dead or revised. There are currently no such studies on UKA; therefore, the next best assessment is a prediction of the "real" long-term outcome, and this is best achieved by survivorship analyses. Ten-year survivorship analysis has always been the gold standard for assessment of a prosthesis. For example, in the United Kingdom there is a 10-year benchmark of no more than 10% failure rate at 10 years.[7] The next step toward better understanding of long-term outcome is to assess 20-year survivorship data. In truth, there are only a few studies available that allow assessment in the second decade; there are many more studies that report follow-up at less than 10 years, and these shorter term survivorship analyses can still provide valuable information that may guide surgical practice.

Lessons Learned from Midterm Assessment

There have been published series with midterm results that have then not reported results at long term. However, there are still valuable lessons that can be learned from these midterm results that are relevant to long-term outcome, and we highlight these here. Kort et al.[8] assessed 130 patients with Phase 3 Oxford UKAs in an eight-surgeon series, with all surgeons performing less than 10 procedures per year. The overall survival is reported at 89%, with a range of follow-up of 2–7 years, but with no indication of how this survival figure was reached. Interestingly, of the 17 failures, they attribute 13 to human error of component malalignment and two further cases of trauma and infection. Thirty-seven patients had preoperative lateral compartment joint space narrowing and one patient had lateral joint space obliteration preoperatively. As a result, this center now closely adheres to the prosthesis guidelines and focuses all the UKAs to be performed by two of their surgeons. This study demonstrates that the indications for surgery, implantation technique, and surgical expertise are all relevant to midterm and therefore long-term outcome. Similarly, in a study of 437 patients with Phase 3 implants, Kuipers et al.[9] reported a cumulative survival of 84.7% (confidence interval [CI], 80.1–89.3%) at 5 years (mean, 2.6 years), with 101 still at risk. Each surgeon in the study performed an average of 8 UKAs per year, and, interestingly, the authors noted that almost a quarter of their revisions were for continuing unexplained pain with no evidence of prosthesis malfunction and no mention as to whether the function improved post-revision. The authors concede these may have been unnecessary revisions. These results reinforce that patient selection and surgical routine are important determinants of early to midterm outcome and therefore must influence long-term outcome. Specifically, integrity of the anterior cruciate ligament (ACL) and preservation of the lateral compartment are important, as outlined in the published guidelines for UKA.[1,10] When the indications are followed, the results can be excellent, as demonstrated by Pandit et al.,[11] who assessed 688 patients with 96.5 cases at risk at 5 years and a cumulative survival rate of 97.3%.

The only comparisons of fixed versus mobile bearings unfortunately do not have long-term follow-up. Confalonieri et al.[12] described a cohort of 40 consecutive patients randomly assigned to a fixed-bearing knee (Allegretto) or a mobile-bearing knee (AMC). There was no statistical difference in the outcome between the two groups, although one of the fixed bearings was revised while none of the mobile bearings were revised and none of the bearings had dislocated. Gleeson et al.[13] randomized 47 patients to a mobile-bearing UKA (Oxford) and 57 to a fixed-bearing UKA (St. Georg Sled). At a mean of 4 years, four knees in the mobile-bearing group and three knees in the fixed-bearing group had been revised.

LONG-TERM OUTCOME

Registry Data
Three registers—the Swedish Knee Arthroplasty Register, the Finnish Arthroplasty Register, and the Australian Orthopaedic Association register—report on specific data for the Oxford UKA at approximately the 10-year time point, and we summarize the most recent outcome data from these registers. Several of the other registers, such as the New Zealand and the Norwegian registers, do not report separate outcome for fixed and mobile, nor in some cases medial and lateral, unicompartmental replacements, and the United Kingdom National Joint Registry presently reports revision rate for specific implants at only 3 years. Therefore, they are not included here. In the 2009

annual report of the Swedish Knee Arthroplasty Register,[14] the cumulative 8-year survival for the Oxford replacement was greater than 91%. The Australian Orthopaedic Association joint registry data from 2009[15] reported a cumulative survival of 87.1% at 8 years. The Finnish Arthroplasty Register reported a 10-year survival of 81% for the Oxford UKA,[16] slightly better than for a fixed-bearing device (79%, Miller-Galante). There is no more detailed information in these reports for mobile-bearing UKA. At other time points, important information has come from the registry data. In 1998, Lewold et al.[17] reported the cause for revision of all unicompartmental replacement in the Swedish Knee Arthroplasty Register up to 10 years. This cited the most common cause for revision as component loosening and the second most common as contralateral compartment progression. Unfortunately, these are merged data for all types of unicompartmental replacement, with the most common being fixed-bearing devices, so the extrapolation to mobile-bearing devices is difficult. Prior to this the same authors did report the cause for revision at 6 years in the Oxford knee.[18] Although these were not long-term data, they did show a proportionally high rate of dislocated bearings and loosening. These observations led one of the coauthors to later describe the absolute importance of good surgical routine, mentioned in the previous section.[6]

Cohort Studies
Ten-Year Studies
Ten-year follow-up of the Oxford prosthesis is reported in nine studies (**Table 18–1**), and there is a wide range in the reported survival. Six of the nine studies at 10 years reported a cumulative survival of 94% or greater; however, three series report a cumulative survival of 85% or less. The inventor series of Murray et al.[19] for the Phase 1 and 2 Oxford knee reported a 10-year cumulative "worst-case" survival rate of 97% (CI, 93–100%). Forty-four knees remained at risk at 10 years, and no failures were due to polyethylene wear or aseptic loosening of the tibial component. Pandit et al.[20] reported the

Table 18-1	Summary of Ten-Year Survival Studies						
						10-Year Survival	
Year	Author	Phase	Number	Mean Age (Years)	Mean Follow-up (Range)	Survival % (95% CI)	At Risk
1998	Murray et al.[19]	1, 2	144	71 (35–91)	7.6 (6–14)	97 (93–100)	44
1999	Kumar and Fiddian[25]	2	100	71	5.6 (1–11)	85 (78–92)	83
2000	Svärd and Price[22]	1, 2	124	70 (51–86)	12.5 (10.1–15.6)	95	97
2002	Emerson et al.[32]	2	50	64	6.8 (2–13)	92 (—)	—
2004	Keys et al.[21]	2	40	68 (40–80)	7.5 (6–10)	100 (—)	6
2004	Rajasekhar et al.[23]	2	135	72 (53–88)	5.8 (2–12)	94 (84–97)	22
2006	Vorlat et al.[26]	2	141	66 (46–89)	5.5 (1–10)	82 (SE 6.9)	80
2009	Mercier et al.[24]	3	43	69 (47–86)	14.9	75 (—)	24
2009	Pandit et al.[20]	3	1000	66 (32–87)	—	96 (—)	—

inventor series of the Phase 3 Oxford knee with 1000 patients and a 96% cumulative revision rate at 10 years. Keys et al.[21] reported their first 40 Phase 3 Oxford UKAs, also with excellent results, supporting the results of the inventor series. The average follow-up was 7.5 years and the survivorship at 10 years was 100% with no losses to follow-up. In another independent series of the Phase 1 and 2 knees, Svärd and Price[22] showed a cumulative survival of 124 patients at 10 years of 95%, with an average follow-up of 12.5 years and no losses to follow-up. Rajasekher et al.[23] showed similar results, with 94% cumulative survival of the Phase 2 knee at 10 years.

Other cohorts do not reveal similar success with the implant. Mercier et al.[24] report an overall survival of 74.7%. However, they specifically draw attention to their broad selection criteria, including ACL-deficient knees and inflammatory arthropathy. When these cases are excluded, the 10-year survival is improved to greater than 85%. In similar fashion, Kumar and Fiddian[25] reported a 10-year survival of 85% (CI, 78–92%) and a mean follow-up of 5.6 years. Again they noted that initial patient selection, such as inflammatory arthropathy, led to four of the seven failures, and functional assessment showed that 98% of all patients were pleased or satisfied with the outcome of their surgery. Vorlat et al.[26] showed the effect of previous high tibial osteotomy (HTO) on the outcome of Oxford UKA. Overall, the cumulative survival at 10 years was 82%; however, four of the failures were in eight patients who had previously undergone HTO (two cases for lateral progression and two for unspecified reasons), and when these were excluded the results improved.

Twenty-Year Studies

There are only two studies that reported 20-year survival (**Table 18–2**). Price and Svärd[27] reported the continuation and further accumulation of the Svärd and Price 10-year study[22] (also reported at 15 years[28]). The strength of this series is that it includes all cases performed with no loss to follow-up. Six hundred eighty-three consecutive knees were assessed and the overall cumulative survival was 92% at 20 years. The most common cause for revision was progression of arthritis in the lateral compartment, although over the 20-year period this only occurred in 10 patients or 1.5% of cases. While previous studies have shown that overcorrection of the varus deformity

may lead to relatively rapid progression of lateral compartment disease,[29] the low rate of progressive lateral arthrosis in this study shows that this is an uncommon feature with the Oxford UKA. This is supported by previous work by Weale et al.[30] In addition, there were no failures attributable to patellofemoral joint problems, which is of note since preoperative patellofemoral disease was not a contraindication to unicompartmental replacement in this study. This study also reinforces the message that adhering to the present-day indications improves outcome since in a subgroup with previous HTO or ACL deficiency (included in the overall results) the failure rate was 71%. The most interesting feature of the Svärd and Price series is the relatively few failures that occur in the second decade. Infection and dislocation appear to be relatively early complications of this procedure, and lateral compartment osteoarthritis and loosening account for the majority of midterm failures. However, only three cases required revision in the second decade, two for lateral progression and one for femoral loosening. Of note, no failures in the second decade were due to polyethylene wear, suggesting that the design features of the implant in reducing contact stress as a design against wear can be successful. The 20-year results of Barrington and Emerson[31] reinforce those of Svärd and Price. Their survivorship was 94% with no revisions for bearing dislocation, tibial subsidence, or polyethylene wear. They also reported excellent functional scores, with mean Knee Society scores improving from 47 preoperatively to 94 postoperatively.

The modes of failure for the 10-year and 20-year studies are listed on **Table 18–3**. Perhaps unsurprisingly, lateral progression becomes a higher proportion of total failures as time progresses, but it still only affects 0.11% per year of follow-up.

Clinical Outcome

Very few long-term clinical outcome data are reported; those that are available are summarized in **Table 18–4**. In assessing the few studies available, it is clear there is no consistency of the clinical outcome assessment used, making generalized interpretation difficult. However, all of the clinical scores significantly improve from postoperation to final follow-up. Price et al.[28] did report robust longitudinal data from 1, 6, and 10 years postoperatively. Interestingly, this shows that the significant increase in clinical scores does not decrease with time;

Table 18-2	Summary of Twenty-Year Survival Studies						
						20-Year Survival	
Year	Author	Phase	Number	Mean Age (Years)	Mean Follow-up (Range)	Survival % (95% CI)	At Risk
2010	Price and Svärd[27]	1, 2, 3	683	69.7	—	92.1 (± 33.2)	15
2010	Barrington and Emerson[31]	2	54	64	16–21	94 (—)	44

Table 18-3   Breakdown of Cause of Revision at 10 and 20 Years

	10-Year Studies* (Study n = 8; Patients n = 4116)		20-Year Studies* (Study n = 2; Patients n = 736)	
Bearing	**0.9**	**(19.5)**	**0.4**	**(8.1)**
Bearing dislocation	0.7	(15.9)	0.3	(5.4)
Bearing fracture	0.1	(2.4)	0.0	(0.0)
Bearing impingement	0.1	(1.2)	0.1	(2.7)
Wear	**0.4**	**(8.5)**	**0.0**	**(0.0)**
Polyethylene wear with major osteolysis	0.0	(0.0)	0.0	(0.0)
Loosening—Total	**1.1**	**(23.2)**	**1.4**	**(27)**
Loosening—not specified	0.2	(4.9)	0.1	(2.7)
Loosening both	0.1	(1.2)	0.3	(5.4)
Femoral loosening	0.2	(4.9)	1.0	(18.9)
Tibial loosening	0.6	(12.2)	0.0	(0.0)
Pain	**0.3**	**(7.3)**	**0.4**	**(8.1)**
Progression	**1.1**	**(23.2)**	**2.2**	**(43.2)**
PFJ progression	0.0	(0.0)	0.0	(0.0)
Lateral progression	1.1	(23.2)	2.2	(43.2)
Infection	**0.4**	**(8.5)**	**0.7**	**(13.5)**
Prosthesis fracture	**0.1**	**(2.4)**	**0.0**	**(0.0)**
ACL rupture	**0.2**	**(3.7)**	**0.0**	**(0.0)**
Plateau fracture	**0.1**	**(1.2)**	**0.0**	**(0.0)**
Recurrent hemarthrosis	**0.1**	**(1.2)**	**0.0**	**(0.0)**
Instability	**0.1**	**(1.2)**	**0.0**	**(0.0)**
TOTAL REVISIONS	**4.6**	**(100)**	**5.0**	**(100)**

*Frequency of revision (proportion of all revisions for this mode).

in other words, patient function is just as good 10 years postoperatively as at 1 year.

SUMMARY

Overall, excellent long-term outcome can be achieved with a mobile-bearing unicompartmental knee replacement. However, this review highlights that patient selection is an important determinant of outcome for this device. In particular, disrupted ACL and previous HTO are important factors, but high body mass index, activity scores, or moderate patellofemoral disease are not contraindications to UKA. There is a low revision rate between 10 and 20 years, which is likely to be a reflection of the "design against wear," which was the keystone of the original design. Earlier complications such as early lateral progression and bearing dislocation can be a problem, although many of these can be overcome by good surgical routine and by frequently performing the procedure. With excellent results between 10 and 20 years, the UKA can be considered as a viable end treatment for medial compartment arthritis with an intact ACL, and these procedures should not be viewed as a mere filler until total knee replacement. Even so, they do remain easier to revise than a total knee replacement; the majority of the reported revisions in these series were to a primary TKA, not a stemmed revision prosthesis. This ease of revision is a factor that may jaundice the reported survival rates from joint registers. Excellent 10-year results can be achieved in series where surgeons have used the correct indications for unicompartmental replacement.

Table 18-4   Summary of the Reported Long-Term Clinical Outcome Studies*

			Clinical Scores									
			AKSS				HSS		OKS		IKS	
			Average		Functional							
Year	Author	Time of Follow-up (Years)	Pre	Post	Pre	Post	Pre	Post	Pre	Post	Pre	Post
1999	Kumar and Fiddian[25]	5.5	62	91	45	71	N/D*	N/D	N/D	N/D	N/D	N/D
2004	Keys et al.[21]	Not specified	37	97	36	87	N/D	N/D	20	40	N/D	N/D
2005	Price et al.[28]	1, 6, and 10	N/D	N/D	N/D	N/D	56.5	Year 1—88.4 Year 6—88.4 Year 10—86	N/D	N/D	N/D	N/D
2006	Vorlat et al.[26]	Not specified	N/D	N/D	N/D	N/D	N/D	N/D	N/D	N/D	N/D	N/D
2009	Mercier et al.[24]	Not specified	N/D	N/D	N/D	N/D	N/D	N/D	N/D	N/D	107.2	145.5
2009	Pandit et al.[20]	Not specified	N/D	N/D	N/D	N/D	N/D	N/D	23	41	N/D	N/D

*N/D, no data.

However, there is variation in reported series, and variation in indications for surgery does appear to be a very important factor in determining outcome.

Although the 20-year data are limited to two studies, it appears the Oxford UKA can be a viable end treatment to medial unicompartmental osteoarthritis and that these procedures should not be viewed as a pre–total knee replacement procedure.

REFERENCES

1. Goodfellow J. Unicompartmental Arthroplasty with the Oxford Knee. Oxford: Oxford University Press, 2006.
2. Rees JL, Price AJ, Beard DJ, et al. Minimally invasive Oxford unicompartmental knee arthroplasty: functional results at 1 year and the effect of surgical inexperience. Knee 2004;11:363-367.
3. Magnussen PA, Bartlett RJ. Cementless PCA unicompartmental joint arthroplasty for osteoarthritis of the knee: a prospective study of 51 cases. J Arthroplasty 1990;5:151-158.
4. Harilainen A, Ylinen P, Sandelin J, Vahvanen V. Survival analysis and predictors of failure in unicompartmental knee replacement using a PCA prosthesis. Knee 1995;1:201-207.
5. Price AJ, Longino D, Rees J, et al. Are pain and function better measures of outcome than revision rates after TKR in the younger patient? Knee 2010;17:196-199.
6. Robertsson O, Knutson K, Lewold S, Lidgren L. The routine of surgical management reduces failure after unicompartmental knee arthroplasty. J Bone Joint Surg [Br] 2001;83:45-49.
7. Medical Devices Agency NIfCE, British Orthopaedic Association. Post-market surveillance of CE marked joint replacement implants including guidance to manufacturers on postmarket clinical studies. EC Medical Devices Directive. London: British Orthopaedic Association, 2000.
8. Kort NP, van Raay JJ, van Horn JJ. The Oxford phase III unicompartmental knee replacement in patients less than 60 years of age. Knee Surg Sports Traumatol Arthrosc 2007;15:356-360.
9. Kuipers B, Kollen B, Kaijser Bots P, et al. Factors associated with reduced early survival in the Oxford phase III medial unicompartment knee replacement. Knee 2010;17:48-52.
10. Kozinn SC, Scott R. Unicondylar knee arthroplasty. J Bone Joint Surg [Am] 1989;71:145-150.
11. Pandit H, Jenkins C, Barker K, et al. The Oxford medial unicompartmental knee replacement using a minimally-invasive approach. J Bone Joint Surg [Br] 2006;88:54-60.
12. Confalonieri N, Manzotti A, Pullen C. Comparison of a mobile with a fixed tibial bearing unicompartmental knee prosthesis: a prospective randomized trial using a dedicated outcome score. Knee 2004;11:357-362.
13. Gleeson RE, Evans R, Ackroyd CE, et al. Fixed or mobile bearing unicompartmental knee replacement? A comparative cohort study. Knee 2004;11:379-384.
14. Lidgren L, Robertsson O, Dahl A. Swedish Knee Arthoplasty Register—Annual Report. Lund: Swedish Knee Arthoplasty Register, 2009, pp 30-34.
15. Graves S. Australian Orthopaedic Association National Joint Registry—Annual Report. Adelaide: Australian Orthopaedic Association, 2009, pp 112-124.
16. Koskinen E, Paavolainen P, Eskelinen A, et al. Unicondylar knee replacement for primary osteoarthritis: a prospective follow-up study of 1,819 patients from the Finnish Arthroplasty Register. Acta Orthop 2007;78:128-135.
17. Lewold S, Robertsson O, Knutson K, Lidgren L. Revision of unicompartmental knee arthroplasty: outcome in 1,135 cases from the Swedish Knee Arthroplasty study. Acta Orthop Scand 1998;69: 469-474.
18. Lewold S, Goodman S, Knutson K, et al. Oxford meniscal bearing knee versus the Marmor knee in unicompartmental arthroplasty for arthrosis: a Swedish multicenter survival study. J Arthroplasty 1995;10:722-731.
19. Murray DW, Goodfellow JW, O'Connor JJ. The Oxford medial unicompartmental arthroplasty: a ten-year survival study. J Bone Joint Surg [Br] 1998;80:983-989.
20. Pandit H, Jenkins C, Beard D, et al. Minimally invasive medial Oxford UKR 10 year survival. Presented at the Annual Meeting of the American Academy of Orthopedic Surgeons, Las Vegas, 2009.
21. Keys GW, Ul-Abiddin Z, Toh EM. Analysis of first forty Oxford medial unicompartmental knee replacement from a small district hospital in UK. Knee 2004;11:375-377.
22. Svärd UC, Price AJ. Oxford medial unicompartmental knee arthroplasty: a survival analysis of an independent series. J Bone Joint Surg [Br] 2001;83:191-194.
23. Rajasekhar C, Das S, Smith A. Unicompartmental knee arthroplasty: 2- to 12-year results in a community hospital. J Bone Joint Surg [Br] 2004;86:983-985.
24. Mercier N, Wimsey S, Saragaglia D. Long-term clinical results of the Oxford medial unicompartmental knee arthroplasty. Int Orthop 2010;34:1137-1143.
25. Kumar A, Fiddian NJ. Medial unicompartmental arthroplasty of the knee. Knee 1999;6:21-23.
26. Vorlat P, Putzeys G, Cottenie D, et al. The Oxford unicompartmental knee prosthesis: an independent 10-year survival analysis. Knee Surg Sports Traumatol Arthrosc 2006;14:40-45.
27. Price AJ Svärd U. A second decade lifetable survival analysis of the Oxford unicompartmental knee arthroplasty. Clin Orthop Relat Res 2011;(469):174-179.
28. Price A, Waite J, Svärd U. Long-term clinical results of the medial Oxford unicompartmental knee arthroplasty. Clin Orthop Relat Res 2005;(435):171-180.
29. Dejour D, Chatain F, Habi S. The role of the femoropatellar articulation and the opposite compartment in the degradation of the functional result of unicompartmental prostheses. [Role de l'articulation femoro-patellaire et du compartiment oppose dans la degradation du resultat fonctionnel des protheses unicompartimentales.] Rev Chir Orthop Reparatrice Appar Mot 1996;82:37-39.
30. Weale AE, Murray DW, Crawford R, et al. Does arthritis progress in the retained compartments after "Oxford" medial unicompartmental arthroplasty? A clinical and radiological study with a minimum ten-year follow-up. J Bone Joint Surg [Br] 1999;81:783-789.
31. Barrington J, Emerson R. The Oxford knee: first report of 20-year follow-up in the US. Presented at the Annual Meeting of the American Academy of Orthopedic Surgeons, New Orleans, 2010.
32. Emerson RH Jr, Hansborough T, Reitman RD, et al. Comparison of a mobile with a fixed-bearing unicompartmental knee implant. Clin Orthop Relat Res 2002;(404):62-70.

CHAPTER 19
Fixed-Bearing Uni: Long-Term Outcomes

Todd C. Kelley and David F. Dalury

KEY POINTS

- The majority of devices traditionally are fixed bearing.
- Fixed bearing is perhaps more flexible in the lateral joint and in the ACL-deficient knee.
- Multiple series show excellent durability in various surgical designs.

INTRODUCTION

Unicompartmental knee arthroplasty (UKA) has been used for several decades to treat arthritis of a single compartment of the tibiofemoral joint that has otherwise failed nonoperative management. The concept is an appealing one: replace only the worn part of the knee joint. The perceived advantages of a UKA compared with a total knee replacement are considered to be a shorter recovery, an earlier return to function, and an increased range of motion. Fixed-bearing UKA has proven successful over the years. Favorable outcomes require proper patient selection, restoration of limb alignment, and careful surgical technique. The previous rigid patient selection criteria for an ideal surgical candidate have been slowly expanding over recent years. Fixed-bearing UKA has been shown to provide excellent patient satisfaction and functional results. Careful review of long-term results is important to justify the continued role of UKA in the treatment of single-compartment knee arthritis.

HISTORICAL BACKGROUND

Modern UKA implants have evolved from the early designs of MacIntosh and McKeever.[1] These prostheses, introduced in the 1950s and 1960s, were metallic hemiarthroplasty implants designed to resurface only the tibial plateau. Early reports of both implants were encouraging; however, metallic hemiarthroplasty never gained popularity due to early loosening and to the advent of metal-to-plastic cemented arthroplasty.[2]

Classic Indications

In 1989, Kozinn and Scott[3] published their classic article detailing the selection criteria for appropriate candidates for UKA. This involves consideration of the patient's age, weight, occupational and recreational demands, range of motion, extent of angular deformity, and intra-articular pathology of the knee. According to their criteria, patients over 60 years old with a low-demand lifestyle are the best candidates. Patients should not be obese; ideally, patients should weigh less than 82 kg (180 pounds). They should have minimal pain at rest, a preoperative range of motion of at least 90°, and no more than a 5° flexion contracture. The angular deformity in the coronal plane should be less than 15° (10° of varus to 15° of valgus) and must be passively correctable to neutral after removal of tibial osteophytes. Intraoperatively, examination of the patellofemoral joint and opposite femoral compartment should not reveal exposed subchondral bone. In addition, the best results are obtained with intact cruciate ligaments. Patients with generalized inflammatory arthropathy are not candidates for UKA. Chondrocalcinosis is considered a relative contraindication for this procedure. Avascular necrosis is not contraindicated as long as adequate healthy bone is available to support the implants.

Expanding Indications: Patient Age, Activity, and Weight

Traditionally, UKA has been used to treat elderly, low-demand patients. However, the indications may be expanding. Pennington et al.[4] in 2003 reviewed the results of UKA in patients 60 years of age or younger. These were all physically active patients. At the time of surgery, all patients were employed and participated in high-demand activities. Forty-five UKAs were reviewed at a mean of 11 years. Only three knees were revised. For the remaining 42 UKAs, 93% were rated as excellent. Survivorship was calculated at 92% at 11 years.

Similarly, Parratte et al.[5] in 2009 reviewed 35 UKAs in patients less than 50 years old. They reported good clinical results and survivorship (80% at 12 years), but also noted that polyethylene wear is the major concern following UKA in this younger age group.

Kozinn and Scott[3] believed that weight in excess of 82 kg should be a contraindication for a UKA. In support of this criterion, Berend et al.[6] reported that body mass index (BMI = kg/m^2) greater than 32 predicted early failure and reduced survivorship. The 82-kg cutoff weight limit continues to be challenged, however. Some cautiously suggest that the cutoff weight limit for a UKA could be raised to 90 kg.[7] Naal et al.[8] reported that BMI had no association with early clinical outcome or implant failure. Tabor et al.[9] also suggested that youth and obesity should not be considered contraindications to UKA. In fact, in their analysis, obese patients had better survivorship than nonobese patients at 20 years.

UKA LONG-TERM RESULTS (Table 19-1)

Much of the published literature combines medial and lateral UKAs. One of the earliest long-term outcome studies of fixed-bearing UKAs was by Marmor in 1988.[10] This included 60 Modular Marmor arthroplasties, 53 medial UKAs, and 7 lateral UKAs. At a minimum of 10 years' follow-up, patients maintained a 70% satisfactory result.

Over the last decade, there have been numerous studies demonstrating the excellent long-term outcomes and survivorship of more modern fixed-bearing UKAs. Squire et al.[11] reviewed 140 consecutive Marmor cemented UKAs with an all-polyethylene tibial component inserted between 1975 and 1982 and published their long-term outcomes. At final follow-up, 34 patients (48 knees) were alive and available for review. Only four patients (four knees) were lost to follow-up. There was a minimum of 15 years' follow-up on 29 patients (40 knees). At this length of follow-up, 12.5% of UKAs required revision. The survivorship analysis showed encouraging results. Using revision surgery for any reason as an end point, survivorship was 84% at 22 years. Using revision surgery for aseptic loosening as an end point, survivorship was 93% at 22 years. Disease progression in the contralateral compartment and tibial subsidence with wear were the major long-term problems. Overall satisfaction, however, was excellent in these patients. In 2002, Argenson et al.[12] reviewed 160 UKAs (145 medial and 15 lateral) with an average of 5.5 years' follow-up (range, 3–9.3 years). Mean patient age was 66 (range, 35–88). Average Hospital for Special Surgery (HSS) score improved from 59 (range, 10–90) to 96 (range, 50–100). Ninety-two percent of these knees were graded as excellent. The 10-year survivorship was 94% with revision for any reason or radiographic loosening as the end point.

Naudie et al.[13] in 2004 reported on their results from 113 medial UKAs. They noted excellent pain relief and restoration of function with a mean follow-up of 10 years. With revision or radiographic loosening as an end point, survivorship was 93% at 5 years and 86% at 10 years. Mean Knee Society knee and function scores improved at final follow-up to 93 and 80

points, respectively. In 2005, Berger et al.[14] reported on 62 consecutive UKAs with a minimum of 10 years' follow-up. Mean postoperative HSS score was 92, with 92% good to excellent results. The 10-year survival rate was 98%. In addition, Berger et al.[15] reported that, at 10 years' follow-up, patellofemoral symptoms were present in only 1.6% of patients. However, at 15 years' follow-up, 10% of patients had moderate to severe patellofemoral symptoms. Although in this series progressive patellofemoral arthritis was the primary mode of failure, clinical results and survivorship were excellent. O'Rourke et al.[16] in 2005 reported on a series of 136 consecutive UKAs with a minimum 21 years' follow-up. With revision for any reason as the end point, survivorship was 84% at 20 years and 72% at 25 years. The patients most at risk for revision were younger at the time of surgery. Although the clinical and functional scores in this group were relatively low at this long-term follow-up, it is important to note that this was a group of elderly patients with multiple medical and orthopaedic comorbidities. Steele et al.[17] reviewed the Bristol database to determine survivorship beyond 10 years of a fixed-bearing UKA. Although the mean Bristol knee score fell from 86 to 79 during the second decade, survivorship was satisfactory into the second decade (85.9% at 20 years and 80% at 25 years).

A review of the literature highlights the important role of implant design in fixed-bearing UKA outcomes. A paper by Eickmann et al.[18] in 2006 reviewed 411 fixed-bearing medial UKAs placed by a single surgeon in the 1980s to 1990s. There was a 9-year survivorship of 80%. This result was highly dependent on implant design. Nine-year survival improved to 94% when tibial component thickness was greater than 7 mm and polyethylene shelf age was less than 1 year. Factors that were associated with revision included younger patient age, thinner tibial component, increased polyethylene insert shelf age, and implant system utilized.

LATERAL UKA RESULTS (Table 19-2)

As lateral compartment osteoarthritis of the knee is relatively rare, results of fixed-bearing UKA for lateral osteoarthritis are limited. Although many series contain results of both medial and lateral unicompartment arthroplasty, there are few published studies of isolated lateral compartment arthroplasty. The limited data suggest that the indications for lateral compartment arthroplasty are not commonly met. Ashraf et al.[19] in 2002 published their experience with the St. Georg Sled in 88 knees. With mean clinical follow-up of 9 years (range, 2–21 years), 15 knees had revision surgery. The 10-year survival rate was 83%. At 15 years, the survival rate was 74.5%. The authors pointed out that these results are acceptable since 4 of the 15 revisions were due to breakage of the implant. After redesign of the implant in 1988, there were no further revisions due to implant failure. At 10 years' follow-up, 78% of patients had

Table 19-1 Long-Term Results of Studies Including Both Medial and Lateral Fixed-Bearing Unicompartmental Knee Arthroplasty

Authors	Year	Implant	Number of Knees in Study	Number of Knees at Follow-up	Patient Age, Mean (Range)	Follow-up, Years (Range)	Results	Comments
Marmor[10]	1988	Marmor	87	60	63 (31–85)	11 (10–13)	70% satisfactory	53 medial, 7 lateral
Squire et al.[11]	1999	Marmor	140	48	68 (51–83)	18 (15.8–21.8) for 29 patients (40 knees)	Average final follow-up: HSS score = 82 Knee Society clinical score = 85 Knee Society functional score = 71	125 medial, 15 lateral 34 patients (48 knees) alive at final follow-up Survivorship = 84% at 22 years using revision for any reason Survivorship = 93% at 22 years using revision for aseptic loosening
Argenson et al.[12]	2002	Miller-Galante	172	160	66 (35–88)	5.5 (3–9.3)	Average HSS score improved from 59 (range, 10–90) to 96 (range, 50–100) 92% excellent, 5% good, 2% fair, 1% poor	145 medial, 15 lateral 10-year survivorship = 94%
Pennington et al.[4]	2003	Miller-Galante	46	45	54 (35–60)	11 (5.6–13.8)	HSS score: 93% excellent	44 medial, 2 lateral All patients were 60 years of age or younger and were all physically active 92% survivorship at 11 years
Naudie et al.[13]	2004	Miller-Galante	113	97	68 (39–87)	10 (3–14)	Mean postoperative Knee Society knee score = 93 Mean postoperative Knee Society function score = 80	All medial UKAs With revision or loosening as the end point, 5-year survivorship = 93%; 10-year survivorship = 86%
Berger et al.[14]	2005	Miller-Galante	62	49	68 (51–84)	12 (10–13)	Mean postoperative HSS score = 92 80% excellent, 12% good, 8% fair	59 medial, 3 lateral With revision or loosening as the end point, 10-year survival rate of 98%; 13-year survival rate of 95.7%
O'Rourke et al.[16]	2005	Marmor	136	19	70.9 (51.1–93.6)	24 (17–28.1)	Average follow-up HSS score = 58 Average follow-up Knee Society clinical score = 72 Average follow-up Knee Society function score = 53	122 medial, 14 lateral 14 patients (19 knees) were alive at 21-year follow-up Only 2 patients lost to follow-up With revision for any reason as the end point, 20-year survival rate of 84%; 25-year survival rate of 72%
Tabor et al.[9]	2005	Marmor	100	95	59 patients older than 60; 36 patients younger than 60	12.1 (0.25–25.5)	Average follow-up Knee Society knee score = 89.3 Average follow-up Knee Society function score = 73.1	5-year survivorship = 93.7% 10-year survivorship = 89.8% 15-year survivorship = 85.9% 20-year survivorship = 80.2% Survival for obese patients at 20 years was better than for nonobese patients
Eickmann et al.[18]	2006	12 different designs	411	N/A	67 (45–89)	9 (0.1–19.3)	N/A	9-year survivorship = 80% Revision related to younger patient age, thin tibial component, increased polyethylene shelf age, and implant system
Steele et al.[17]	2006	St. Georg Sled	203	N/A	67.1 (35.7–85)	14.8 (10–29.4)	Mean Bristol knee score fell from 86 to 79 during the second decade	Survivorship at 20 years = 85.9% Survivorship at 25 years = 80%
Parratte et al.[5]	2009	Miller-Galante	35	35	46 (41–49)	9.7 (5–16)	Mean postoperative Knee Society knee score = 97 Mean postoperative Knee Society function score = 89	All medial Survivorship at 12 years = 80.6%

Table 19-2	Long-Term Results of Lateral Fixed-Bearing Unicompartmental Knee Arthroplasty							
Authors	Year	Implant	Number of Knees in Study	Number of Knees at Follow-up	Patient Age, Mean (Range)	Follow-up, Years (Range)	Results	Comments
Ashraf et al.[19]	2002	St. George Sled	88	83	69 (35-81)	9 (2-21)	78% good to excellent at 10 years	Survivorship = 83% at 10 years; 74% at 15 years
Pennington et al.[20]	2006	Miller-Galante	29	29	68 (52-86)	12.4 (3.1-15.6)	All with excellent or good results	Placed tibial component in 10-15° of internal rotation for improved implant contact in extension
Sah and Scott[21]	2007	1990s: PFC 2001: PFC Sigma 2002-2004: Preservation UKR	49	48	61 (37-84)	5.2 (2-15)	All patients mean postoperative Knee Society score = 89 Primary osteoarthritis patients scored higher than posttraumatic arthritis patients	Used medial approach for possible need to convert to total knee arthroplasty
Argenson et al.[23]	2008	Marmor (15) Alpina (1) Miller-Galante (20) ZUK (4)	40	38	61 (34-79)	12.6 (3-23)	23 enthusiastic 9 satisfied 1 no change 4 not satisfied	Survivorship = 92% at 10 years; 84% at 16 years

excellent or good results. The authors noted that the surgeries were performed by multiple surgeons, suggesting that these results are reproducible.

Pennington et al.[20] in 2006 discussed the concept of the "screw-home" mechanism in relation to proper positioning of the tibial component. The authors stressed the importance of positioning of the tibial component in 10–15° of internal rotation. This modification to the tibial component positioning was made after multiple observations of the femoral component overriding the anterior-medial aspect of the tibial component with knee extension. Placing the tibial component in 10–15° of internal rotation allows centerline articulation of the components throughout the entire range of motion. They further reported on 29 consecutive lateral unicompartmental arthroplasties using this modification, with a mean follow-up of 12.4 years (range, 3.1–15.6 years). There were no revisions, and the HSS score was excellent or good in all cases.

In 2007, Sah and Scott[21] published their midterm results on 49 lateral UKAs through a medial approach.[22] The average follow-up was 5.2 years (range, 2–15 years). Surgeries were performed for either primary osteoarthritis or posttraumatic arthritis. Mean postoperative Knee Society scores improved to 89 and there were no revisions. Of note, the mean postoperative knee and function scores were significantly higher for patients with primary osteoarthritis than patients with posttraumatic arthritis. Interestingly, while the authors noted that 102 knees were originally scheduled for lateral unicompartmental arthroplasty, only 49 of the knees actually received a lateral unicompartmental arthroplasty. For the remaining 53 cases, the initial plan was aborted after direct visualization of all compartments, and the case was converted to a total knee arthroplasty. In the authors' opinion, the familiar medial arthrotomy used in this study allows for an easy conversion to total knee arthroplasty if necessary.

Argenson et al.[23] in 2008 reported long-term results of 40 lateral unicompartmental arthroplasties with an average 12.6-year follow-up. Indications for surgery included a preoperative range of knee flexion over 100°, full extension, and a stable knee in the frontal and sagittal planes. In the later years of the study, they preformed preoperative varus/valgus stress radiographs to evaluate the medial compartment and to determine correction of the deformity. At final follow-up, 62% of patients were enthusiastic, 24% were satisfied, and 14% reported no change or were not satisfied. There were only four revisions for symptomatic osteoarthritis progression. Survivorship of the implants was 92% at 10 years and 84% at 16 years.

CONCLUSION

A review of the literature regarding fixed-bearing UKA confirms the importance of proper patient selection. While there has been some cautious expansion of traditional indications in terms of patient age, activity, and weight, published studies continue to emphasize the importance of alignment, preoperative range of motion, and limited disease in other compartments. In general, mild to moderate disease appears to be well tolerated in the patellofemoral joint, and the majority of authors feel an intact anterior cruciate ligament is an advantage for a fixed-bearing UKA. Careful surgical technique (good cementation, removal of loose cement and bone fragments, and appropriate implant-to-implant alignment) is paramount. Utilization of a well-designed implant with accurate instrumentation, modern polyethylene design, and good fixation is important. Recent studies of fixed-bearing UKA demonstrate long-term (over 10 years) survival rates of 90%.

Patient selection criteria are paramount, and improved surgical technique, instrumentation, and implants contribute to the longevity of the fixed-bearing UKA. The relatively recent surge of interest in "minimally invasive" surgery has led to an increase in the use of UKA. Currently there are inadequate data to comment on how that will influence UKA results. Further study is necessary.

REFERENCES

1. Jamali AA, Scott RD, Rubash HE, Freiberg AA. Unicompartmental knee arthroplasty: past, present, and future. Am J Orthop 2009; 38:17-23.
2. Scott RD, Joyce MJ, Ewald FC, Thomas WH. McKeever metallic hemiarthroplasty of the knee in unicompartmental degenerative arthritis: long-term clinical follow-up and current indications. J Bone Joint Surg [Am] 1985;67:203-207.
3. Kozinn SC, Scott R. Unicondylar knee arthroplasty. J Bone Joint Surg [Am] 1989;71:145-150.
4. Pennington DW, Swienckowski JJ, Lutes WB, Drake GN. Unicompartmental knee arthroplasty in patients sixty years of age or younger. J Bone Joint Surg [Am] 2003;85:1968-1973.
5. Parratte S, Argenson JN, Pearce O, et al. Medial unicompartmental knee replacement in the under-50s. J Bone Joint Surg [Br] 2009; 91:351-356.
6. Berend KR, Lombardi AV Jr, Mallory TH, et al. Early failure of minimally invasive unicompartmental knee arthroplasty is associated with obesity. Clin Orthop Relat Res 2005;(440):60-66.
7. Deshmukh RV, Scott RD. Unicompartmental knee arthroplasty: long-term results. Clin Orthop Relat Res 2001;(392):272-278.
8. Naal FD, Neuerburg C, Salzmann GM, et al. Association of body mass index and clinical outcome 2 years after unicompartmental knee arthroplasty. Arch Orthop Trauma Surg 2009;129:463-468.
9. Tabor OB Jr, Tabor OB, Bernard M, Wan JY. Unicompartmental knee arthroplasty: long-term success in middle-age and obese patients. J Surg Orthop Adv 2005;14(2):59-63.
10. Marmor L. Unicompartmental arthroplasty of the knee with a minimum ten-year follow-up period. Clin Orthop Relat Res 1988; (228):171-177.
11. Squire MW, Callaghan JJ, Goetz DD, et al. Unicompartmental knee replacement: a minimum 15 year follow-up study. Clin Orthop Relat Res 1999;(367):61-72.
12. Argenson JN, Chevrol-Benkeddache Y, Aubaniac JM. Modern unicompartmental knee arthroplasty with cement: a three to ten-year follow-up study. J Bone Joint Surg [Am] 2002;84: 2235-2239.
13. Naudie D, Guerin J, Parker DA, et al. Medial unicompartmental knee arthroplasty with the Miller-Galante prosthesis. J Bone Joint Surg [Am] 2004;86:1931-1935.
14. Berger RA, Meneghini RM, Jacobs JJ, et al. Results of unicompartmental knee arthroplasty at a minimum of ten years of follow-up. J Bone Joint Surg [Am] 2005;87:999-1006.
15. Berger RA, Meneghini RM, Sheinkop MB, et al. The progression of patellofemoral arthrosis after medial unicompartmental replacement: results at 11 to 15 years. Clin Orthop Relat Res 2004;(428): 92-99.
16. O'Rourke MR, Gardner JJ, Callaghan JJ, et al. The John Insall Award. Unicompartmental knee replacement: a minimum twenty-one-year follow-up, end-result study. Clin Orthop Relat Res 2005;(440): 27-37.
17. Steele RG, Hutabarat S, Evans RL, et al. Survivorship of the St Georg Sled medial unicompartmental knee replacement beyond ten years. J Bone Joint Surg [Br] 2006;88:1164-1168.
18. Eickmann TH, Collier MB, Sukezaki F, et al. Survival of medial unicondylar arthroplasties placed by one surgeon 1984–1998. Clin Orthop Relat Res 2006;(452):143-149.
19. Ashraf T, Newman JH, Evans RL, Ackroyd CE. Lateral unicompartmental knee replacement survivorship and clinical experience over 21 years. J Bone Joint Surg [Br] 2002;84:1126-1130.
20. Pennington DW, Swienckowski JJ, Lutes WB, Drake GN. Lateral unicompartmental knee arthroplasty: survivorship and technical considerations at an average follow-up of 12.4 years. J Arthroplasty 2006;21:13-17.
21. Sah AP, Scott RD. Lateral unicompartmental knee arthroplasty through a medial approach: study with an average five-year follow-up. J Bone Joint Surg [Am] 2007;89:1948-1954.
22. Sah AP, Scott RD. Lateral unicompartmental knee arthroplasty through a medial approach: surgical technique. J Bone Joint Surg [Am] 2008;90(Suppl 2 Pt 2):195-205.
23. Argenson JN, Parratte S, Bertani A, et al. Long-term results with a lateral unicondylar replacement. Clin Orthop Relat Res 2008;(466): 2686-2693.

SECTION 5
Patella and Hybrid Options

CHAPTER 20
Patellofemoral Arthroplasty: Indications and Outcomes

Jeffrey H. DeClaire

KEY POINTS

- Initial management of patellofemoral arthritis will consist of conservative measures, including appropriate physical therapy to restore patellofemoral mechanics, nonsteroidal anti-inflammatory medications combined with injection treatment, weight reduction, and activity modification. When nonsurgical treatment is ineffective and pain becomes disabling, surgical alternatives may be considered.
- Patellofemoral arthroplasty and total knee arthroplasty remain the most predictable treatment alternatives for isolated degenerative arthritis of the patellofemoral joint. With the development of new implant designs and improved surgical technique, patellofemoral arthroplasty can provide a more conservative approach with the ability to retain the medial and lateral menisci, as well as the anterior and posterior cruciate ligaments.
- Appropriate patient selection remains the key factor in achieving high long-term success rates with patellofemoral arthroplasty. The procedure can be considered in patients with primary end-stage osteoarthritis, isolated to the patellofemoral joint. In addition, patients with posttraumatic degenerative arthritis or advanced chondromalacia of either the patellar surface, trochlear surface, or both can also be considered candidates for patellofemoral arthroplasty.
- Patellofemoral arthroplasty is contraindicated in patients with any evidence of tibiofemoral arthritis or advanced chondromalacia in the medial or lateral compartments.
- The surgical technique for patellofemoral arthroplasty is slightly different than that used in total knee arthroplasty.
- Because most patients with patellofemoral arthritis will have preexisting quadriceps insufficiency, it is extremely important to begin the development of the quadriceps muscle preoperatively.

INTRODUCTION

Osteoarthritis limited to the patellofemoral joint has been a disabling condition for many patients, and a very challenging clinical entity to treat. The incidence of isolated patellofemoral arthritis has continued to increase and will continue to create greater demands for more definitive treatment options.[1] Davies and colleagues reported in a radiologic study that isolated patellofemoral arthritis was found in 9.2% of 206 knees in 174 consecutive patients older than 40 years of age.[2] Another study by McAlindon and associates found that as many as 24% of women and 11% of men over the age of 55 with symptomatic knee arthritis had isolated degenerative arthritis of the patellofemoral articulation.[3] Initial management of patellofemoral arthritis will consist of conservative measures, including appropriate physical therapy to restore patellofemoral mechanics, nonsteroidal anti-inflammatory medications combined with injection treatment, weight reduction, and activity modification. When nonsurgical treatment is ineffective and pain becomes disabling, surgical alternatives may be considered.

Nonarthroplasty options for patellofemoral arthrosis have typically provided incomplete relief, with short-term fair to good results in 20–75% of patients. Arthroscopy with débridement and marrow stimulation procedures have had limited short-term results, with only 40–60% of patients with satisfactory results.[4] Osteochondral allograft procedures, autologous chondrocyte implantation, with or without tibial tubercle osteotomy, have also had inconsistent success, with unsatisfactory short-term results reported as high as 25–30%.[5,6] Although patellectomy has been considered a surgical alternative, it results in significant alteration of the patellofemoral biomechanics and will significantly decrease both the quadriceps force and the extensor moment arm. Experimentally, this has been shown to reduce extension power by 25–60%, which can require an increase in quadriceps force of 15–30% to achieve adequate extension torque.[7,8] Extension lag and decreased knee flexion after patellectomy are common and are frequently associated with residual knee pain and instability resulting in a failure rate as high as 45%.[9] In addition, tibiofemoral joint reactive forces have been shown to increase as much as 250% after patellectomy, which therefore will increase the risk of progressive degenerative arthritis of the tibiofemoral joint space.[10]

Patellofemoral arthroplasty and total knee arthroplasty continue to remain the most predictable treatment alternatives for isolated degenerative arthritis of the patellofemoral joint. Although total knee arthroplasty is a successful treatment option for some patients, it may not be desirable in all patients.[11] Patellofemoral arthroplasty can provide a more conservative approach, and it may be more appropriate in the properly selected patient. In contrast to total knee arthroplasty, patellofemoral arthroplasty will address only the affected area of pathology, with the ability to preserve the tibiofemoral joint space, medial and lateral menisci, and both the anterior and posterior cruciate ligaments. More normal knee kinematics and physiologic motion can therefore be preserved with patellofemoral arthroplasty. With the development of new implant designs, and improved surgical technique, more consistent and predictable clinical success can be achieved.

INDICATIONS/CONTRAINDICATIONS

In the past, success with patellofemoral arthroplasty has been inconsistent and unpredictable. This has largely been related to poor implant design, lack of good surgical instrumentation, and poor patient selection. Appropriate patient selection remains the key factor in achieving high long-term success rates with patellofemoral arthroplasty. The procedure can be considered in patients with primary end-stage osteoarthritis, isolated to the patellofemoral joint. In addition, patients with posttraumatic degenerative arthritis or advanced chondromalacia of either the patellar surface, trochlear surface, or both can also be considered candidates for patellofemoral arthroplasty. Patellar or trochlear dysplasia can also be successfully treated with patellofemoral arthroplasty. Slight tilt or subluxation observed on preoperative tangential radiographs can successfully be treated with patellofemoral arthroplasty. It is extremely important to address any patellar malalignment abnormalities, either preoperatively or intraoperatively. Patellar instability or chronic recurrent patellar dislocation is considered a contraindication to patellofemoral arthroplasty unless the condition has been successfully treated prior to surgery.[12] It is important to understand that patellofemoral arthroplasty is a resurfacing procedure and will not correct any preexisting rotational or angular malalignment of the knee. This is a unique difference from total knee arthroplasty in that patellofemoral arthroplasty will not correct or change the mechanical or anatomic axis, as well as femoral or tibial rotation. Preoperative alignment assessment is also critical in determining the likelihood for the future development of degenerative arthritis of the tibiofemoral joint space and/or patellar maltracking, subluxation, and dislocation.

Patellofemoral arthroplasty is contraindicated in patients with any evidence of tibiofemoral arthritis or advanced chondromalacia. This is important to identify preoperatively, as the most common cause for long-term failure, or the need for conversion of patellofemoral arthroplasty to total knee arthroplasty, is progressive degenerative arthritis of the tibiofemoral joint space.[13] In addition, uncorrected patellar instability combined with severe patellofemoral malalignment will present an increased risk for early failure and usually is best treated with total knee arthroplasty.[14] More recent emerging technology has allowed for chondral abnormalities of the medial or lateral femoral condyles to be addressed simultaneously at the time of patellofemoral arthroplasty.[15] Clinical experience, however, is limited at this time and such combined procedures should be used only in carefully selected clinical conditions. Patellofemoral arthroplasty is also not appropriate in patients with inflammatory arthritis or chondral calcinosis of the weight-bearing surfaces of the tibiofemoral joint space or menisci. Patients with chronic anterior knee pain that cannot be directly attributed to the patellofemoral joint space are also poor candidates for this procedure. It is also very important that the patient has realistic expectations regarding the extent of pain relief, the duration of recovery, and the allowable postoperative activities following patellofemoral arthroplasty in order to achieve high success rates.

Patellofemoral arthroplasty has been found to be most suitable for the younger or middle-aged patient (55–60 years), providing a more definitive resolution without the need for performing a total knee arthroplasty.[16] Typically, the younger patients have been told to live with their severe disability because they were "too young" for total knee arthroplasty as the only option. It is difficult to recommend the sacrifice of both the medial and lateral compartments, as well as the anterior cruciate ligament and the posterior cruciate ligament, to treat the arthritic patellofemoral compartment if an equally successful and less destructive alternative can be found. Patellofemoral arthroplasty can therefore offer a reasonable treatment option for patients with severe disabling degenerative arthritis isolated to the patellofemoral joint, yet who are too young for total knee arthroplasty, as well as being a less destructive option for the older patient. In the appropriately selected patient, long-term survivorship has been reported as high as 98% with an average follow-up of 17 years.[17] It can also be utilized as an interim step when total knee arthroplasty may not be the ideal treatment option due to age or other clinical circumstances.[16] Conversion of patellofemoral arthroplasty to total knee arthroplasty has been shown by several authors to be equally successful as primary total knee arthroplasty without the need for bone grafting, special augments, or a varus-valgus constrained revision knee implant.[17] Older patients (60–85 years) are also good candidates, as this can provide a more conservative and less invasive approach than total knee arthroplasty.[12,18]

CLINICAL EVALUATION AND PREOPERATIVE PLANNING

A full preoperative evaluation should be undertaken, including a very detailed history and physical examination to verify that the symptoms and clinical findings are isolated to the patellofemoral joint. The history should focus on any elements of prior patellar instability with previous history of recurrent subluxation and/or dislocation. It is extremely important that the symptomatology be localized to the anterior compartment of the knee, and that it originates from the degenerative process of the chondral surfaces of the patellofemoral joint, and is not related to the peripatellar soft tissue structures. Many times these patients will have had prior surgical procedures, with arthroscopy being the most common surgical intervention performed. This sometimes may include lateral release, chondroplasty, and prior realignment procedures. Pain should be primarily isolated to the patellofemoral joint and will frequently be associated with retropatellar crepitus. Patellofemoral pain is often exacerbated by activities such as stair climbing, rising from a chair, sitting with the knee flexed, squatting, and walking on uneven ground. Leslie and Bentley have found that the clinical triad of quadriceps wasting greater than 2 cm, chronic effusion, and retropatellar crepitance are the best physical predictors of articular cartilage breakdown of the patellofemoral joint.[19]

Physical examination should also include a full assessment of the ligament structures to rule out any associated instabilities. Retropatellar crepitance and associated effusion are common, as well as retropatellar pain with squatting. Any associated medial or lateral joint line tenderness should be a suspicion for possible diffuse involvement of the cartilage chondral breakdown and/or the possibility for meniscal pathology. Peripatellar soft tissue causes for pain should also be thoroughly evaluated, such as pesanserine bursitis, medial and lateral retinacular tendinitis, prepatellar bursitis, patellar tendinitis, or referred pain from the back or ipsilateral hip. Careful assessment of patellar alignment, including assessment of the Q angle and patellar tracking, is also extremely important. As mentioned previously, minor patellar tilt or subluxation can typically be addressed preoperatively or intraoperatively; however, significant patellar malalignment with elements of recurrent dislocation and subluxation should be considered a contraindication to this procedure. There are limited data in the literature regarding the performance of patellofemoral arthroplasty and patellar realignment simultaneously. Anterior or posterior cruciate ligament insufficiency is not a contraindication to patellofemoral arthroplasty; however, cruciate ligament reconstruction should be addressed prior to patellofemoral arthroplasty to reduce the risk of anterior knee pain and instability. This is also important in order to preserve the articular cartilage and meniscal structures within the tibiofemoral joint space.

Standing weight-bearing radiographs are essential for evaluation of the femorotibial joint space; these should include a standing bilateral anteroposterior view, a 45° flexion posteroanterior view, and lateral and skyline views[20] (**Fig. 20–1**). A long-leg standing weight-bearing (1.37 cm) axial alignment radiograph is also necessary to further evaluate the anatomic and mechanical axis of the knee (**Fig. 20–2**). Mild changes of the tibiofemoral joint space may be accepted; however, if there are any concerns for early degeneration of the chondral surface of the medial or lateral compartments, or associated meniscal pathology, then further evaluation is required either arthroscopically or at the time of surgery. Lateral radiographs are helpful in demonstrating degenerative changes of the patellofemoral joint but more useful for the assessment of patella alta or patella baja. Tangential radiographic views or skyline views are helpful in confirming the presence of severe degenerative change of the patellofemoral joint, but sometimes may not accurately identify the severity of the degeneration. It is not uncommon to observe some apparent joint space preservation with minimal or no osteophytes in the presence of severe articular cartilage loss (**Fig. 20–3**).

Arthroscopic evaluation has been helpful in this setting when there are questions as to the severity and degree of cartilage degeneration, as well as any other concerns for intra-articular pathology (**Fig. 20–4**). The clinical success of arthroscopy for isolated osteoarthritis of the patellofemoral joint has been unpredictable, but it can have value in evaluating the severity of the chondral change if this is not clearly defined on the preoperative radiographic evaluation, or there is uncertainty for the indication to perform a patellofemoral arthroplasty. Other areas of concern, such as early degeneration of the tibiofemoral joint space and meniscal pathology, may also be evaluated at the time of arthroscopic evaluation. This evaluation is extremely critical, as this will certainly play into the future prognosis and long-term success of patellofemoral arthroplasty. Photographs from prior arthroscopic treatment can also be of extreme value in a thorough evaluation of the knee to validate whether the degenerative process is isolated to the patellofemoral joint.

Preoperative education and physical therapy are also extremely helpful in the success of patellofemoral arthroplasty. Many of these patients will have significant quadriceps atrophy because of long-standing knee pain and altered

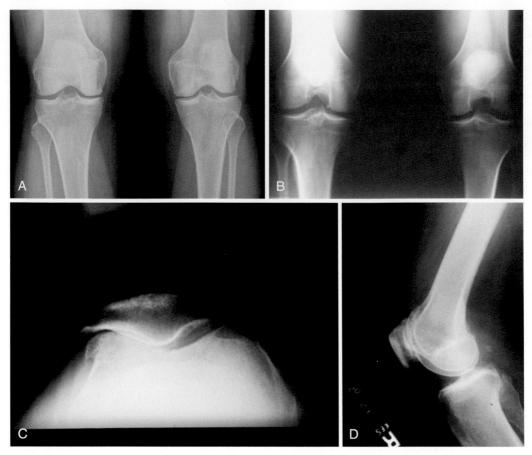

Figure 20-1 Standing anteroposterior **(A)**, bilateral standing 45° midflexion **(B)**, sunrise **(C)**, and lateral **(D)** views showing isolated patellofemoral arthritis.

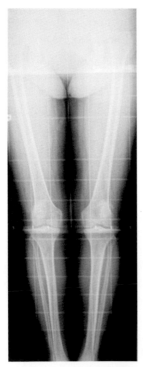

Figure 20-2 The long-leg standing weight-bearing axial alignment view is critical in evaluating the anatomic and mechanical axis of the knee.

patellofemoral mechanics. Reestablishment of appropriate quadriceps strength prior to surgical intervention will significantly improve the postoperative recovery.

SURGICAL TECHNIQUE

Setup and Equipment

The procedure is approached in a manner similar to that of total knee arthroplasty, utilizing general or regional anesthesia. A short-acting spinal anesthetic with light sedation is preferable, as this will allow for a more successful approach with pain management. This has also been very beneficial in initiating early weight bearing and recovery of quadriceps muscle function within hours after the procedure. After induction of anesthesia, the patient is positioned in the supine position, with a small bolster placed at the foot of the bed to allow for knee flexion between 70° and 90° (**Fig. 20–5**). Hyperflexion is not necessary and can sometimes hinder the exposure of the distal femur. The surgical instrumentation is relatively simple and follows the same principles as total knee arthroplasty (**Fig. 20–6**). Intramedullary instrumentation is used for the anterior femoral resection, followed by preparation of the trochlea with a simple motorized rasp.

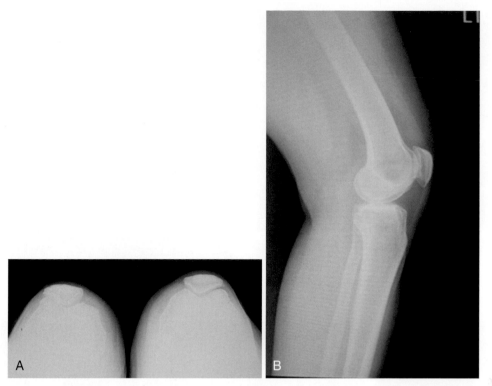

Figure 20-3 **(A)** Bilateral sunrise view of a 54-year-old female with isolated patellofemoral degenerative arthritis of the left knee with some preservation of the joint space. **(B)** Lateral view of the same patient.

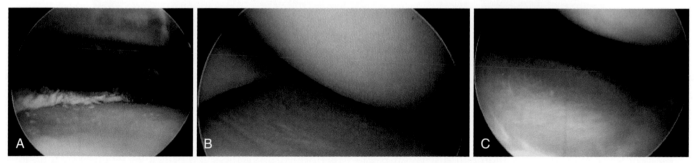

Figure 20-4 **(A)** Arthroscopic view of the patellofemoral joint of the patient in Figure 20-3 revealing severe grade IV degenerative changes on both the patellar and trochlear surfaces. **(B)** Arthroscopic view of the medial compartment of the same patient revealing intact articular surfaces and a normal medial meniscus. **(C)** Arthroscopic view of the lateral compartment showing a normal lateral meniscus and normal articular cartilage.

Technical Description

The surgical exposure for patellofemoral arthroplasty is slightly different than that used in total knee arthroplasty. Care must be taken to evaluate, observe, and protect the normal anatomy throughout the procedure. The skin incision is made just medial to the midline in order to minimize problems with point-loading during kneeling[20] (**Fig. 20–7**). The incision should extend from approximately 1–2 cm above the superior pole of the patella to just 1 cm below the joint line. It is not necessary to extend the incision distally as much as would be performed in a total knee arthroplasty as most of

the exposure will focus on the anterior and distal femur. The joint capsule and synovium can be opened using a standard short medial patellar arthrotomy or a midvastus approach (**Fig. 20–8**). A small mini-arthrotomy is ideal, as this will facilitate exposure for referencing the anterior cortex during the procedure. Care is taken to minimize resection of the fat pad and be cautious of the anterior horn of the lateral and medial menisci, as well as the intermeniscal ligament.

Prior to proceeding with the patellofemoral arthroplasty, it is important to perform a thorough inspection of the entire joint to make certain there are still appropriate indications

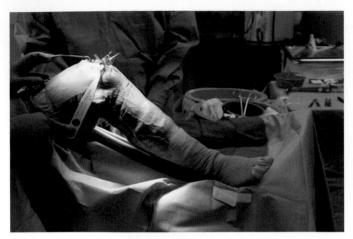

Figure 20-5 Patient positioning with knee flexion between 70° and 90°.

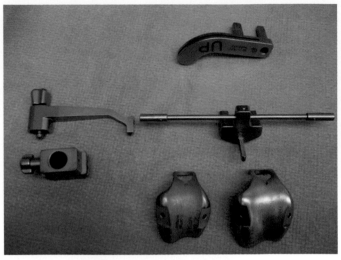

Figure 20-6 Surgical instrumentation.

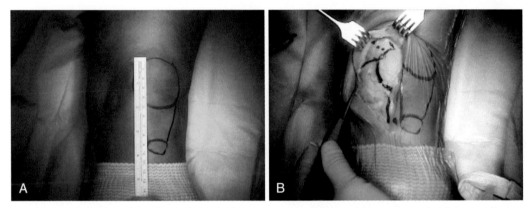

Figure 20-7 **(A)** An anteromedial skin incision is made beginning 1-2 cm proximal to the superior pole of the patella extending to just below the joint line. **(B)** The deep fascial layer is exposed for either a midvastus or medial arthrotomy.

for the procedure (**Fig. 20–9**). A thorough discussion prior to surgery is essential in order to prepare the patient that, if significant degenerative changes are noted in the medial or lateral weight-bearing areas or any other significant pathology is identified, a total knee arthroplasty can be performed simultaneously. If a femoral condylar defect is noted in addition to isolated patellofemoral arthritis, then an osteochondral plug can be harvested from the relatively healthy area of the trochlea or from the intercondylar notch (**Fig. 20–10**). It is important to assess the size of the condylar defect, as there is still limited clinical experience with this combined approach, keeping in mind that progressive degeneration of the femorotibial joint space can be the cause of short-term failure.

With the leg in full extension, resection of the patella can be performed first in order to facilitate the exposure of the distal femur for preparation of the trochlea. This will also avoid eversion of the patella, which will minimize the soft tissue trauma to the extensor mechanism. Patellar resection is performed using the same principles followed in total knee arthroplasty, with a measured resection approach. Using a towel clip, the patella can be easily everted and stabilized for preparation (**Fig. 20–11**). Removing the surrounding synovial tissue from the periphery of the patella is helpful in accurately identifying the level of resection. If necessary, the infrapatellar fat pad can be partially excised to also facilitate exposure. Once the periphery of the patella is cleared of synovial tissue to define its margins, a measured resection can be performed. As in total knee arthroplasty, it is extremely important to restore the native patellar thickness to avoid overstuffing the patellofemoral joint, which can affect patellar articulation, patellar tracking, and range of motion. The patella should be measured using calipers in all four quadrants in order to retain the normal patellar height in the most accurate manner, and to avoid an oblique level of resection (**Fig. 20–12**). Transverse patellar osteotomy can be performed utilizing a freehand method or instrument method, depending on the surgeon's

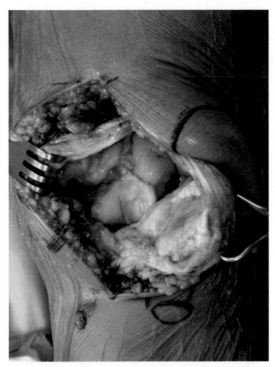

Figure 20-8 The arthrotomy is performed, taking care not to incise the articular cartilage, the medial or lateral menisci, or the transverse intermeniscal ligament.

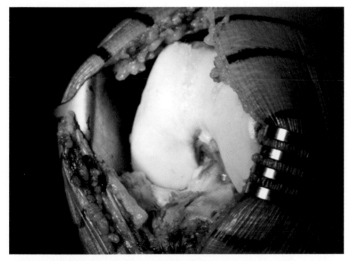

Figure 20-9 A thorough evaluation of the entire joint is performed to verify preservation of the articular cartilage of the medial and lateral compartments, the medial and lateral menisci, and the anterior and posterior cruciate ligaments.

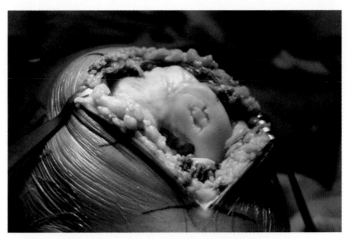

Figure 20-10 Osteochondral defect identified on the medial femoral condyle that can be treated with autogenous osteochondral grafting. An osteochondral donor plug can be harvested from a healthy area of the unaffected trochlea.

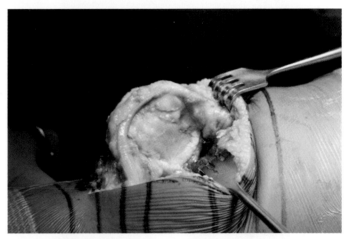

Figure 20-11 With the leg in full extension, the patella can be prepared first by using a towel clip to evert and stabilize the patella. Removal of the peripatellar synovium from the periphery of the patella can more accurately identify the appropriate level of resection.

preference (**Fig. 20–13**). The resection level should be parallel, and once again, assessment should be made with the caliper in all four quadrants to avoid the risk of an oblique cut, which could contribute to patellar mal-tracking (**Fig. 20–14**). Sizing of the patella can then be performed in the usual manner, taking care to medialize the patella to enhance patellar tracking (**Fig. 20–15**). If there is a portion of the lateral patellar facet not covered by the patellar component, removal of this bone should be performed in order to avoid any potential source of impingement, which may occur during articulation (**Fig. 20–16**). The thickness of the patella should then be reassessed following insertion of the prosthetic component trial. Ideally the goal is to have the thickness of the remaining patella and the patellar prosthesis equal to the appropriate patellar thickness.

Once the patella has been appropriately prepared, it can be easily displaced into the lateral gutter, thereby avoiding eversion of the patella with much less surgical trauma or injury to the quadriceps extensor mechanism. A custom-designed patellar retractor has been developed to facilitate the

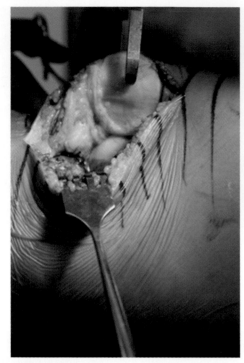

Figure 20-12 Patellar thickness is measured with the caliper, with assessment of both the medial and lateral facets.

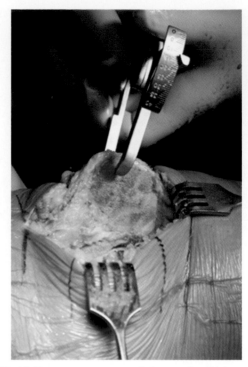

Figure 20-14 Repeat assessment of the patellar thickness is made following resection to verify appropriate thickness and symmetric resection of bone.

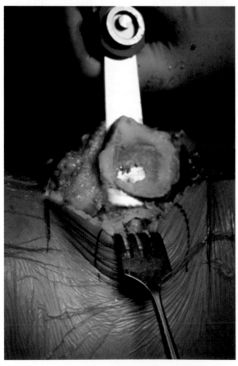

Figure 20-13 Transverse osteotomy can be performed using a freehand technique or instrumented method, depending on the surgeon's preference.

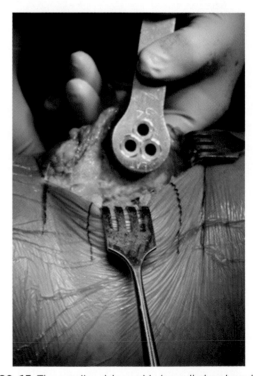

Figure 20-15 The patellar sizing guide is applied and medialized for improved patellar tracking. Three lug holes are drilled that are standardized to allow for interchangeability of the component for determining the exact size.

retraction of the patella, as well as protect the resected surface throughout the procedure (**Fig. 20–17**). The knee is then flexed and held in a position between 70° and 90° of flexion. It is important to note that hyperflexion should be avoided as this can cause greater difficulties with exposure of the distal femur due to the increased tension that is applied across the extensor mechanism the further the knee is flexed. A drill hole is made into the center of the intercondylar notch, in the

trochlear groove, approximately 1–2 cm anterior to the roof of the intercondylar notch (**Fig. 20–18**). Marrow elements are suctioned in order to minimize the risk of fat embolization when the fluted intramedullary rod is inserted for placement of the anterior cutting guide. The intramedullary rod is inserted and securely anchored to the distal femur (**Fig. 20–19**). The patellofemoral alignment guide block is then inserted over the intramedullary rod with the arrow of the guide block pointing toward the knee. The rotational alignment for the anterior resection can be achieved using Whiteside's line, as exposure of the medial and lateral epicondyles can sometimes be difficult (**Fig. 20–20**). If adequate exposure has been obtained, the transepicondylar axis can also be used, positioning the handles of the alignment rod parallel to the epicondylar axis (**Fig. 20–21**). It is important to note that there should be no additional external rotation added to the alignment of the anterior resection, keeping in mind that this is a resurfacing procedure, which is not designed to correct rotational or angular alignment. The alignment guide block is then secured in place to the intramedullary rod using the small fixation knob. Femoral rotation has now been set, and the patellofemoral alignment rod can be removed. The anterior resection guide is then inserted with appropriate referencing of the anterior cortex in order to provide a minimal amount of bone resection (**Fig. 20–22**). An angel wing can also

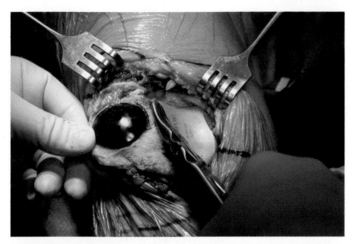

Figure 20-16 Excess bone from the lateral facet is removed to avoid a potential source of bone impingement.

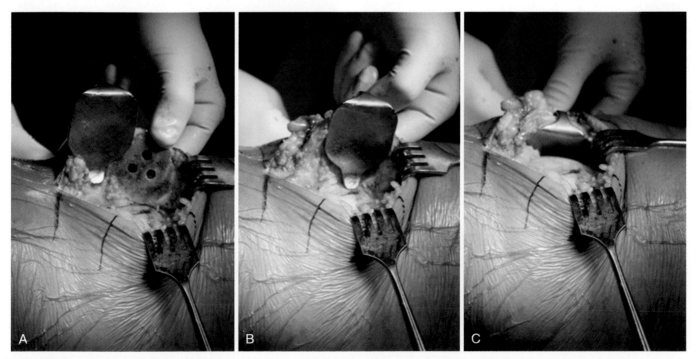

Figure 20-17 (A) A custom-designed patellar retractor is used to protect the resected patellar surface and to facilitate displacement of the patella into the lateral gutter for exposure of the distal femur. **(B and C)** The patellar surface is protected and displaced into the lateral gutter without eversion.

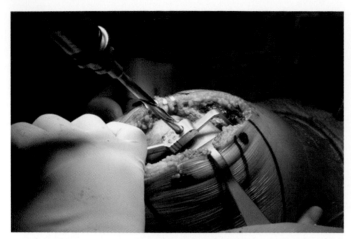

Figure 20-18 The intramedullary drill hole is made 1-2 cm above the roof of the intercondylar notch centered in the trochlear groove.

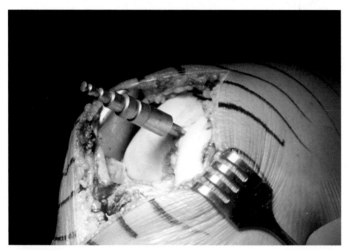

Figure 20-19 The intramedullary rod is inserted and securely anchored to the distal femur.

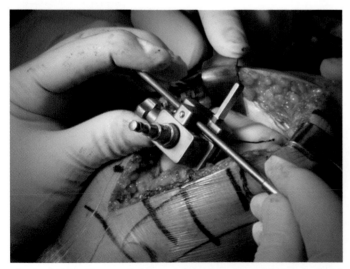

Figure 20-20 The patellofemoral alignment guide block is inserted over the intramedullary rod. The rotational alignment is established by referencing Whiteside's line or the transepicondylar axis.

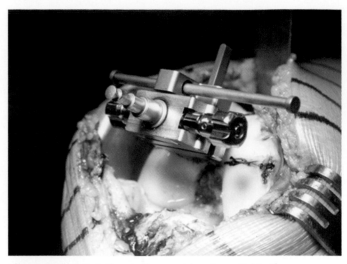

Figure 20-21 Rotational alignment is set parallel to the transepicondylar axis using the alignment rod.

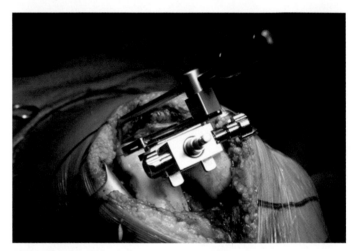

Figure 20-22 Depth of resection of the anterior femur is established by referencing the most prominent point of the lateral femur. This allows for a very conservative level of bone resection.

be used as a secondary reference to help ensure that the implant will sit flush once the anterior resection has been made without risk for notching. The anterior cut is then made through the slot in the resecting guide using an oscillating saw in the usual manner (**Fig. 20–23**).

Once the anterior resection has been made, correct femoral component sizing can then be performed utilizing the trial templates (**Fig. 20–24**). It is extremely important to achieve maximum coverage of the anterior femur. The largest femoral component should therefore be used in order to create complete coverage of the anterior femur without medial or lateral overhang. Once the appropriate size has been chosen, the intercondylar notch portion of the trial component can be outlined with methylene blue to correctly identify the cartilage to be resected (**Fig. 20–25**). Using a conical or a motorized

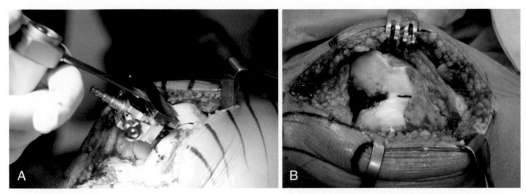

Figure 20-23 (A) An oscillation saw is used to resect the anterior femur at the appropriate level with the correct rotation. **(B)** The depth of resection of the anterior femur should be assessed and should be flush with the anterior cortex of the femur.

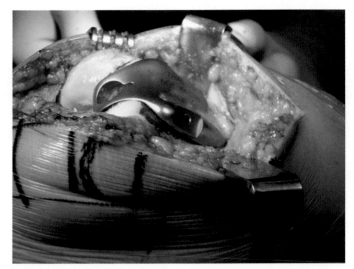

Figure 20-24 Correct femoral component sizing is performed utilizing the trial templates. The largest femoral component should be used to achieve maximum coverage of the anterior femur without creating overhang of the component.

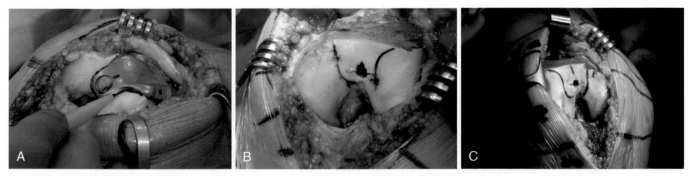

Figure 20-25 (A-C) Methylene blue is used to outline the intercondylar notch area to identify the area of articular cartilage to be removed.

rasp, the articular cartilage can be removed in the designated area of the trochlear groove to accommodate the implant (**Fig. 20–26**). It is important to note that only minimal rasping is required, so as not to inset the intercondylar portion of the implant to the bone. The implant is designed as an onlay prosthesis, and therefore will fit 1–2 mm proud of the intercondylar bone surface. This is a critical point, as this prosthesis will allow the patellar component to articulate with the femoral component without contacting the articular cartilage during flexion. This has been one of the concerns with long-term success, as early articular erosion has been identified with other implant designs. Multiple cement fixation drill holes are made to assure appropriate cement penetration for component fixation (**Fig. 20–27**). Using the trial template, the drill hole is then created to accommodate the central peg of the prosthetic component (**Fig. 20–28**). Trial reduction can then be performed

to make certain that restoration of normal patellofemoral mechanics and alignment has been achieved (**Fig. 20–29**). There should be no evidence of patellar tilt or subluxation throughout the full range of motion with the usual "no-touch technique" as utilized in total knee arthroplasty. If any increase in patellar tilt or mild subluxation is identified, this can be addressed successfully by performing a lateral release. With appropriate patient selection and surgical technique, proximal realignment at the time of surgery should be unnecessary in most cases and ideally identified preoperatively.

Preparation of the anterior femoral surface as well as the patellar surface can then be made in the usual manner before application of bone cement and implantation of the patellofemoral component. Cement is applied to both the trochlear component and the prepared surface of the femur to assure adequate cement penetration (**Fig. 20–30**). Manual pressure is

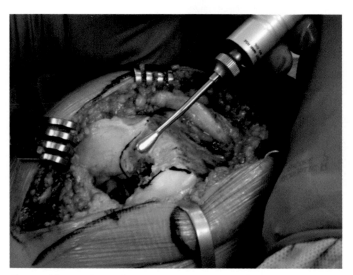

Figure 20-26 The articular cartilage of the trochlea is removed with a conical rasp or a motorized rasp to expose the subchondral bone. This requires only a minimal amount of rasping as the implant is designed as an onlay prosthesis.

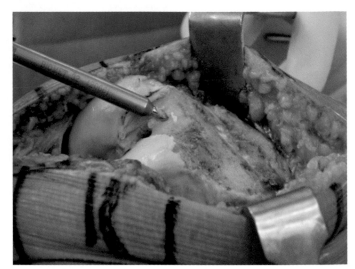

Figure 20-27 Multiple cement fixation drill holes are made in the subchondral bone of the trochlea to assure appropriate cement penetration.

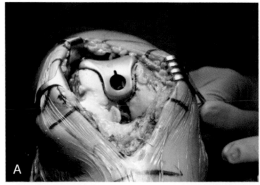
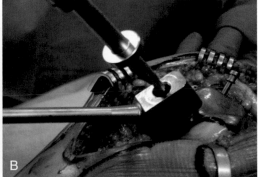

Figure 20-28 With the trial template secured to the femur **(A)**, the drill hole is created to accommodate the central peg of the trochlear component **(B)**.

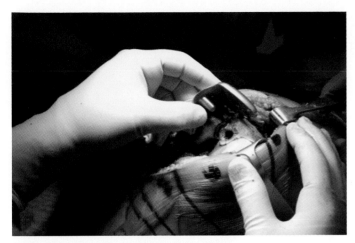

Figure 20-29 Trial reduction can be performed to assure appropriate patellar tracking and alignment using a "no-touch technique." Any residual lateral tilt or subluxation can be addressed at this time.

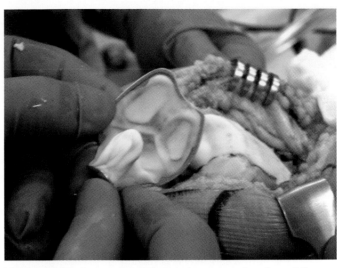

Figure 20-30 Cement is applied to the prepared surface of the femur with digital pressurization to assure adequate cement penetration. It is also applied to the undersurface of the prosthesis and the central peg.

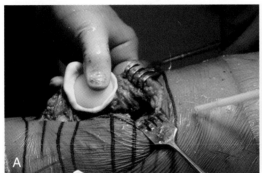

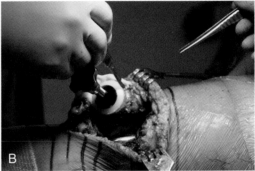

Figure 20-31 (A) The patella is prepared in a similar manner with meticulous attention to the removal of all cement to avoid any possibility of third body wear. **(B)** Patella preparation is completed with pressurization of the bone cement using a patellar clamp until the cement cures.

applied to the trochlear component, while a patellar clamp is used for the patellar component until the cement cures (**Fig. 20–31**). Meticulous attention to detail is important in order to remove all excreted cement and avoid any possibility of third body wear. Final assessment for patellar alignment and tracking can then be made, followed by thorough lavage of the wound and standard closure of the arthrotomy, as well as the subcutaneous layer and a subcuticular closure of the skin (**Fig. 20–32**). The unique design of this component with a central peg eliminates any concerns for the transitional area into the notch that can sometimes cause impingement or interfere with tracking of the patella in deep flexion (**Fig. 20–33**). Postoperative radiographs are performed in order to confirm appropriate implant position and alignment (**Fig. 20–34**).

POSTSURGICAL FOLLOW-UP

Because most patients with patellofemoral arthritis will have preexisting quadriceps insufficiency, it is extremely important to begin the development of the quadriceps muscle preoperatively. Appropriate pain management is essential in the early postoperative phase in order to restore quadriceps function and to prevent shutdown of the extensor mechanism. Intra-articular injection performed at the time of surgery with a "pain cocktail" has been helpful in minimizing pain in the early postoperative phase[21] (**Fig. 20–35**). Quadriceps isometric exercises, straight leg raises, and range-of-motion exercises are started immediately on the day of surgery. The use of a continuous passive motion machine is helpful during the hospitalization, but may not be necessary

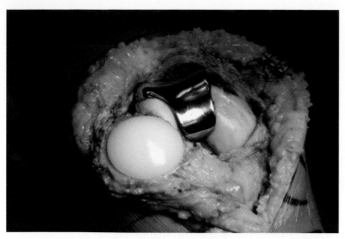

Figure 20-32 Final intraoperative view of the patellofemoral prosthesis showing appropriate alignment of the components. Notice the preservation of the fat pad and the minimal exposure of the tibial-femoral joint space.

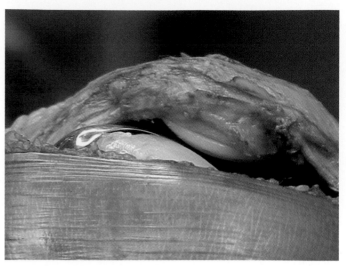

Figure 20-33 Patellofemoral articulation showing appropriate alignment and patellar tracking with a "no-touch technique." Also note that the patellar component does not articulate with the articular cartilage in deep flexion.

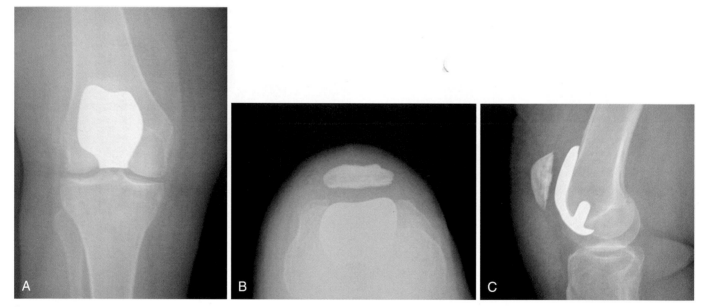

Figure 20-34 Postoperative weight-bearing anteroposterior **(A)**, sunrise **(B)**, and lateral **(C)** radiographs showing accurate alignment and positioning of the components.

for all patients. Full weight bearing is permitted immediately, and patients are encouraged to begin weight bearing on the day of surgery with the use of crutches, walker, or a cane. Ketorolac (Toradol) 15 mg intravenously has been extremely helpful in controlling the inflammatory response when given preoperatively, in addition to every 6 hours for the first 24 hours postoperatively, in patients without allergy to nonsteroidal anti-inflammatories. Thromboembolism prophylaxis is used similar to that for total knee arthroplasty, with warfarin (Coumadin) being utilized during the hospital stay. The majority of patients will continue with enteric-coated aspirin (325 mg twice daily) for 4–6 weeks, unless there is an increased risk for thromboembolism or increased bleeding tendency where aspirin cannot be utilized. In these situations, warfarin is used for 2 weeks. Intravenous antibiotics are used for the first 24 hours in order to prevent infection. When quadriceps strength returns, patients are allowed to progress with unrestricted activities, with recommendation to avoid excessive loading and deep flexion, and high-impact activities.

Table 20-1	Clinical Results of Patellofemoral Arthroplasty (PFA)			
Series	Average Age	No. of PFAs	Implant Design	Follow-up
Argenson et al. (1995)	57 (range, 19-82)	66	Autocentric	84% good to excellent 5.5 yr (range, 2-10 yr)
Kooijman et al. (2003)	50 (range, 20-77)	45	Richards II	86% good to excellent 17 yr (range, 15-21 yr)
Lonner et al.	44 (range, 28-59)	25	Avon trochlea, Nexgen patella	96% good to excellent 6 mo (1 mo to 1 yr)
Ackroyd et al. (2007)	NA	109	Avon	95.8% good to excellent 5.2 yr (range, 5-8 yr)
Cartier et al. (2005)	65 (range, 23-89)	72	Richards I & II	85% good to excellent 4 yr (range, 2-12 yr)
Blazina et al. (1979)	39 (range, 19-81)	57	Richards I & II	85% good to excellent 2 yr (range, 8-42 mo)
Arciero et al.	62 (range, 33-86)	25	Richards II CSF-Wright	85% good to excellent 5.3 yr (range, 3-9 yr)
Smith et al. (2002)	72 (range, 42-86)	45	Lubinus	69% good to excellent 4 yr (range, 2-6 yr)
Merchant et al. (2004)	49 (range, 30-81)	15	LCS	93% good to excellent 3.8 yr (range, 2.3-5.5 yr)

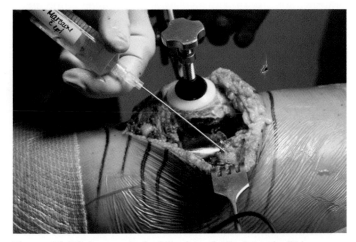

Figure 20-35 Intra-articular injection of a "pain cocktail" is performed prior to closure. Both the deep capsular layer and the subcutaneous layers are injected.

CLINICAL RESULTS

Inconsistent results for patellofemoral arthroplasty have been largely related to poor component design, lack of instrumentation, and poor patient selection. Many techniques relied on a freehand method of bone preparation, creating greater variability in component placement and depth of bony resection. New design concepts have been implemented to allow for a more accurate method of bone preparation with an instrumented technique and improved patient selection. Most studies have reported good to excellent results in approximately 80–90% of cases at short- and midterm follow-up (**Table 20–1**). McKeever, in 1955, was the first to describe good results following patellar resurfacing using a metal prosthesis

fixed with a screw.[22] Subsequently, other authors reported varied results using this technique. Blazina et al., in 1979, were the first to describe resurfacing of both the patella and trochlear surface.[23] Various publications over the years, however, have had success rates varying from 44% to 90%. Kooijman et al.[24] reported excellent or good results in 86% of cases with a mean follow-up of 17 years. In the patient group without ongoing tibiofemoral arthritis, the survivorship increased to 98%. In 1988, Arciero et al.[25] reported on 20 patellofemoral arthroplasties with 85% satisfactory results, and in 2006 Ackroyd et al. reported a 95.8% survivorship at 5 years' follow-up with no cases of failure of the prosthesis.[26] Poor component design and inconsistent patient selection criteria have also contributed to early failures of patellofemoral arthroplasty. Original descriptions of the procedure did not include strict inclusion criteria for patient selection, and had numerous technical pitfalls with little emphasis based on realignment of the extensor mechanism of the knee. Consequently, early designs showed disappointing results. Over the years, with the development of new implant designs, improved surgical instrumentation, and more accurate patient selection criteria, the clinical success of patellofemoral arthroplasty has improved significantly.[18]

When compared to total knee arthroplasty, patellofemoral arthroplasty has the potential advantage of retaining the menisci and the cruciate ligaments, and thereby retaining more natural kinematics of the knee joint with a less invasive procedure. The main reasons for early failure have been persistent malalignment, wear, impingement, and progressive degeneration of the tibiofemoral joint space. In the past 5 years, newer implant designs have been introduced that can more accurately reproduce patellofemoral joint function. Ackroyd et al. reported on 306 patellofemoral arthroplasties in 240 patients with a high level of pain relief and improved function. In 5 years of follow-up, there was no significant deterioration in function or progression of pain, and there were no late complications attributed to the arthroplasty.[26] Disease progression in the tibiofemoral joint space occurred in 14 patients (16 knees, 5%) requiring conversion in 10 of these patients (11 knees, 3.6%), and anterior knee pain was recorded in 14 knees (4%). There were no failures secondary to mechanical loosening. In 2006, Sisto and Sarin reported on 25 custom patellofemoral arthroplasties, with intention to recreate the patient's own anatomy and to address any inherent problems associated with designed implants.[27] Computed tomography scanning was utilized to construct a three-dimensional model of the patient's femoral groove, which then allowed for the creation of a cobalt chrome custom implant. Subsequent follow-up was 73 months (6 years), and all 25 implants were in place and functioning well. The Knee Society Functional Score was 89 points, and the Knee Society objective score was 91 points, with 18 excellent and 7 good results. No patient had required additional surgery or had component loosening.

Patellofemoral arthroplasty can produce consistently good-quality functional results in the appropriately selected patient with the major advantage of preservation of the tibiofemoral joint, as well as the medial and lateral menisci and cruciate ligaments. Early results with new prosthetic designs have been encouraging, with the ability to restore considerable improvement in function and range of motion, as well as significant decrease in pain. Patient selection for patellofemoral arthroplasty remains one of the key factors in achieving high success rates. Lonner, in 2004, showed that the results of patellofemoral arthroplasty can be optimized by accurate alignment and positioning of the prosthesis combined with appropriate balance of the soft tissue structures to enhance more normal patellar tracking. He noted that implant design may also play a factor in patellofemoral complications.[18] It is also important to note that the incidence of patellar complications was found to be reduced from 17% with a first-generation implant to 4% with a second-generation implant.

COMPLICATIONS

Early failure for patellofemoral arthroplasty has been primarily related to persistent pain secondary to patellar snapping and instability. Further surgical intervention sometimes is necessary, which may involve an arthroscopic approach or possibly revision surgery to improve soft tissue alignment and/or to revise the trochlear prosthesis. Many of these problems have been related to implant design features, as well as extensor mechanism malalignment that was not accurately identified

preoperatively. There has been a substantial improvement in contemporary design that has reduced the tendency for patellar maltracking or dysfunction due to the improvement in the prosthetic trochlear geometry. Soft tissue impingement resulting in residual anterior knee pain and/or patellar instability may occur in a small percentage of patients, and is similar in frequency to that seen in total knee arthroplasty. The long-term concerns of component subsidence, loosening, and polyethylene wear have been extremely uncommon, occurring in less than 1% of published cases combined. Component loosening of the trochlea has been more common in the cementless design. Progressive degenerative arthritis of the tibiofemoral joint space has been the most common cause for failure of patellofemoral arthroplasty, occurring in approximately 20% of knees at 15 years' follow-up. If revision to total knee arthroplasty is necessary, the procedure can be performed in a similar fashion as a standard primary total knee arthroplasty (**Fig. 20–36**). The all-polyethylene patellar component can usually be retained, and a standard total knee arthroplasty can be performed without the need for stems, augments, bone grafting, and use of a varus-valgus constrained component. The clinical outcomes following conversion to total knee arthroplasty have been encouraging, with clinical results comparable to those for primary total knee arthroplasty.[17]

TIPS AND PEARLS

- Patient selection remains the key factor in the success of patellofemoral arthroplasty. Accurate diagnosis confirming that the degenerative process is isolated to the patellofemoral joint is essential.
- Imaging studies should always include bilateral standing anteroposterior radiographs, as well as a 45° midflexion view to accurately assess the tibiofemoral joint space for any preexisting degenerative changes that may jeopardize the clinical outcome. Lateral and bilateral tangential views of the patellae are also critical.
- The use of arthroscopy can be very important in accurately determining the indications for patellofemoral arthroplasty. It can provide additional diagnostic capabilities to further evaluate the articular surfaces of the tibiofemoral joint space, the medial and lateral menisci, and the anterior and posterior cruciate ligaments. In addition, it will also provide a very accurate assessment of the severity of degeneration of the patellofemoral joint space.
- Patients with a high Q angle (more than 20° in females, 15° in males) or clinical evidence of patellar malalignment, subluxation, or dislocation should undergo surgical correction with tibial tubercle anteromedialization prior to or during patellofemoral

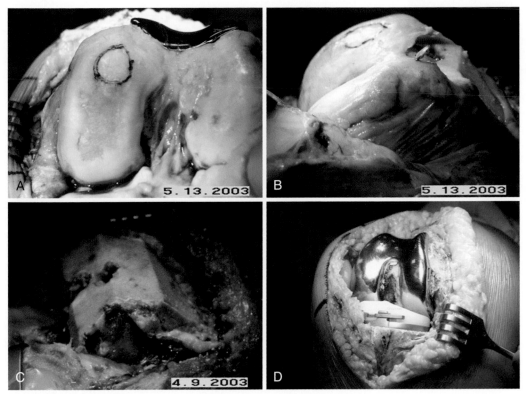

Figure 20-36 (A) A 52-year-old male with progressive degenerative arthritis of the tibial-femoral compartment 10 years after patellofemoral joint replacement. **(B)** View of the distal femur with the trochlear component removed without significant bone loss. **(C)** Final preparation of the distal femur. Note that the trochlear area is without bone loss, and is prepared in the usual manner for a primary cruciate-retained total knee arthroplasty. **(D)** Final implantation of a cruciate-retained total knee arthroplasty.

arthroplasty. Remember, patellofemoral arthroplasty will not correct any angular or rotational malalignment.

- Careful selection of implant design and instrumentation is important in the clinical success of patellofemoral arthroplasty. Conservative resection of bone and an anatomic transitional area in the intercondylar notch are important key factors. In general, onlay-type components are more applicable for all trochlear shapes, regardless of

trochlear dysplasia, and have a more predictable success rate with a lower incidence of patellar subluxation, patellar catching, and snapping than the inlay design.

- Preoperative physical therapy, combined with an early progressive postoperative rehabilitation program, focusing on restoring quadriceps muscle function, along with a preemptive multimodal pain management program, will greatly enhance early recovery.

REFERENCES

1. Kurtz S, Ong K, Lau E, et al. Projections of primary and revision hip and knee arthroplasty in the United States from 2005 to 2030. J Bone Joint Surg [Am] 2007;89:780-785.
2. Davies AP, Vince AS, Shepstone L, et al. The radiologic prevalence of patellofemoral osteoarthritis. Clin Orthop Relat Res 2002;(402):206-212.
3. McAlindon RE, Snow S, Cooper C, et al. Radiographic patterns of osteoarthritis of the knee joint in the community: the importance of the patellofemoral joint. Ann Rheum Dis 1992;51:844-849.
4. Federico DJ, Reider B. Results of isolated patellar debridement for patellofemoral pain in patients with normal patellar alignment. Am J Sports Med 1997;25:663-669.
5. Fulkerson JP. Anteromedialization of the tibial tubercle for patellofemoral malalignment. Clin Orthop Relat Res 1983;(177):176-181.
6. Minas T, Chiu R. Autologous chondrocyte implantation. Am J Knee Surg 2000;13:41-50.
7. Ackroyd CE, Polyzoides AJ. Patellectomy for osteoarthritis: a study of 81 patients followed from two to twenty-one years. J Bone Joint Surg [Br] 1978;60:353-357.
8. Kaufer H. Mechanical function of the patella. J Bone Joint Surg [Am] 1971;53:1151-1156.
9. Laskin RS, Palletta G. Total knee replacement in the patient who had undergone patellectomy. J Bone Joint Surg [Am] 1995;77:1708-1712.
10. Dinham JM, French PR. Results of patellectomy for osteoarthritis. Postgrad Med 1972;48:590.
11. Laskin RS, Van Steijn M. Total knee replacement for patients with patellofemoral arthritis. Clin Orthop Relat Res 1989;(367):89-95.
12. Grelsarner RP. Current concepts review: patellofemoral arthritis. J Bone Joint Surg [Am] 2006;188:1849-1859.

13. Lonner JH. Patellofemoral arthroplasty. *In* Lotke JL, Lonner JH (eds). Knee Arthroplasty, 3rd ed. Philadelphia: Lippincott Williams & Wilkins, 2009, pp 343-359.

14. Mont MA, Haas S, Mullick T, et al. Total knee arthroplasty for patellofemoral arthritis. J Bone Joint Surg [Am] 2002;84: 1977-1981.

15. Lonner JH, Mehta S, Booth RE. Ipsilateral patellofemoral arthroplasty and autogenous osteochondral femoral condylar transplantation. J Arthroplasty 2007;22:1103-1136.

16. Gioe TJ, Novak C, Sinner P, et al. Knee arthroplasty in the young patient: survival in a community registry. Clin Orthop Relat Res 2007;(464):83.

17. Lonner JH, Jasko JG, Booth RE. Revision of a failed patellofemoral arthroplasty to a total knee arthroplasty. J Bone Joint Surg [Am] 2006;88:2337-2342.

18. Lonner JH. Patellofemoral arthroplasty: the impact of design on outcomes. Orthop Clin North Am 2008;39:347-354.

19. Leslie IJ, Bentley G. Arthroscopy in the diagnosis of chondromalacia patellae. Ann Rheum Dis 1978;37:540-547.

20. Yacoubian SV, Scott RD. Skin incision translation in total knee arthroplasty: the difference between flexion and extension. J Arthroplasty 2007;22:353-355.

21. Busch CA, Shore BJ, Bhandari R, et al. Efficacy of periarticular multimodal drug injection in total knee arthroplasty: a randomized trial. J Bone Joint Surg [Am] 2006;88:949-963.

22. McKeever DC. Patellar prosthesis. J Bone Joint Surg [Am] 1955; 37:1074.

23. Blazina M, Fox JM, Deo Pizzo W, et al. Patellofemoral replacement. Clin Orthop Relat Res 1979;(144):98-102.

24. Kooijman HJ, Driessen APPM, van Horn JR. Long-term results of patellofemoral arthroplasty. J Bone Joint Surg [Br] 2003;85:836-840.

25. Arciero R, Toomey H. Patellofemoral arthroplasty: a three to nine year follow-up study. Clin Orthop Relat Res 1988;(236):60.

26. Ackroyd CE, Newman JF, Elderidge J, Webb M. The Avon patellofemoral arthroplasty: two to five year results. J Bone Joint Surg [Br] 2003;85(Suppl 11):162-163.

27. Sisto DJ, Sarin VK. Custom patellofemoral arthroplasty of the knee. J Bone Joint Surg [Am] 2006;88:1475-1480.

SUGGESTED READING

Carrier P, Sanouiller JL, Grelsamer R. Patellofemoral arthroplasty. J Arthroplasty 1990;5:49.

Fulkerson JP. Disorders of the Patellofemoral Joint. Baltimore: Williams & Wilkins, 1996.

Harrington KD. Long term results for the McKeever patellar resurfacing prosthesis used as a salvage procedure for severe chondromalacia patella. Clin Orthop Relat Res 1992;(279):201-213.

Hendrix MRG, Ackroyd CE, Lonner JH. Revision patellofemoral arthroplasty: 3-7 year follow-up. J Arthroplasty 2008;23:977-983.

Jackson RW, Kunkel SS, Taylor GJ. Lateral retinacular release for patellofemoral pain in the older patient. Arthroscopy 1991;7:283-286.

Krajca-Radcliffe JB, Coker TP. Patellofemoral arthroplasty: a 2 to 18 year follow-up study. Clin Orthop Relat Res 1996;(330):143.

Levitt RL. A long term evaluation of patellar prosthesis. Clin Orthop Relat Res 1973;(97):153-157.

Merchant AC. Early results with a total patellofemoral joint replacement arthroplasty prosthesis. J Arthroplasty 2004;19:829-836.

Rosenberg TD, Paulos LE, Parker RD, et al. The forty-five degree posteroanterior flexion weight-bearing radiograph of the knee. J Bone Joint Surg [Am] 1988;70:1479-1483.

Sisto DJ. Patellofemoral degenerative joint desease. *In* Fu FH, Harner DC, Vince K (eds). Knee Surgery. Baltimore: Williams & Wilkins, 1994, pp 1203-1221.

Tauro B, Ackroyd CE, Newman JH, et al. The Lubinus patellofemoral arthroplasty: a five to ten year prospective study. J Bone Joint Surg [Br] 2001;83:696.

CHAPTER 21
Long-Term Patellofemoral Progression

*Jared R.H. Foran, Neil P. Sheth, and Craig J. Della Valle**

KEY POINTS

- The natural history of the patellofemoral articulation after unicompartmental arthroplasty is poorly understood, and the majority of unicompartmental literature fails to adequately address and describe patellofemoral progression.
- The preoperative status of the patellofemoral articulation does not appear to affect the early to midterm results of Oxford mobile-bearing unicompartmental arthroplasty.
- The rate of long-term radiographic progression of patellofemoral degeneration is as high as 65%, but the majority of progression is low grade and rarely requires revision.
- Revision for patellofemoral progression appears to be less common than revision for adjacent tibiofemoral degeneration.
- Well-designed, long-term studies specifically addressing the clinical and radiographic progression of patellofemoral articulation are needed.

INTRODUCTION

Long-term survivorship of unicompartmental knee arthroplasty (UKA) is predicated on preoperative patient selection, obtaining proper limb alignment while avoiding overcorrection, and appropriate component position and sizing. An aspect of implant survivorship that is poorly understood is the natural history of arthritis progression in the adjacent tibiofemoral and/or patellofemoral compartments. However, one of the most common reasons cited for UKA failure is pain in one or more of the un-resurfaced compartments.[1] The incidence and sequelae of patellofemoral compartment degeneration following UKA has been incompletely delineated. The purpose of this chapter is to summarize the natural history of patellofemoral compartment degeneration, and to describe the contribution of this degeneration to the long-term survival of UKA.

PREEXISTING PATELLOFEMORAL ARTHROSIS

The contribution of preexisting radiographic patellofemoral arthrosis and/or anterior knee pain to the survivorship of UKA has been described, yet remains a source of debate. Intuitively, preexisting patellofemoral arthritis and/or anterior knee pain should compromise the results of UKA, and many authors consider either of these findings to be contraindications to UKA.[2,3] However, several studies have contradicted this assumption. In one short-term study, Beard et al.[4] performed an intraoperative evaluation of the patellofemoral articulation in 824 medial UKAs using the Oxford (Biomet; Bridgend, United Kingdom) prosthesis. They noted full-thickness trochlear or patellar cartilage loss in 128 knees (13%). With minimum 1-year follow-up, the knees with cartilage loss did not have significantly worse Oxford scores or Knee Society scores, although patients with full-thickness patellar loss did have significantly worse Knee Society Functional Scores. Additionally, increasing severity of patellofemoral degeneration did not worsen the outcome. In another prospective study, Beard et al.[5] evaluated the outcomes of 100 UKAs (Oxford, Biomet). Although 54% of knees had preoperative anterior knee pain and 54% had preoperative radiographic patellofemoral degeneration (including 10% with joint space obliteration), these knees had outcomes similar to the 46% without preoperative pain or degeneration. Knees with lateral patellofemoral degeneration faired slightly worse than knees with medial patellofemoral degeneration, but each of these groups still had good overall outcomes. The authors concluded that neither medial patellofemoral joint degeneration nor anterior knee pain should be considered a contraindication to Oxford UKA. Kuipers et al.[6] also assessed the effect of preoperative patellofemoral joint involvement and reported on 437 Oxford UKAs evaluated at a mean of 2.6 years (range,

*The authors have not received any financial support for the work and have no other financial or personal connections to the work presented in this manuscript. Dr. Foran is on the governing/editorial board of an AAOS publication. Dr. Della Valle performs consulting services for Angiotech, Smith and Nephew, Biomet, and Kinamed and has received research support from Zimmer.

Table 21-1 Studies That Include Patients with Preoperative Radiographic Patellofemoral Arthritis, but without Postoperative Documentation of Patellofemoral Disease Progression

Author	Year	# of Pts.	# of UKAs	Medial	Lateral	Follow-up Time (yr)			Prosthesis Design	# of Failures	% of Total	Reasons for Failures		
						Mean	Min.	Max.				Patello-femoral	Adjacent Tib-Fem	Non-DJD Etiology
Jones[18]	1981	179	207	n/a	n/a	2.6	n/a	n/a	multiple	23	11%	1	3	19
Hasegawa[17]	1998	60	77	77	0	7	5	9	PCA	9	12%	0	1	8
Murray[20]	1998	114	144	144	0	7.6	n/a	13.8	Oxford	5	3%	0	2	3
Vorlat[23]	2000	38	41	38	3	4.8	2	8.3	Oxford	3	7%	0	2	1
Svard[22]	2001	103	124	124	0	12.5	10.1	15.6	Oxford	6	5%	0	0	6
Steele[21]	2006	174	203	203	0	14.8	10	29.4	St. Georg Sled	16	8%	1	6	11
Biswal[16]	2009	87	128	118	10	5.7	3	8	Allegretto	9	7%	0	3	6
Lustig[19]	2009	134	144	84	60	5.2	2	13.3	Uni-HLS Evolution	11	8%	0	5	6

0.1–7.9 years). The authors found that preoperative patellofemoral osteoarthritis was not associated with decreased implant survival. In fact, they noted a paradoxical 70% reduction in revision risk for patients with preoperative patellofemoral osteoarthritis.

The longer term results of preexisting patellofemoral degeneration on the outcomes of UKA are less clear. There are several longer term outcome studies in which patellofemoral degeneration was not considered to be an absolute contraindication to UKA.[7-15] Most of these failed to demonstrate significant differences in failure rates among those patients with and without preexisting patellofemoral arthrosis. However, Argenson et al.[8] studied 160 UKAs (Miller-Galante; Zimmer, Warsaw, IN) for a mean of 5.5 years (range, 3–9.3 years) and found that two of their five revisions were secondary to patellofemoral arthritis. These authors noted that both of the revisions for patellofemoral arthritis also had preexisting patellofemoral degeneration. As a result of their findings, the authors now consider extensive loss of cartilage in the patellofemoral joint found on preoperative radiograph or intraoperative inspection to be a contraindication to UKA.

A substantial number of studies include patients with patellofemoral arthrosis as part of the inclusion criteria for UKA, but fail to mention the status of the patellofemoral joint clinically or radiographically at follow-up.[16-23] These are shown in **Table 21-1**. Svard and Price,[22] for example, reported the long-term results of 124 medial UKAs using the Oxford mobile-bearing prosthesis. In their cohort, "the state of the patellofemoral compartment was not used as a criterion for selection and no patient was rejected because of patellofemoral degeneration." Six knees (4.8%) were revised for reasons unrelated to the patellofemoral compartment. However, there was no mention that the patellofemoral compartment was included as part of the follow-up evaluation. In the majority of these studies (see Table 21-1), there were no failures that were secondary to patellofemoral arthritis, and in two studies, only one failure was due to patellofemoral complications. It is

therefore tempting to conclude that the inclusion of preoperative patellofemoral degeneration does not negatively affect outcomes. However, in each of these studies, there is no clear indication that the clinical or radiographic status of the patellofemoral joint was evaluated as one of the outcome measures. It may be that there truly were no complications attributable to the patellofemoral joint. Alternatively, it is possible that the authors were not looking for patellofemoral complications, given a bias that the patellofemoral joint is not a relevant source of pain in these patients. Therefore, we are guarded with respect to our interpretation of these reports and believe that meaningful conclusions regarding the extent to which preoperative patellofemoral involvement affects UKA longevity cannot be drawn based on these studies.

LONG-TERM PATELLOFEMORAL ARTHRITIC PROGRESSION

We reviewed the literature for UKA outcome studies, with a specific emphasis on reports with long-term follow-up. Although there were several studies that specifically address patellofemoral complications following UKA, a surprising number of studies did not specifically include the status of the patellofemoral joint as part of their clinical and/or radiographic follow-up criteria.[11,17,22-43] In these studies, it is difficult to conclude whether patellofemoral degeneration was simply not a source of clinical complication, or whether the patellofemoral joint actually impacted the results of UKA but was overlooked in the study design. As such, meaningful conclusions regarding the natural history of the patellofemoral articulation following UKA cannot be drawn from these studies.

Table 21-2 lists another large subset of studies in which it is difficult to draw conclusions regarding the fate of the patellofemoral joint following UKA.[21,44-50] In each of these outcome studies, the authors indicated that failures occurred secondary to "progression of disease" but, unfortunately, failed to differentiate if that progression occurred in the un-resurfaced

Table 21-2		**Long-Term Studies Demonstrating Radiographic Evidence of Adjacent Compartment Degeneration, but without Delineation of Tibiofemoral or Patellofemoral Compartment Progression**												
						Follow-up Time (yr)						Reasons for Failures		
Author	Year	# of Pts.	# of UKAs	Medial	Lateral	Mean	Min.	Max.	Prosthesis Design	# of Failures	% of Total	Patello-femoral	Adjacent Tib-Fem	Non-DJD Etiology
Marmor[46]	1988	51	60	53	7	11	10	13	Marmor	21	35%	1	2	11
Scott[49]	1991	100	86	88	12	n/a	8	12	Mark I and Mark II	13	15%	0	2	11
Weale[50]	1994	34	42	n/a	n/a	n/a	12	17	St. Georg Sled	5	12%	n/a	n/a	n/a
Ansari[44]	1997	n/a	461	461	0	4	1	17	multiple	20	4%	0	9	11
Gioe[45]	2003	427	516	474	42	10	n/a	n/a	multiple	39	8%	0	2	19
O'Rourke[48]	2005	103	136	122	14	n/a	21	n/a	Marmor	19	14%	n/a	n/a	10
Steele[21]	2006	174	203	203	0	14.8	10	29.4	St. Georg Sled	16	8%	1	6	11
Newman[47]	2009	23	24	n/a	n/a	15	15	15	St. Georg Sled	4	17%	0	2	1

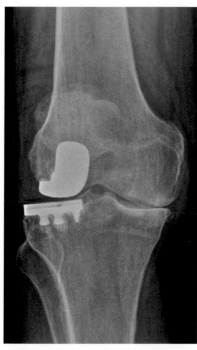

Figure 21-1 An anteroposterior standing radiograph of a patient 4 years after a right lateral UKA. Note the progression of degenerative changes in the adjacent tibiofemoral compartment. The patient remains clinically asymptomatic and has thus not required a revision procedure.

tibiofemoral compartment or in the patellofemoral compartment (**Fig. 21–1**). Steele et al.[21] reported on 203 medial UKAs (St. Georg Sled; Waldemar-Link, Hamburg, Germany) with a mean follow-up of 14.8 years (range, 10–29.4 years). The most common reason for failure in this cohort was "progression in another compartment." Seven of 16 failures were secondary to progression. At least one revision was required because of progression of disease in both the lateral and patellofemoral compartments, but the authors did not specify the location of

progression of the other six failures. O'Rourke et al.[48] described the minimum 21-year results of 136 UKAs (Marmor; Richards Orthopaedics, Memphis, TN). In this series, the overall revision rate was 14.9% (19 knees) and the majority of revisions (9 knees) were secondary to "disease progression." Again, the location of progression was not explicitly stated. The authors did, however, report that 75 knees (59%) had radiographic patellofemoral arthritis and 66 knees (52%) had contralateral tibiofemoral progression. Although progression occurred in both compartments, it is unclear if the progressions that lead to failure occurred in the tibiofemoral compartment, patellofemoral compartment, or both. Similarly, Gioe et al.[45] reported on the 5- and 10-year survivorship of 516 UKAs (474 medial, 42 lateral) using prostheses from multiple manufacturers. A total of 39 failures were identified. The most common reason for revision was "progression of arthritis in the uninvolved compartments," which accounted for 51.3% of the failures. Again, the location of the progression was not delineated. Thus, once again, the fate of the patellofemoral compartment is inconclusive based on these reports.

Fortunately, a subset of studies have evaluated the clinical and radiographic progression of disease specifically in the patellofemoral compartment[7-15,51-66] (**Table 21–3**). These studies had follow-up ranging from an average of 2 years to 14.9 years and included both medial and lateral UKAs using a variety of implants. Although the all-cause failure rate ranged from 0% to 30%, in general very few failures were secondary to patellofemoral progression. In fact, in nearly two thirds of these studies the majority of failures were related to causes other than progression of disease (in either compartment). Price et al.[14] followed 114 medial UKAs (Oxford) for a minimum of 10 years and found that 16 of 23 failures were unrelated to disease progression and the other 7 failures were due to progression in the lateral compartment. Hernigou and Deschamps[55] reported 22 total failures out of 99 UKAs (Lotus;

Table 21-3 All Studies That Specifically Evaluate the Status of the Patellofemoral Joint at Follow-up (List Includes Studies That Did Not Grade the Severity of Disease Progression)

Author	Year	# of Pts.	# of UKAs	Medial	Lateral	Follow-up Time (yr)			Prosthesis Design	# of Failures	% of Total	Reasons for Failures			PF % of Total	Time to Failure (yr)	# with X-ray PF Progression	% of Total
						Mean	Min.	Max.				Patello-femoral	Adjacent Tib-Fem	Non-DJD Etiology				
Bae[9]	1983	60	72	68	4	3.9	2	8	Marmor and Modular II	1	1%	1	0	0	100%	n/a	n/a	n/a
Kennedy[56]	1987	n/a	100	100	0	4.3	2	10.3	Marmor	5	5%	1	1	3	20%	2.42	n/a	n/a
Klemme[11]	1994	30	33	28	5	5.7	2	9.3	Marmor	4	12%	0	0	4	0%	n/a	0	0%
Bert[54]	1998	97	100	94	6	10.1	9.5	12.2	Biomet (MBUKA)	12	12%	0	10	2	0%	n/a	0	0%
Lewold[57]	1998	n/a	14,722	13,436	1336	n/a	n/a	n/a	multiple	1135	8%	29	299	807	3%	n/a	n/a	n/a
Tabor[65]	1998	58	67	61	6	9.7	5	20	Marmor-like	11	16%	0	4	7	0%	n/a	n/a	n/a
Squire[64]	1999	103	140	125	15	17	15	21.2	Marmor	14	10%	0	7	7	0%	n/a	91	65%
Weale[66]	2000	38	43	39	4	n/a	5	n/a	St. Georg Sled	0	0%	0	0	0	0%	n/a	1	2%
Ackroyd[7]	2002	322	408	408	0	6.4	n/a	21	St. Georg Sled	25	6%	1	8	16	4%	n/a	n/a	n/a
Argenson[8]	2002	147	160	145	15	5.5	3	9.3	Miller-Galante	5	3%	2	1	2	40%	1, 1.7	96	60%
Hernigou[55]	2002	80	99	74	25	14	10	20	Lotus	22	22%	1	3	18	5%	11	29	29%
Pennington[62]	2003	41	46	44	2	11	5.6	13.8	MG	3	7%	0	0	3	0%	n/a	19	41%
Berger[53]	2004	48	59	59	0	13	11	15	MG	4	7%	2	0	0	50%	7, 12	21	36%
Khan[10]	2004	n/a	30	26	4	n/a	10	n/a	St. Georg Sled	2	7%	0	0	2	0%	n/a	2	7%
Lisowski[13]	2004	28	30	n/a	n/a	2.5	2.1	3.0	Oxford Phase 3	0	n/a	0	0	0	0%	n/a	15	50%
Berger[52]	2005	51	62	59	3	n/a	10	n/a	MG	2	3%	2	0	0	0%	7, 11	21	34%
Price[14]	2005	89	114	114	0	n/a	10	n/a	Oxford	23	30%	0	7	16	0%	n/a	11	10%
Price[15]	2005	447	564	564	0	n/a	n/a	n/a	Oxford	24	4%	0	10	14	0%	n/a	n/a	n/a
Li[58]	2006	n/a	28	28	0	2	n/a	n/a	Miller-Galante	0	0%	0	0	0	0%	n/a	10	37%
Li[58]	2006	n/a	28	28	0	2	n/a	n/a	Oxford	2	7%	0	0	2	0%	n/a	10	38%
Pennington[61]	2006	24	29	0	29	12.4	3.1	15.6	MG	0	0%	0	0	0	0%	n/a	0	0%
Argenson[51]	2008	39	40	0	40	12.6	3	23	multiple	5	13%	1	3	1	20%	2.4	5	13%
Koskinen[12]	2009	42	46	46	0	7	2.7	13.1	Miller-Galante II	8	17%	0	3	5	0%	n/a	4	9%
Mercier[59]	2009	40	43	43	0	14.9	1	18	Oxford	13	30%	0	3	10	0%	n/a	13	30%
Parratte[60]	2009	31	35	35	0	9.7	5	16	Miller-Galante	6	17%	1	1	4	3%	8.1	6	17%
Saenz[63]	2010	113	144	144	0	3	2	4.5	Stryker UKA (EIUS)	16	11%	4	0	12	25%	n/a	4	3%

Howmedica, Benoist Girard, Herouville Saint Clair, France), of which 18 failed secondary to etiologies unrelated to progression, 3 failed from progression in the adjacent tibiofemoral compartment, and 1 failed from progression in the patellofemoral compartment. Overall, when failure was due to disease progression, it most commonly occurred in the un-resurfaced tibiofemoral compartment.

When the studies in Table 21–3 are taken in summation, revision for progression in the adjacent tibiofemoral compartment was nearly eight times more common than revision for patellofemoral progression (there were 360 revisions for tibiofemoral progression versus 45 revisions for patellofemoral progression). No revisions were performed for patellofemoral progression in any of the knees that received the Oxford mobile-bearing prosthesis despite the fact that all four of the studies that involved the Oxford UKA reported radiographic patellofemoral progression ranging from 10% to 50% of knees. It is also interesting to note that two of these four studies included patients with preoperative radiographic patellofemoral osteoarthritic changes. In contradistinction, 9 of 20 studies involving fixed-bearing devices (excluding studies that included both fixed- and mobile-bearing designs) reported knees that required revision for patellofemoral progression. All but five of these studies excluded knees with preoperative patellofemoral degeneration. Berger et al.[53] followed 59 medial UKAs (Miller-Galante) for a mean of 13 years (range, 11–15 years) and noted that the only two revisions in the cohort had failed secondary to progressive patellofemoral degeneration (7 and 12 years). Two additional patients had moderate or severe patellofemoral symptoms. Interestingly, at 10 years only 1.6% of patients had patellofemoral symptoms, but this increased to 10% at 15 years. Saenz et al.[63] followed 144 medial UKAs (EIUS UKA; Stryker, Mahwah, NJ). Although they had a short average follow-up of only 3 years (range, 2–4.5 years), there were four knees with patellofemoral degeneration that required revision. No knees

required revision for adjacent tibiofemoral progression, and 12 required revision for reasons unrelated to progression. The reason for early patellofemoral failure in this cohort is unclear, but it is a noticeable outlier. Preoperatively, the authors excluded patients with any anterior knee pain, but did not specifically note if preoperative radiographic degeneration was accepted.

As seen in Table 21–3, although the overall failure rate secondary to patellofemoral progression was low, the incidence of radiographic progression was notably higher, ranging from 0% to 65%. It is notable that five of the studies quantified the percentage of knees with radiographic patellofemoral progression, but did not grade the severity of the progression. Three of these five studies report progression greater than or equal to 50% (50%, 60%, and 65%), which represents the highest incidences reported. Because progression can range from simple osteophytes to full-thickness changes, the clinical significance of these ungraded changes is uncertain (**Fig. 21–2**). Furthermore, despite the high rate of radiographic progression, revision for patellofemoral progression was reported in only one of these studies (two knees).[8]

In the studies that did grade the radiographic patellofemoral progression, the grade was typically low. For example, although Pennington et al.[62] reported progression in 19 of 46 knees (41%), all were classified as Berger grade I (osteophytes only). Similarly, Argenson et al.[51] reported progression in 5 of 40 knees (13%) and all of these were Ahlbäck grade I changes (joint space narrowing < 3 mm). Hernigou and Deschamps[55] performed a thorough radiographic analysis on 99 UKAs with a mean follow-up of 14 years (range, 10–20 years). In addition to the 29 knees (29%) that developed patellofemoral osteoarthritis, 28 knees had impingement of the femoral component on the patella. They found that impingement occurred with an oversized or anteriorly placed femoral component. Impingement led to patellar notching and erosion, and was associated with a higher incidence of patellofemoral symptoms than

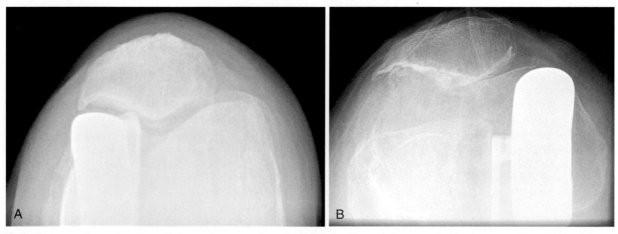

Figure 21-2 Skyline radiographs of patellofemoral progression after UKA showing mild osteoarthritic changes **(A)** and full-thickness cartilage loss **(B)**.

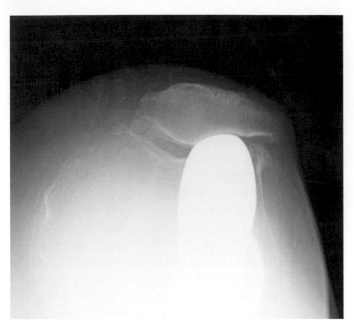

Figure 21-3 Skyline radiograph of a patient with a previously performed medial UKA. Note the impingement of the femoral component on the patella resulting in a groove in the articular surface of the un-resurfaced patella. This patient presented with severe anterior knee pain and underwent conversion to a total knee arthroplasty.

knees with patellofemoral osteoarthritis without impingement (**Fig. 21–3**). One knee (1%) required revision because of patellar impingement. In the series by Berger et al.,[52] all four knees with grade 4 patellofemoral changes had associated patellar impingement.

CONCLUSION

Clinical success following unicompartmental knee arthroplasty is very closely associated with proper patient selection. The debate continues as to whether preexisting patellofemoral joint degeneration has a definite impact on long-term favorable outcomes after UKA, although the inclusion of patients with preexisting patellofemoral osteoarthritis does not appear to affect the early results of the Oxford mobile-bearing UKA. The literature does support the fact that adjacent compartment degeneration, both tibiofemoral and/or patellofemoral, is common at long-term follow-up. However, as it pertains specifically to the patellofemoral joint, low-grade changes were most commonly encountered and rarely required a revision procedure.

Long-term prospective studies are still needed to specifically evaluate the fate of the patellofemoral joint following UKA. Future studies need to clearly document the status of the patellofemoral articulation as well as the prevalence of anterior knee pain preoperatively, identify patients with full-thickness cartilage defects intraoperatively, detail the clinical and radiographic degeneration of the joint with special attention to grading the severity of degeneration, and assess whether patellofemoral joint arthrosis should be considered a risk factor for revision surgery. Clinical trials that include these elements will help determine the incidence of patellofemoral complications following UKA, and will improve our ability to choose the correct patient and achieve clinical success.

REFERENCES

1. Borus T, Thornhill T. Unicompartmental knee arthroplasty. J Am Acad Orthop Surg 2008;16:9-18.
2. Kozinn SC, Scott R. Unicondylar knee arthroplasty. J Bone Joint Surg [Am] 1989;71:145-150.
3. Stern SH, Becker MW, Insall JN. Unicondylar knee arthroplasty: an evaluation of selection criteria. Clin Orthop Relat Res 1993;(286):143-148.
4. Beard DJ, Pandit H, Gill HS, et al. The influence of the presence and severity of pre-existing patellofemoral degenerative changes on the outcome of the Oxford medial unicompartmental knee replacement. J Bone Joint Surg [Br] 2007;89:1597-1601.
5. Beard DJ, Pandit H, Ostlere S, et al. Pre-operative clinical and radiological assessment of the patellofemoral joint in unicompartmental knee replacement and its influence on outcome. J Bone Joint Surg [Br] 2007;89:1602-1607.
6. Kuipers BM, Kollen BJ, Bots PC, et al. Factors associated with reduced early survival in the Oxford phase III medial unicompartment knee replacement. Knee 2010;17:48-52.
7. Ackroyd CE, Whitehouse SL, Newman JH, Joslin CC. A comparative study of the medial St Georg sled and kinematic total knee arthroplasties: ten-year survivorship. J Bone Joint Surg [Br] 2002;84:667-672.

8. Argenson JN, Chevrol-Benkeddache Y, Aubaniac JM. Modern unicompartmental knee arthroplasty with cement: a three to ten-year follow-up study. J Bone Joint Surg [Am] 2002;84:2235-2239.
9. Bae DK, Guhl JF, Keane SP. Unicompartmental knee arthroplasty for single compartment disease: clinical experience with an average four-year follow-up study. Clin Orthop Relat Res 1983;(176):233-238.
10. Khan OH, Davies H, Newman JH, Weale AE. Radiological changes ten years after St. Georg Sled unicompartmental knee replacement. Knee 2004;11:403-407.
11. Klemme WR, Galvin EG, Petersen SA. Unicompartmental knee arthroplasty: sequential radiographic and scintigraphic imaging with an average five-year follow-up. Clin Orthop Relat Res 1994;(301):233-238.
12. Koskinen E, Paavolainen P, Eskelinen A, et al. Medial unicompartmental knee arthroplasty with Miller-Galante II prosthesis: mid-term clinical and radiographic results. Arch Orthop Trauma Surg 2009;129:617-624.
13. Lisowski LA, Verheijen PM, Lisowski AE. Oxford Phase 3 unicompartmental knee arthroplasty (UKA): clinical and radiological results of minimum follow-up of 2 years. Orthop Traumatol Rehabil 2004;6:773-776.

14. Price AJ, Dodd CA, Svard UG, Murray DW. Oxford medial unicompartmental knee arthroplasty in patients younger and older than 60 years of age. J Bone Joint Surg [Br] 2005;87:1488-1492.

15. Price AJ, Waite JC, Svard U. Long-term clinical results of the medial Oxford unicompartmental knee arthroplasty. Clin Orthop Relat Res 2005;(435):171-180.

16. Biswal S, Brighton RW. Results of unicompartmental knee arthroplasty with cemented, fixed-bearing prosthesis using minimally invasive surgery. J Arthroplasty 2010;25:721-727.

17. Hasegawa Y, Ooishi Y, Shimizu T, et al. Unicompartmental knee arthroplasty for medial gonarthrosis: 5 to 9 years follow-up evaluation of 77 knees. Arch Orthop Trauma Surg 1998;117:183-187.

18. Jones WT, Bryan RS, Peterson LF, Ilstrup DM. Unicompartmental knee arthroplasty using polycentric and geometric hemicomponents. J Bone Joint Surg [Am] 1981;63:946-954.

19. Lustig S, Paillot JL, Servien E, et al. [Cemented all polyethylene tibial insert unicompartimental knee arthroplasty: a long term follow-up study]. Orthop Traumatol Surg Res 2009;95:12-21.

20. Murray DW, Goodfellow JW, O'Connor JJ. The Oxford medial unicompartmental arthroplasty: a ten-year survival study. J Bone Joint Surg [Br] 1998;80:983-989.

21. Steele RG, Hutabarat S, Evans RL, et al. Survivorship of the St Georg Sled medial unicompartmental knee replacement beyond ten years. J Bone Joint Surg [Br] 2006;88:1164-1168.

22. Svard UC, Price AJ. Oxford medial unicompartmental knee arthroplasty: a survival analysis of an independent series. J Bone Joint Surg [Br] 2001;83:191-194.

23. Vorlat P, Verdonk R, Schauvlieghe H. The Oxford unicompartmental knee prosthesis: a 5-year follow-up. Knee Surg Sports Traumatol Arthrosc 2000;8:154-158.

24. Aleto TJ, Berend ME, Ritter MA, et al. Early failure of unicompartmental knee arthroplasty leading to revision. J Arthroplasty 2008;23:159-163.

25. Ashraf T, Newman JH, Evans RL, Ackroyd CE. Lateral unicompartmental knee replacement survivorship and clinical experience over 21 years. J Bone Joint Surg [Br] 2002;84:1126-1130.

26. Bergenudd H. Porous-coated anatomic unicompartmental knee arthroplasty in osteoarthritis: a 3- to 9-year follow-up study. J Arthroplasty 1995;10(Suppl):S8-S13.

27. Carr A, Keyes G, Miller R, et al. Medial unicompartmental arthroplasty: a survival study of the Oxford meniscal knee. Clin Orthop Relat Res 1993;(295):205-213.

28. Cartier P, Sanouiller JL, Grelsamer RP. Unicompartmental knee arthroplasty surgery: 10-year minimum follow-up period. J Arthroplasty 1996;11:782-788.

29. Christensen NO. Unicompartmental prosthesis for gonarthrosis: a nine-year series of 575 knees from a Swedish hospital. Clin Orthop Relat Res 1991;(273):165-169.

30. Fehring TK, Odum SM, Masonis JL, Springer BD. Early failures in unicondylar arthroplasty. Orthopedics 2010;33:11.

31. Gulati A, Chau R, Simpson DJ, et al. Influence of component alignment on outcome for unicompartmental knee replacement. Knee 2009;16:196-199.

32. Hamilton WG, Collier MB, Tarabee E, et al. Incidence and reasons for reoperation after minimally invasive unicompartmental knee arthroplasty. J Arthroplasty 2006;21(6 Suppl 2):98-107.

33. Heck DA, Marmor L, Gibson A, Rougraff BT. Unicompartmental knee arthroplasty. A multicenter investigation with long-term follow-up evaluation. Clin Orthop Relat Res 1993;(286):154-159.

34. Hernigou P, Deschamps G. Alignment influences wear in the knee after medial unicompartmental arthroplasty. Clin Orthop Relat Res 2004;(423):161-165.

35. Jeer PJ, Keene GC, Gill P. Unicompartmental knee arthroplasty: an intermediate report of survivorship after the introduction of a new system with analysis of failures. Knee 2004;11:369-374.

36. Kort NP, van Raay JJ, Cheung J, et al. Analysis of Oxford medial unicompartmental knee replacement using the minimally invasive technique in patients aged 60 and above: an independent prospective series. Knee Surg Sports Traumatol Arthrosc 2007;15:1331-1334.

37. Koskinen E, Paavolainen P, Eskelinen A, et al. Unicondylar knee replacement for primary osteoarthritis: a prospective follow-up study of 1,819 patients from the Finnish Arthroplasty Register. Acta Orthop 2007;78:128-135.

38. Newman JH, Ackroyd CE, Shah NA. Unicompartmental or total knee replacement? Five-year results of a prospective, randomised trial of 102 osteoarthritic knees with unicompartmental arthritis. J Bone Joint Surg [Br] 1998;80:862-865.

39. Robertsson O, Lidgren L. The short-term results of 3 common UKA implants during different periods in Sweden. J Arthroplasty 2008;23:801-807.

40. Schai PA, Suh JT, Thornhill TS, Scott RD. Unicompartmental knee arthroplasty in middle-aged patients: a 2- to 6-year follow-up evaluation. J Arthroplasty 1998;13:365-372.

41. Swank M, Stulberg SD, Jiganti J, Machairas S. The natural history of unicompartmental arthroplasty: an eight-year follow-up study with survivorship analysis. Clin Orthop Relat Res 1993;(286):130-142.

42. Walton MJ, Weale AE, Newman JH. The progression of arthritis following lateral unicompartmental knee replacement. Knee 2006;13:374-377.

43. Whittaker JP, Naudie DD, McAuley JP, et al. Does bearing design influence midterm survivorship of unicompartmental arthroplasty? Clin Orthop Relat Res 2010;(468):73-81.

44. Ansari S, Newman JH, Ackroyd CE. St. Georg sledge for medial compartment knee replacement: 461 arthroplasties followed for 4 (1–17) years. Acta Orthop Scand 1997;68:430-434.

45. Gioe TJ, Killeen KK, Hoeffel DP, et al. Analysis of unicompartmental knee arthroplasty in a community-based implant registry. Clin Orthop Relat Res 2003;(416):111-119.

46. Marmor L. Unicompartmental arthroplasty of the knee with a minimum ten-year follow-up period. Clin Orthop Relat Res 1988;(228):171-177.

47. Newman J, Pydisetty RV, Ackroyd C. Unicompartmental or total knee replacement: the 15-year results of a prospective randomised controlled trial. J Bone Joint Surg [Br] 2009;91:52-57.

48. O'Rourke MR, Gardner JJ, Callaghan JJ, et al. The John Insall Award. Unicompartmental knee replacement: a minimum twenty-one-year followup, end-result study. Clin Orthop Relat Res 2005;(440):27-37.

49. Scott RD, Cobb AG, McQueary FG, Thornhill TS. Unicompartmental knee arthroplasty: eight- to 12-year follow-up evaluation with survivorship analysis. Clin Orthop Relat Res 1991;(271):96-100.

50. Weale AE, Newman JH. Unicompartmental arthroplasty and high tibial osteotomy for osteoarthrosis of the knee: a comparative study with a 12- to 17-year follow-up period. Clin Orthop Relat Res 1994;(302):134-137.

51. Argenson JN, Parratte S, Bertani A, et al. Long-term results with a lateral unicondylar replacement. Clin Orthop Relat Res 2008;(466):2686-2693.

52. Berger RA, Meneghini RM, Jacobs JJ, et al. Results of unicompartmental knee arthroplasty at a minimum of ten years of follow-up. J Bone Joint Surg [Am] 2005;87:999-1006.

53. Berger RA, Meneghini RM, Sheinkop MB, et al. The progression of patellofemoral arthrosis after medial unicompartmental replacement: results at 11 to 15 years. Clin Orthop Relat Res 2004;(428):92-99.

54. Bert JM. 10-year survivorship of metal-backed, unicompartmental arthroplasty. J Arthroplasty 1998;13:901-905.

55. Hernigou P, Deschamps G. Patellar impingement following unicompartmental arthroplasty. J Bone Joint Surg [Am] 2002;84:1132-1137.

56. Kennedy WR, White RP. Unicompartmental arthroplasty of the knee: postoperative alignment and its influence on overall results. Clin Orthop Relat Res 1987;(221):278-285.

57. Lewold S, Robertsson O, Knutson K, Lidgren L. Revision of unicompartmental knee arthroplasty: outcome in 1,135 cases from the Swedish Knee Arthroplasty study. Acta Orthop Scand 1998;69:469-474.

58. Li MG, Yao F, Joss B, et al. Mobile vs. fixed bearing unicondylar knee arthroplasty: a randomized study on short term clinical outcomes and knee kinematics. Knee 2006;13:365-370.

59. Mercier N, Wimsey S, Saragaglia D. Long-term clinical results of the Oxford medial unicompartmental knee arthroplasty. Int Orthop 2010;34:1137-1143.

60. Parratte S, Argenson JN, Pearce O, et al. Medial unicompartmental knee replacement in the under-50s. J Bone Joint Surg [Br] 2009;91:351-356.

61. Pennington DW, Swienckowski JJ, Lutes WB, Drake GN. Lateral unicompartmental knee arthroplasty: survivorship and technical considerations at an average follow-up of 12.4 years. J Arthroplasty 2006;21:13-17.

62. Pennington DW, Swienckowski JJ, Lutes WB, Drake GN. Unicompartmental knee arthroplasty in patients sixty years of age or younger. J Bone Joint Surg [Am] 2003;85:1968-1973.

63. Saenz CL, McGrath MS, Marker DR, et al. Early failure of a unicompartmental knee arthroplasty design with an all-polyethylene tibial component. Knee 2010;17:53-56.

64. Squire MW, Callaghan JJ, Goetz DD, et al. Unicompartmental knee replacement: a minimum 15 year followup study. Clin Orthop Relat Res 1999;(367):61-72.

65. Tabor OB Jr, Tabor OB. Unicompartmental arthroplasty: a long-term follow-up study. J Arthroplasty 1998;13:373-379.

66. Weale AE, Murray DW, Baines J, Newman JH. Radiological changes five years after unicompartmental knee replacement. J Bone Joint Surg [Br] 2000;82:996-1000.

CHAPTER 22
Hybrid Arthroplasty: Two-Compartment Approach

Lindsey Rolston

KEY POINTS

- Hybrid arthroplasty allows surgeons to address medial and patellofemoral arthritis with a monolithic femoral component while maintaining both cruciate ligaments.
- The design rationale, surgical technique, and midterm results are discussed.
- A review of patient selection and complications is included.

SETUP AND EQUIPMENT

Total knee arthroplasty (TKA) continues to be a safe and effective surgical procedure for arthritis of the knee, remaining the gold standard for treatment.[1,2] However, from the author's experience of performing TKAs for over 15 years, several observations are apparent. First, not all total knee replacement patients are happy with their postoperative function. The work of Phil Noble[3] suggests that upward of 50% of TKA patients describe some form of functional deficit, particularly side-to-side movement. Such outcomes highlight the necessity of the anterior cruciate ligament (ACL) and how it may relate to functional satisfaction subsequent to knee arthroplasty. The second observation was that the ACL and the posterior cruciate ligament (PCL) were oftentimes healthy and undamaged at the time of the surgery. It was unsettling to realize that contemporary surgical techniques required the undue resection of these structures. The final observation was the documented combination of wear of the medial compartment and the patellofemoral joint (PFJ), coupled with a nonsymptomatic lateral compartment.[4] Resection of the entire articular surface represented further unnecessary sacrifice of healthy tissue.

The idea of partial knee arthroplasty to allow retention of the lateral compartment and the cruciate ligaments is not new. Unicompartmental knee arthroplasty (UKA) and patellofemoral arthroplasty (PFA) have both been performed now for nearly 30 years.[5,6] Replacing the medial compartment alone during UKA, while ignoring arthritic changes at the PFJ, has been recognized as a satisfactory surgical option.[7] However, there is significant evidence that osteoarthritis (OA) may progress postoperatively, potentially compromising clinical outcome.[8,9] One potential solution is the addition of a PFA to an existing UKA. However, mating these two implants can be technically challenging, via the introduction of three discontinuous zones between the articular cartilage and the implant. In addition to technical considerations, procedure cost must also be considered. The use of two procedures instead of one to address bicompartmental knee disease unnecessarily increases surgical cost. Seven years ago, a monolithic implant was designed to simultaneously replace the medial and the PFJ compartments of the knee (Journey Deuce Bi-Compartmental Knee System; Smith and Nephew, Inc., Memphis, TN) (**Fig. 22–1**). This device conserves both the ACL and PCL, in addition to sparing the nonsymptomatic lateral compartment. The all-polyethylene or metal-backed medial tibial baseplate is unicompartmental. Initial expectations included a smaller incision, potentially shorter recovery times postoperatively, less pain, reduced blood loss, and improved stability and function.

APPROACH

The development of less invasive arthroplasty techniques has been of interest for many years, despite concerns of reduced surgical visualization.[10] Assuming relative ease of insertion and acceptable clinical outcomes, it is the author's opinion that minimally invasive procedures are preferred. With the Deuce knee, the surgeon does not need to visualize the lateral compartment, other than momentarily to assess its integrity. The surgical technique allows for a relatively small incision and ease of insertion. Standard medial-parapatellar arthrotomy has been used for 80% of the author's patients. Typically, this only involves a 1-inch split into the quadriceps. In 20% of patients, the author has used a midvastus approach without difficulty. This approach is typically reserved for those patients who have not undergone surgery previously, are less muscular, and are more flexible. When comparing the exposure of TKA to that of the Deuce knee, the potential benefits of this procedure are less dependent on incision length. Rather, the conservation of healthy tissue appears to be most important. Specifically, one is not exposing the lateral compartment or the lateral geniculate artery, which can increase pain and reduce postoperative function if not coagulated. Approximately 50% less bone is excised with the Deuce knee compared to traditional TKA. Moreover, the surgeon is able to avoid subluxing the tibia forward, placing a retractor in the lateral gutter, or everting the patella. The resulting reduction in blood loss and tissue tension may further improve postoperative surgical outcome. Surgeons are encouraged to make whatever exposure is necessary to perform the procedure without struggling, as incision length and violation of the quadriceps are not of primary concern with regard to recovery. Furthermore, liberal incision length may reduce risk of malalignment, skin slough, and retained cement.[11,12] A comparison of TKA exposure versus that of the Deuce knee is provided in **Figure 22–2**.

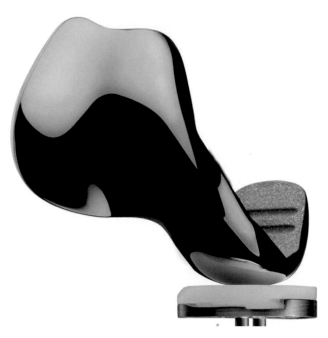

Figure 22-1 Journey Deuce Bi-Compartmental Knee System (Smith and Nephew, Inc., Memphis, TN).

TECHNICAL DESCRIPTION (SEE VIDEO 22-1)

The technique for Deuce implantation begins with tibial preparation, which is similar to that of UKA. The Deuce tibial cutting block utilizes one pin to fixate the cutting block to the tibia, with a second pin utilized for fixation extending under the lateral tibial condyle. The initial pin is placed as a negative stop for the vertical and horizontal resection. This prevents stress risers under the tibial spine or in a vertical direction, helping prevent fracture. The two pins in these locations not only act to fixate the block but also avoid placement of pins in the subchondral bone, which could result in subchondral collapse of the tibial baseplate and subsequent failure of the procedure. A conservative tibial cut of 2–4 mm is made. In most instances, a resection of 2 mm off the lowest point of the tibial articular surface is ideal. If a neutrally aligned knee with medial and PFJ compartment wear exists, a 4-mm cut on the tibia is utilized to prevent overcorrection and overloading of the lateral compartment. A conservative tibial cut is recommended, allowing for neutral varus/valgus placement with a slope of 2–4°. Bicompartmental knee arthroplasty (BKA) with

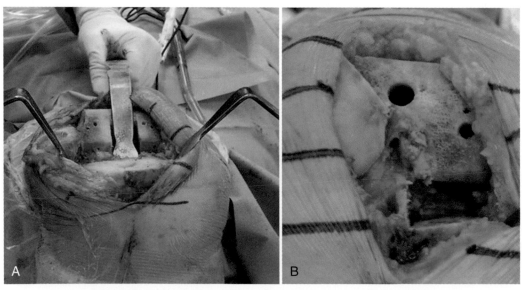

Figure 22-2 Comparison of TKA **(A)** and Deuce knee **(B)** exposures.

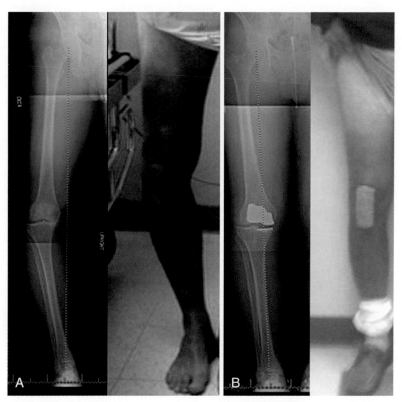

Figure 22-3 Restoration of knee alignment before and after implantation of the Deuce knee: preoperative **(A)** and postoperative **(B)**.

the Deuce knee has been shown to support knee alignment restoration.[13] As with UKA, it is important to place the tibial base on the cortical rim without overhang, and to position the component as far laterally as possible without violating the ACL attachment on the tibia. This allows for maximal load to be distributed across the tibia. Spacer blocks allow for the determination of proper knee flexion and extension. Bone cuts similar to that for TKA are made, allowing for correction of extensive varus deformity. In contrast to UKA, balancing the knee in extension can be performed independent of flexion, supporting extensive deformity correction (**Fig. 22–3**).[13,14] Mating the transition zone between the trochlea and lateral femoral condyle was the largest initial technical concern. With revised instrumentation, the author is able to make this process occur in a reproducible manner.

After the cuts have been made, trial implants are used just as in TKA (**Fig. 22–4**). The patellar component and preparation are the same as those utilized for TKA. A lateral retinacular peel and partial lateral facetectomy are utilized to balance the PFJ articulation. It is even more critical with BKA to perform proper balancing of the PFJ articulation to prevent contact of the lateral facet of the patella with the native lateral femoral condyle at the transition zone. The technical considerations that have been observed in TKA regarding balancing the PFJ need to be highlighted with BKA. In addition to balancing the soft tissue restraints of the lateral retinaculum,

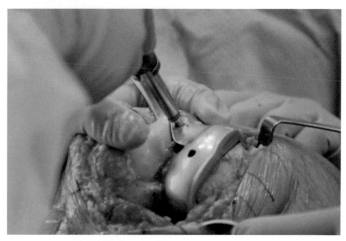

Figure 22-4 Deuce knee trial implants in situ.

shifting the monolithic implant laterally as far as possible without overhang is essential to allowing the proper tracking of the patella within the trochlear groove. The trochlear groove is the same as that of the Genesis II Total Knee System (Smith and Nephew), an implant with a proven track record for PFJ function and excellent clinical outcomes.[15,16] Both onlay and inset patella components have been used with good results. However, it is the author's preference to use a 7.5-mm-thickness three-peg-only patella. This allows for conservation of the patella cut, as well as adequate coverage and positioning of the patella with the implant.

Rotation of the femoral component is also an important aspect of PFJ mechanics. Maintaining proper rotation or adding a degree or two of external rotation allows for optimization of PFJ function. Because the femoral component is monolithic, the consequence of rotation of the implant needs to be considered as it relates to medial versus PFJ compartment balancing. This increased external rotation can potentially place the tibiofemoral contact area more medially, whereas internal rotation of the implant can adversely affect PFJ mechanics. The rotation of the femoral implant is determined by the anterior-posterior line of the trochlear groove, as well as the medial epicondylar axis. Identifying the epicondylar axis remains difficult. Therefore, the anterior-posterior line remains the mainstay for determination of rotation of the femoral implant.

SPECIAL CONSIDERATIONS, INDICATIONS, AND PATIENT SELECTION

First and foremost, a symptomatic lateral compartment is a contraindication to Deuce implantation. The history and physical examination are critical in determining the origin of lateral knee pain. Pain at the lateral facet of the patella is often related to PFJ arthritis and can be successfully treated. However, true lateral joint line pain will not be addressed by this procedure, regardless of how pristine the lateral compartment may look radiographically. Such cases may benefit from preoperative magnetic resonance imaging (MRI) and/or arthroscopy to address lateral compartment pathology. An intact ACL is preferred. However, the author has a series of patients without an ACL who have had successful outcomes; ACL deficiency has been observed in 6.38% of patients. If patients present with symptomatic instability, it is preferable to either perform ACL reconstruction at the time of surgery, or convert to TKA. For patients who are ACL deficient, but have lower activity levels and are asymptomatic, proceeding with BKA will not affect clinical outcome. Finally, as in UKA or PFA, inflammatory arthritis is an additional contraindication.

In difficult cases where flexion contracture is beyond 10°, conversion to TKA may be necessary. Flexion contracture can be improved with releases of the hamstring tendons medially and capsular tissue posteriorly and excision of posterior osteophytes in the medial aspect of the knee. Adequate bone quality is preferred. There are minimal limits on the extent of varus deformity that can be corrected, which is unlike UKA. Because actual bone cuts are made and the knee can be balanced in flexion independent of extension, a medial release up to 20° of varus can be performed. This occurs while achieving good stability and functional outcome postoperatively.

| Box 22-1 | **Beware of Patella Baja** |

- Avoid knees status post–closing wedge high tibial osteotomy.
- A CLOSING WEDGE CREATES A PATELLA BAJA.
- Patella baja brings the patella in contact with native cartilage and transition zone.

One common question revolves around patient selection: Who is the ideal candidate? Is it the young active patient who can appreciate the stability of the knee gained by retaining the cruciate ligaments, in addition to reduced bone resection? Alternatively, is it the elderly patient fearful of the pain and rehabilitation following TKA? After performing 800 of these procedures, it is the opinion of the author that age and activity level are not critical in determining candidacy. Each of these patient groups can benefit equally from BKA with the Deuce knee. Appropriate preoperative physical examination is critical. The location of pain is the most important factor. As the patients refer to a lateral aspect of their knee, it is essential to pinpoint whether this is the lateral facet of the patella, or whether this is true lateral joint line tenderness. The patients who point to the lateral facet of the patella are still candidates for Deuce, as the PFJ is resurfaced. If patients have true lateral joint line pain, it will not be addressed if the lateral compartment is not resurfaced. Lack of radiographic evidence of lateral OA will not help determine candidacy if any lateral pain exists. In such a case, it is appropriate to consider MRI or arthroscopy prior to determining the implant choice. ACL integrity, flexion contracture, patellar tracking, and lateral compartment narrowing must also be considered during the physical examination.

Clearly, a lateral notch osteophyte on the lateral condyle can and should be excised in each and every case. The necessary excision of this "kissing lesion" is not a contraindication to implantation of the Deuce. Full-thickness lesions of the weight-bearing rail of the lateral femoral condyle should not be accepted; in this case, conversion to TKA is recommended. Additional special considerations include the neutrally aligned knee with medial compartment arthrosis and an open lateral compartment. Most medial compartment arthritic knees result in varus deformity. Occasionally, based on the anatomy of the femur and tibia, radiographs may reveal medial and PFJ arthritis with a nonsymptomatic lateral compartment. When this occurs, it is critical to resect more bone on the tibial side to avoid overcorrection. Patella baja may result from high tibial valgus osteotomy (**Box 22–1**). In this instance the patella is brought in contact with the native cartilage in the transition zone, which is not optimal. Moreover, the closing wedge high tibial osteotomy results in a neutrally aligned medial compartment that is at risk for overcorrection. In both cases, conversion to TKA is necessary.

POSTSURGICAL FOLLOW-UP

As previously noted, one of the potential benefits of Deuce implantation is improved recovery. By conserving healthy tissue and minimizing joint trauma during surgery, postoperative function may be improved. Early evidence supports this hypothesis. In a gait study of 8 BKA patients and 10 controls,[17] the Deuce was found to support normal frontal plane mechanics and extensor moments about the knee during walking. At 1.2 years following surgery, Deuce patients had largely returned to normal function. Regarding clinical outcomes, the author has collected postoperative data during a single-surgeon survey of 400 Deuce and 152 TKA patients matched for body mass index and age (65 years for Deuce; 66 years for TKA). The average follow-up for the Deuce group is 29 months versus 22 months for TKA. The average total Knee Society score for the Deuce currently exceeds that of the TKA group at nearly every interval through 3 years, surpassing 90 by 6 months (**Fig. 22–5**). This is likewise the case for range of motion at every interval through 3 years (**Fig. 22–6**).

In addition to clinical outcome, the author has surveyed early functional outcomes. Included in this survey were the number of days the patient utilized any assistive devices, time to return to driving, discontinuation of all pain medicine, length of hospital stay, length of incision, average tourniquet time, and whether the patient needed a blood transfusion. In the author's experience, Deuce patients discontinue their use of assistive devices 10 days earlier than TKA patients. They are able to return to driving 13 days earlier than TKA patients and discontinue their pain medicine 9 days earlier. The length of hospital stay is 2.5 days for Deuce versus 3.5 days for TKA. The average tourniquet time is 7 minutes shorter for Deuce, as compared to TKA. Only 1.87% of patients required a blood transfusion with Deuce versus 36% with TKA. At 43 months' follow-up, there is a 1.3% revision rate. Complications have included the following: 3 manipulations, 3 cases of infection (1 acute, 2 chronic), 1 loose all-polyethylene tibial component, 1 partial lateral meniscectomy, 1 medial tibial plateau fracture, 1 loose patella, 2 liner locking mechanism failures, and 1 tibial baseplate fracture.

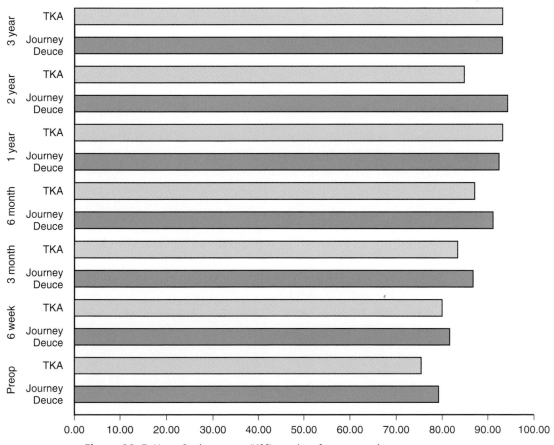

Figure 22-5 Knee Society score (KSS) results of postoperative surgeon survey.

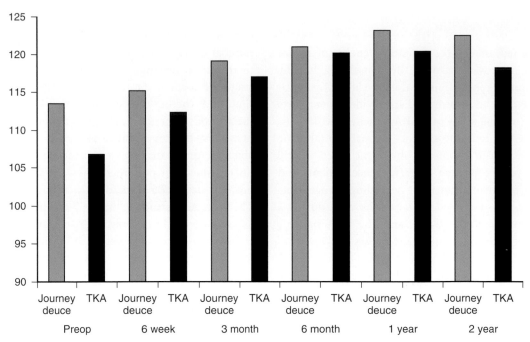

Figure 22-6 Range-of-motion (ROM) results of postoperative surgeon survey.

To date, over 5000 Deuce knees have been implanted over the course of 7 years; 800 are attributed to the author. Early postoperative clinical outcomes have been acceptable. However, in order to verify the long-term safety and efficacy of the Deuce knee, additional studies are necessary.

TIPS AND PEARLS

Optimal results with any type of partial knee arthroplasty are dependent upon a multitude of factors. After performing 800 Deuce procedures, the author has observed no femoral failures. This largely parallels the TKA literature. When considering UKA or BKA, the tibial side of the arthroplasty seems to be the weak link. The first recommendation is to minimize the depth of the tibial resection. Reasons for this include the fact that the subchondral bone plate is a more rigid plate of bone on which to apply a baseplate. The proximal tibia below 4 mm becomes softer and less able to resist the forces on the medial aspect. In addition, a partial knee arthroplasty is often utilized in younger patients who may be at risk for future revision arthroplasty. Preservation of this tibial bone is critical to the success of any future revision procedure.

The importance of balancing the knee is essential in reducing excessive stress on the medial tibial baseplate. Therefore, correction of a large varus deformity is recommended. This counters common instruction for UKA, where release and correction of such deformity is avoided. However, in the

author's experience during BKA, it is also important not to overcorrect the deformity and place the weight-bearing line onto the lateral joint. Holding the knee in full extension after the femoral and tibial inserts are cemented allows the cement to cure in the same line as the maximal stress that will be encountered. This is the case for all knee arthroplasty procedures, but cannot be overemphasized during BKA.

Recovery following partial knee arthroplasty is multifactorial. Appropriate pain management is critical. In the author's experience, a pain cocktail has been most useful. Femoral and/or sciatic nerve blocks have been a recommended method of pain management. However, blocks can compromise weight bearing in the affected limb for 1–2 days, potentially increasing fall risk during ambulation. Oftentimes these patients are discharged during this same time interval, and therefore this femoral and/or sciatic nerve block may inhibit proper therapy and recovery.

CONCLUSIONS

The author's experience with the Deuce knee suggests that this device can be effectively utilized to treat BKA patients with symptomatic medial and PFJ compartments. While TKA is an effective treatment for bicompartmental disease, evidence supports improved functional outcomes following BKA with the Deuce.[17] This appears to be due primarily to ACL preservation and reduced bone resection, tissue distress, and blood loss during implantation. Moreover, the author's survey of 800

Deuce patients supports the stability of the Deuce knee at 2.5 years follow-up. BKA is a viable procedure for a significant number of OA patients.[8,9] Although additional research is necessary to address mid- to long-term outcomes, the current procedure will likely have a place in the orthopaedics reconstructive market for years to come.

REFERENCES

1. Hart JA. Joint replacement surgery. Med J Aust 2004;180: S27-S30.
2. Kurtz S, Mowat F, Ong K, et al. Prevalence of primary and revision total hip and knee arthroplasty in the United States from 1990–2002. J Bone Joint Surg [Am] 2005;87:1487-1497.
3. Noble PC, Conditt MA, Cook KF, Mathis KB. The John Insall Award. Patient expectations affect satisfaction with total knee arthroplasty. Clin Orthop Relat Res 2006;(452):35-43.
4. Ledingham J, Regan M, Jones A, Doherty M. Radiographic patterns and associations of osteoarthritis of the knee in patients referred to hospital. Ann Rheum Dis 1993;52:520-526.
5. Borus T, Thornhill T. Unicompartmental knee arthroplasty. J Am Acad Orthop Surg 2008;16:9-18.
6. Leadbetter WB, Ragland PS, Mont MA. The appropriate use of patellofemoral arthroplasty: an analysis of reported indications, contraindications, and failures. Clin Orthop Relat Res 2005; (436):91-99.
7. Kendrick BJ, Rout R, Bottomley NJ, et al. The implications of damage to the lateral femoral condyle on medial unicompartmental knee replacement. J Bone Joint Surg [Br] 2010;92:374-379.
8. Berger RA, Meneghini RM, Sheinkop MB, et al. The progression of patellofemoral arthrosis after medial unicompartmental replacement: results at 11 to 15 years. Clin Orthop Relat Res 2004; (428):92-99.
9. Hernigou P, Deschamps G. Patellar impingment following unicompartmental arthroplasty. J Bone Joint Surg [Am] 2002;84:1132-1137.
10. Khanna A, Gougoulias N, Longo UG, Maffulli N. Minimally invasive total knee arthroplasty: a systemic review. Orthop Clin North Am 2009;40:479-489.
11. Berenc KR, Lombardi AV. Avoiding the potential pitfalls of minimally invasive total knee surgery. Orthopedics 2005;289:1326-1330.
12. Dalury DF, Dennis DA. Mini-incision total knee arthroplasty can increase risk of component malalignment. Clin Orthop Relat Res 2005;(440):77-81.
13. Rolston L, Siewart K. Assessment of knee alignment after bicompartmental knee arthroplasty. J Arthroplasty 2009;24:1111-1114.
14. Emerson RH, Higgins LL. Unicompartmental knee arthroplasty with the Oxford prosthesis in patients with medial compartment arthritis. J Bone Joint Surg [Am] 2008;90:118-122.
15. Bourne RB, Laskin RS, Guerin JS. Ten-year results of the first 100 Genesis II total knee replacement procedures. Orthopedics 2007; 30:S83-S85.
16. Crockarell JR, Hicks JM, Schroeder RJ, et al. Total knee arthroplasty with asymmetric femoral condyles and tibial tray. J Arthroplasty 2010;25:108-113.
17. Wang H, Dugan E, Frame J, Rolston L. Gait analysis after bi-compartmental knee replacement. Clin Biomech 2009;24: 751-754.

CHAPTER 23
Modular Bicompartmental Knee Arthroplasty

Jess H. Lonner

KEY POINTS

- Modular bicompartmental knee arthroplasty is an effective consideration for patients with bicompartmental disease, when there is reasonable range of knee motion, minimal deformity, and stable ligaments.
- Unlike a monolithic femoral component, a modular approach to bicompartmental knee arthroplasty allows independent component sizing and alignment, without having to compromise either.
- Short-term outcomes are good, but durability depends on meticulous surgical technique and use of soundly designed unicompartmental and patellofemoral arthroplasties.

INTRODUCTION

Isolated unicompartmental knee arthroplasty (UKA) and patellofemoral arthroplasty (PFA) are effective for localized arthritis; however, arthritis commonly affects both the medial (or lateral) and patellofemoral compartments, and traditionally total knee arthroplasty (TKA) has been performed in those circumstances. While some have suggested that patellofemoral arthritis and symptoms can be ignored when performing UKA,[1,2] others have not replicated that approach. Additionally, the presence of grade 3 or 4 chondromalacia in the medial or lateral compartments is a contraindication to PFA when treating patellofemoral arthritis, making TKA the conventional treatment.[3]

A disruptive evolutionary approach to tissue-sparing partial knee arthroplasty was introduced several years ago in the form of a monolithic bicompartmental knee arthroplasty, which resurfaces the medial and patellofemoral compartments, sparing the cruciate ligaments and lateral compartment.[4] While the initial reception to the concept of bicompartmental knee arthroplasty was lukewarm, it is gaining interest and relevance as techniques improve, designs change, and results emerge. Two generic methods of bicompartmental knee arthroplasty are currently available— my preference is a modular approach, utilizing separate and unlinked UKAs and PFAs; the alternative, discussed in other chapters of this book, is either an off-the-shelf or custom monolithic prosthesis with a linked trochlear and unicondylar femoral segment. This chapter discusses the rationale for use of an unlinked modular bicompartmental knee arthroplasty and its clinical results.

RATIONALE FOR BICOMPARTMENTAL KNEE ARTHROPLASTY

The rationale behind this strategy to knee arthroplasty is twofold. First, a large segment of patients undergoing TKA have isolated bicompartmental arthritis involving the medial (or lateral) and patellofemoral compartments and have no significant deformity, excellent motion, and intact cruciate ligaments. One radiographic study of 470 knees evaluated for osteoarthritis found that 50% had arthritis affecting both the medial and patellofemoral compartments, but sparing the lateral compartment, and that tricompartmental arthritis was rare.[5] Often these patients are treated with TKA. While this is highly effective in providing considerable pain relief and survivorship, TKA patients often do not achieve the desired level of function and normalcy.[6] This may be related to the altered kinematics of the knee following TKA, which tend to be relatively normal after UKA, PFA, and bicompartmental knee arthroplasty due to the retention of the anterior cruciate ligament and anatomic structures in the other compartments.[7-9] Second, a number of knees treated with isolated patellofemoral or unicompartmental tibiofemoral arthroplasty will develop progressive arthritis in an un-resurfaced compartment of the knee over a period of time and are often converted to TKAs rather than adding a partial knee arthroplasty to the degenerated compartment. Staged modular bicompartmental arthroplasty may be a valid treatment method in these situations. However, despite its intuitive, rational philosophy, few data exist regarding how patients may fair if a modular stepwise approach to resurfacing is utilized rather than conversion to TKA in these patients.

INDICATIONS FOR BICOMPARTMENTAL KNEE ARTHROPLASTY

The indications for this procedure are similar to those used for UKA or PFA, with the addition of arthritis or painful chondromalacia in the "second" compartment (**Fig. 23–1**). Therefore, it can be used for patients with medial or lateral compartment and patellofemoral degenerative joint disease or painful chondromalacia, provided there is full extension (or less than a 5° flexion contracture), "good" range of motion (typically greater than 90° of flexion), minimal deformity, functional cruciate and collateral ligament stability, and an intact and painless "third" compartment. Further details of the indications for isolated unicompartmental and patellofemoral arthroplasty are given in their respective chapters in this book. While some surgeons may prefer to restrict this surgery to patients who are young and active, I have had great success in elderly patients and offer it to appropriate candidates without applying arbitrary age restrictions. Some surgeons have advocated isolated medial unicompartmental arthroplasty with a mobile-bearing implant design for bicompartmental arthritis involving the medial and patellofemoral compartments, in essence disregarding the arthritis and symptoms in the patellofemoral compartment.[1,2] Berend et al.[1] and Beard et al.[2] have found that neither preoperative patellofemoral arthritis nor pain negatively impacts the results of the unicompartmental arthroplasty using a mobile-bearing implant. On the contrary, others have found that failures due to anterior knee pain will predictably occur when resurfacing only the medial compartment of the knee when there is also patellofemoral arthritis. Since the data regarding mobile-bearing knees in bicompartmental arthritis have not been replicated in other series (particularly those using fixed-bearing implants), and the rational explanation for the apparent absence of patellofemoral symptoms is elusive, my preference is to treat patients with bicompartmental arthritis and symptoms involving both the medial (or lateral) and patellofemoral compartments with modular bicompartmental arthroplasty (**Figs. 23–2 and 23–3**).

RATIONALE FOR UNLINKED MODULAR BICOMPARTMENTAL KNEE ARTHROPLASTY

Currently, two monolithic bicompartmental knee arthroplasty implants are available, both with little or no published clinical results. The Journey Deuce (Smith & Nephew, Memphis, TN) is a noncustomized implant that resurfaces the trochlear and medial femoral condylar femoral surfaces with a linked component that mates with a medial unicompartmental tibial component and an all-polyethylene patellar button; the iDuo (ConforMIS, Burlington, MA) is a custom-designed implant that resurfaces the patellofemoral compartment and either the medial or lateral compartments, also linking the trochlear and femoral condylar segments. While early experience with the monolithic device has raised awareness of the role of bicompartmental knee arthroplasty in general, there are some challenges associated with use of an "off-the-shelf" monolithic bicompartmental arthroplasty for trochlear-medial femoral condylar resurfacing.

With this philosophical approach to bicompartmental resurfacing, the varus-valgus alignment of the component is determined by the apposition of the lateral transitional edge of the trochlear component with the lateral femoral condyle. Given the variability in coronal alignment and morphology of the distal femur, there will be concomitant variability in how the implant can be aligned to ensure that the lateral edge

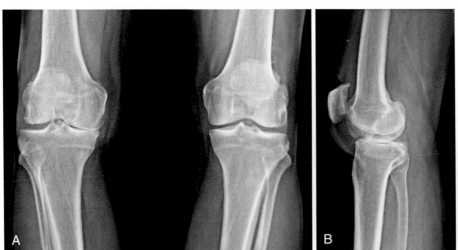
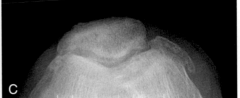

Figures 23-1 Preoperative anteroposterior **(A)**, lateral **(B)**, and sunrise **(C)** radiographs of a 60-year-old man with bicompartmental knee arthritis.

of the trochlear prosthesis is flush with the lateral femoral condyle. This may compromise sizing and alignment of the condylar portion of the prosthesis. Certainly, an analysis of radiographs of the monolithic implant will show variability in the trochlear and condylar orientation relative to the distal femur with some components in varus, others in valgus, and others in neutral alignment relative to the femoral mechanical axis (**Fig. 23–4**). This malalignment can have detrimental implications for durability and functional outcomes. Except in ideal morphologies of the distal femur, it is rare to have

both segments of the prosthesis (i.e., the trochlear and condylar segments) aligned and sized perfectly with a non-customized monolithic prosthesis. Whether compromise in the alignment or position has deleterious implications on patellar tracking and midterm performance of the implant is not yet known; however, it may explain why one series of 42 monolithic bicompartmental knee arthroplasties reported 12% revisions and 25% anterior knee pain at short-term follow-up.[10]

The inherent challenges and concerns regarding use of a monolithic bicompartmental knee arthroplasty are further highlighted by a study of 117 computed tomography scans that identified considerable variability in the geometric relationships between the trochlear and medial or lateral femoral condylar surfaces.[11] This study strengthens the argument for an unlinked modular approach to bicompartmental knee arthroplasty to optimize alignment and sizing of its individual components. Thus, the alternative approach to bicompartmental knee arthroplasty, and my personal preference, is a modular unlinked trochlear and medial femoral condylar prosthesis, which allows the individual compartmental resurfacing procedures to be performed "independent" of each other, ensuring appropriate orientation and alignment of the individual components relative to the critical axial and rotational axes of the distal femur, without having to compromise implant position based on how the component is positioned in the other compartment (see Figs. 23–2 and 23–3). This also allows size interchangeability between compartments to accommodate potential variability in femoral geometry and aspect ratios between patients and

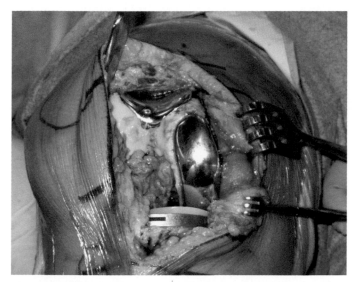

Figure 23-2 Intraoperative photograph of modular bicompartmental knee arthroplasty.

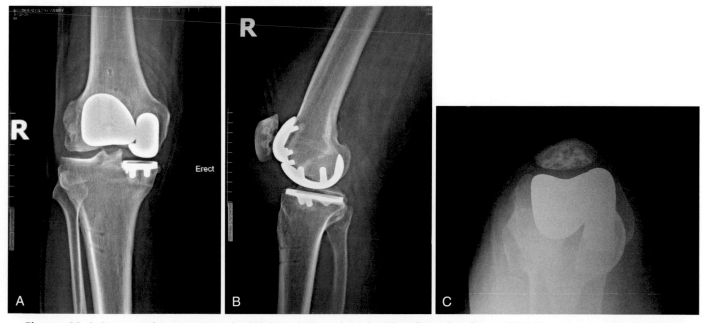

Figures 23-3 Postoperative anteroposterior **(A)**, lateral **(B)**, and sunrise **(C)** radiographs after modular bicompartmental arthroplasty.

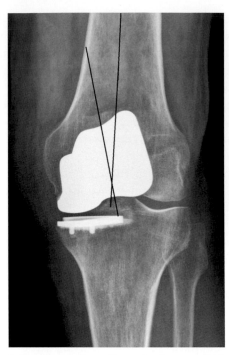

Figure 23-4 Anteroposterior radiograph of a monolithic bicompartmental knee arthroplasty showing the difficulty of achieving accurate alignment of both the trochlear and condylar portions of the prosthesis. In this case, while the femoral condylar segment appears to be appropriately aligned relative to the mechanical axis, the trochlear portion is directed toward the medial cortex, which may compromise patellar tracking.

compartments of the knee. The modular approach to bicompartmental resurfacing is also highly compatible with robotic assistance for bone preparation and three-dimensional preoperative planning.[12]

When performing modular bicompartmental resurfacing, the gap between the transitional edge of the trochlear component and the proximal edge of the femoral component of the unicompartmental arthroplasty may vary in size. This distance may be as little as 1 mm and as large as 10 mm depending on the distal femoral shape and size (see Fig. 23–2). Problems with the transitional gap between the trochlear and condylar prostheses have not been observed with independent resurfacing, provided the implants are appropriately positioned flush with or recessed approximately 1 mm relative to the articular cartilage. Prominent edges could result in patellar prosthesis catching or snapping over the implants and should therefore be avoided. Implant edge prominence can result from technical errors or trochlear implant design features.[13] Malaligned, malpositioned, improperly sized trochlear components or those that do not rest flush with the condylar surfaces can impact patellar tracking and have consequences relative to patellar tracking and short- and long-term success of bicompartmental arthroplasty.

CLINICAL RESULTS OF MODULAR BICOMPARTMENTAL KNEE ARTHROPLASTY

Gait analysis and isokinetic strength tests indicate that normal knee mechanics and gait are restored after bicompartmental knee arthroplasty.[9] Early clinical results of bicompartmental knee arthroplasty have shown excellent pain relief and knee function and restoration of appropriate knee alignment.[4,14-18] Recipients can commonly rise independently and ascend stairs reciprocally.[9,16] However, since the procedure is relatively new, long-term outcomes have still to be established.

There have been several recent reports on the results of modular unlinked bicompartmental knee arthroplasty. Heyse et al. reported on nine knees in nine patients with an average age at surgery of 64 ± 5 years treated with medial UKA and PFA.[15] Three procedures were performed in a staged fashion, with a mean of 5 years between UKA and PFA. At a mean follow-up of 12 ± 5 years (range, 4–17 years), no revision surgeries were necessary, although one asymptomatic patient had substantial progression of lateral arthritis. The Knee Society knee score increased from 39 ± 24 preoperatively to 92 ± 10 ($p = .007$), and the Knee Society Functional Score increased from 30 ± 9 preoperatively to 83 ± 18 ($p = .002$), at latest follow-up ($p = .002$). Mean range of motion increased from 107° to 121° ($p = .04$), and all patients were satisfied or very satisfied.[15] Mahoney et al. reported on short-term experience with 17 unlinked UKAs and PFAs, observing mild or no pain and greater than 120° of flexion in all patients.[16] In that series, all patients were able to rise unassisted and ascend stairs in a reciprocal manner. There were no cases of incompatibility between the UKA or PFA components.[16] John et al. reviewed the initial 30 consecutive modular unlinked bicompartmental UKA/PFAs performed by this author and found that, at a minimum 1-year follow-up (range, 1–2.5 years), the WOMAC pain score decreased from 11.0 to 2.8 ($p = .0001$), the WOMAC function score decreased from 13.6 to 3.2 ($p = .0008$), the WOMAC total score decreased from 24.6 to 6.0 ($p = .0001$), range of motion increased from 122° to 138° ($p = .0001$), and Knee Society Functional and Knee scores increased from 56 to 92 and 40 to 88, respectively ($p = .0001$). There were no perioperative complications and no radiographic evidence of loosening, polyethylene wear, or progressive arthritis of the lateral tibiofemoral compartment.[17]

Despite these encouraging results, the outcomes of bicompartmental knee arthroplasty can be compromised by poor implant design, component malalignment or malposition, improper patient selection, and progressive arthritis of the un-resurfaced compartment. In a series by Parratte et al., 6 of 77 knees treated with combined medial UKA and PFA developed asymptomatic progression of lateral compartment osteoarthritis at a mean 12-year follow-up. No revisions were necessary for arthritis progression, and in those surviving prostheses, there was substantial improvement in pain, function, and knee scores. However, in that series 27 knees failed at a mean of 8 years (range, 11 months to 22 years) due to aseptic loosening of the trochlear component ($n = 20$) and the tibial component ($n = 7$). Of the trochlear components that failed, 15 were cementless. Despite these failures, those authors continue to advocate for modular bicompartmental knee arthroplasty, recognizing that cementless trochlear component fixation, crude instrumentation and techniques, and poor polyethylene quality and implant designs were responsible for aseptic loosening in the series.[14] The high rate of trochlear component failures in isolated PFAs with the same design used in the series by Parratte et al.[14] was noted in previous series.[19] Further study with newer techniques and designs will determine whether long-term durability compares to that of TKA. Certainly contemporary reports of improved early functionability and outcomes with bicompartmental knee arthroplasty are encouraging.[4,12,17]

STAGED BICOMPARTMENTAL RESURFACING

Another novel concept to consider is a staged approach to bicompartmental arthroplasty for progressive arthritis after unicompartmental or patellofemoral arthroplasty. After UKA, the development or progression of symptomatic patellofemoral arthritis may occur in 7–10% of patients at 10–15 years.[20,21] Additionally, after PFA 10–25% of patients may develop progressive tibiofemoral arthritis at 7–16 years.[19,22-24] Typically these patients are treated with revision to TKA. It makes intuitive sense that, in those patients with an isolated

patellofemoral or unicompartmental arthroplasty, progressive degeneration of one of the un-resurfaced compartments of the knee can be treated with staged single-compartment resurfacing, rather than conversion to TKA, thereby performing a staged modular bicompartmental arthroplasty. However, despite one study that included three patients who underwent staged modular bicompartmental knee arthroplasty,[15] there are no published data that review the results of this method of treatment as an alternative to revision to TKA.

CONCLUSION

In appropriately selected patients with bicompartmental knee arthritis of the medial or lateral and patellofemoral compartments (or painful chondromalacia in the "second" compartment), modular bicompartmental knee arthroplasty is a legitimate alternative to TKA and may be more effective than UKA or PFA alone in these situations. While modular bicompartmental knee arthroplasty is appealing as a conservative and kinematics-preserving approach to knee arthritis, sound surgical technique and use of quality prostheses will be important determinants of success. Modular bicompartmental knee arthroplasty using unlinked unicompartmental and patellofemoral knee prostheses allows greater flexibility in sizing and alignment of components that cannot be achieved with monolithic prostheses, and thereby allows more accurate restoration of compartmental anatomy. Using a modular bicompartmental arthroplasty rather than a monolithic prosthesis makes intuitive sense; however, no studies have established whether one approach is superior to the other.

REFERENCES

1. Berend KR, Lombardi AV, Adams JB. Obesity, young age, patellofemoral disease, and anterior knee pain: identifying the unicondylar arthroplasty patient in the United States. Orthopedics 2007;5(Suppl): 19-23.

2. Beard DJ, Pandit H, Ostlere S, et al. Preoperative clinical and radiological assessment of the patellofemoral joint in unicompartmental knee replacement and its influence on outcome. J Bone Joint Surg [Br] 2007;89:1602-1607.

3. Lonner JH. Patellofemoral arthroplasty. J Am Acad Orthop Surg 2007;15:495-506.

4. Rolston L, Bresch J, Engh G, et al. Bicompartmental knee arthroplasty: a bone-sparing, ligament-sparing, and minimally invasive alternative for active patients. Orthopedics 2007;30(8 Suppl):70-73.

5. Ledingham J, Regan M, Jones A, Doherty M. Radiographic patterns and associations of osteoarthritis of the knee in patients referred to hospital. Ann Rheum Dis 1993;52:520-526.

6. Noble PC, Gordon MJ, Weiss JM, et al. Does total knee replacement restore normal knee function? Clin Orthop Relat Res 2005;(435): 157-165.

7. Patil S, Colwell CW Jr, Ezzet KA, D'Lima DD. Can normal knee kinematics be restored with unicompartmental knee replacement? J Bone Joint Surg [Am] 2005;87:332-338.

8. Suggs JF, Park SE, Steffensmeier S, et al. Function of the anterior cruciate ligament after unicompartmental arthroplasty: an in vitro robotic study. J Arthroplasty 2004;19:224-229.

9. Wang H, Dugan E, Frame J, Rolston L. Gait analysis after bi-compartmental knee replacement. Clin Biomech 2009;24: 751-754.

10. Tria AJ Jr. Bicompartmental arthroplasty of the knee. Instr Course Lect 2010;59:61-73.

11. Banks SA, Abbasi A, Van Vorhis R, et al. Morphology of the distal femur for bicompartmental arthroplasty. Presented at the Annual Meeting of the American Academy of Orthopedic Surgeons, 2010.

12. Lonner JH. Modular bicompartmental knee arthroplasty with robotic arm assistance. Am J Orthop 2009;38(2 Suppl):28-31.

13. Lonner JH. Patellofemoral arthroplasty: the impact of design on outcomes. Orthop Clin North Am 2008;39:347-354.

14. Paratte S, Pauly V, Aubaniac JM, Argenson JN. Survival of bicompartmental knee arthroplasty at 5–23 years. Clin Orthop Relat Res 2010;(468):64-72.

15. Heyse TJ, Khefacha A, Cartier P. UKA in combination with PFR at average 12-year follow-up. Arch Orthop Trauma Surg 2010;130: 1227-1230.

16. Argenson JN, Parratte S, Bertani A, et al. The new arthritic patient and arthroplasty options. J Bone Joint Surg [Am] 2009;91(Suppl 5): 43-48.

17. John T, Sheth N, Lonner JH. Modular bicompartmental arthroplasty of the knee. Presented at the Annual Meeting of the Knee Society, September 2010.

18. Rolston L, Siewert K. Assessment of knee alignment after bicompartmental knee arthroplasty. J Arthoplasty 2009;24:1111-1114.

19. Argenson JN, Flecher X, Parratte S, Aubaniac JM. Patellofemoral arthroplasty: an update. Clin Orthop Relat Res 2005;(440):50-53.

20. Kahn OH, Davies H, Newman JH, Weale AE. Radiological changes ten years after St. Georg Sled unicompartmental knee replacement. Knee 2004;11:403-407.

21. Berger RA, Meneghini RM, Sheinkop MB, et al. The progression of patellofemoral arthrosis after medial unicompartmental replacement: results at 11 to 15 years. Clin Orthop Relat Res 2004;(428): 92-99.

22. Cartier P, Sanouiller JL, Khefacha A. Long-term results with a first patellofemoral prosthesis. Clin Orthop Relat Res 2005;(436): 47-54.

23. Nicol SG, Loveridge JM, Weale AE, et al. Arthritis progression after patellofemoral joint replacement. Knee 2006;13:290-295.

24. Kooijman HJ, Driessen APPM, VanHorn JR. Long-term results of patellofemoral arthroplasty: a report of 56 arthroplasties with 17 years of follow-up. J Bone Joint Surg [Br] 2003;85:836-840.

SECTION 6
Complications

SECTION 4
Complications

CHAPTER 24
Failure Modes of Unicompartmental Arthroplasty

Jack M. Bert

KEY POINTS

- Unicompartmental arthroplasty is a common surgical procedure in the patient with unicompartmental disease.
- Midterm and long-term survivorship of unicompartmental arthroplasty is highly variable, and multiple factors contribute to failed procedures.
- This chapter describes the most common mechanisms of failed unicompartmental replacement and attempts to explain their etiology of failure.

INTRODUCTION

Unicompartmental knee arthroplasty (UKA) has become a common surgical procedure for unicompartmental osteoarthritis both nationally and internationally in the middle-aged and older patient. Midterm and long-term survivorship of UKA is highly variable. From 1998 to 2005, the incidence of performance of UKA increased at a rate of 32.5% compared to an increase in the performance of total knee arthroplasty of 9.4% during the same period.[1] In the past 30 years, multiple authors have reported on the indications and contraindications for UKA.[2–23]

INDICATIONS

The classic indications for UKA include:
1. Patients with a relatively sedentary occupation
2. Those patients with less than 10° of mechanical varus deformity
3. Patients with range of motion greater than 90° without a flexion contracture
4. Those patients with osteoarthritis or posttraumatic arthritis
5. Nonobese patients
6. Those patients with unicompartmental pain only

The "one-finger test" has been reported as a useful indicator as to the location of the pain correlative with the patient's radiographs exhibiting single-compartment osteoarthritis.[3]

CONTRAINDICATIONS

Contraindications have included:
1. Rheumatoid arthritis
2. Nonlocalized or generalized knee pain
3. Patients with decreased range of motion with a flexion contracture
4. Patients with an active lifestyle (runner or impact-loading sports)
5. Those patients with knee instability
6. Severe exogenous obesity

Operating on patients who exhibit contraindications can result in reduced survivorship of UKA.[2,3]

ETIOLOGY OF FAILURES

Furthermore, failures of UKA can occur as a result of:
1. Poor surgical and/or cement technique
2. Inappropriate component design
3. Excessive tibial bone removal
4. Component malalignment
5. Component failure
6. Performing UKA on inappropriately selected patients who have exceeded recommended indications[2,3]

Some designs that are no longer utilized exhibited exceedingly high failure rates as a result of component design and polyethylene failure.[24,25] Furthermore, using all-polyethylene tibial (APT) components in elderly patients with increased posterior tibial slope and removal of significant amounts of tibial bone have resulted in increased medial tibial collapse with subsidence of the tibial component in some patients.[26] Despite recent articles indicating that metal backing reduces strains across the cement-bone interface,[27] the longest published survivorship has utilized APT components with specific undersurface macrostructure on both the inferior portion of the APT component and its eccentric post. However, it has been emphasized that minimal tibial bone was removed in those cases that exhibited the longest survivorship.[19,28]

THE IMPORTANCE OF SURGICAL TECHNIQUE (SEE VIDEO 24-1)

Surgical technique is critical when performing UKA, and accounts for failures regardless of the prosthesis utilized. Surgical recommendations include lateralization of the femoral component when doing medial UKA to account for external rotation during extension of the knee (**Fig. 24–1**). When using an all-polyethylene component, it is important to implant the widest tibial component possible from the medial tibial cortex to the anterior cruciate ligament, resting on the medial tibial cortex (**Fig. 24–2**). Using a Steinmann pin through the intercondylar notch to retract the patella and facilitate exposure is helpful. Appropriate cement technique is critical and involves drilling, using pulse lavage, and drying the surfaces prior to applying the cement (**Fig. 24–3**). The cement should be applied in its doughy stage as well.[29] This allows for improved fixation of both the femoral and tibial components.[30] When choosing APT components, laboratory studies have confirmed that a dovetail undersurface macrostructure of the tibial component provides the greatest resistance to lift-off and shear stresses (**Fig. 24–4**). Waffle undersurface patterns tend to result in the worst resistance to lift-off and shear stress application.[31,32]

COMPLICATIONS OF SURGICAL TECHNIQUE

It is critical to avoid removal of too much tibial bone in order to prevent fracture and/or subsidence of the tibial component. Fractures have been reported (**Figs. 24–5 and 24–6**) through the tibial pin sites, resulting in difficult revision scenarios.[33–35]

Early medial collapse has been reported with significant medial bone removal, and an 11% rate of subsidence of the medially placed APT components has been reported with 2.5-year follow-ups. Upon radiographic review of these patients, the tibial component lacked peripheral support and there was significant bone removal.[26] As originally reported by Bloebaum et al.,[36] the majority of the proximal tibia, when resecting approximately 6–11 mm below the articular surface, is

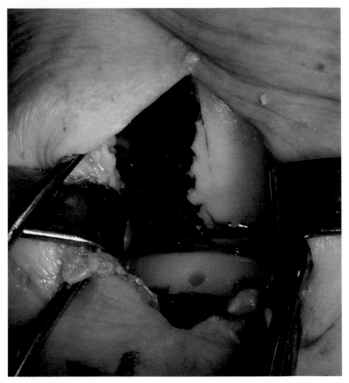

Figure 24-2 APT tibial component resting on medial tibial cortex.

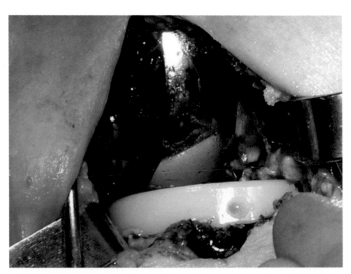

Figure 24-1 Lateralization of femoral component in medial UKA.

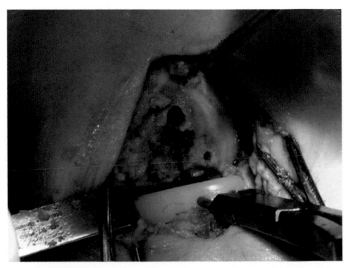

Figure 24-3 Drilling of femur prior to cementing status post pulse lavage and drying.

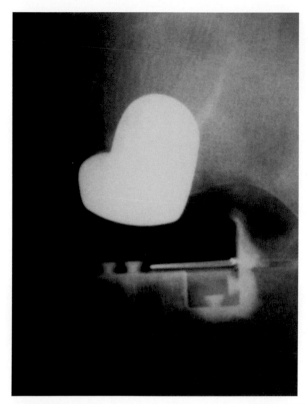

Figure 24-4 Dovetail interface structure on undersurface of tibial APT component.

highly porous cancellous bone consisting predominantly of air. When viewing these resected specimens through the electron microscope, it is apparent that up to 80% of the proximal tibia is cancellous bone at these levels, as demonstrated by polarized (**Fig. 24–7A**) and nonpolarized (**Fig. 24–7B**) electron microscopic views of the proximal tibia.[36] Furthermore, the posteromedial and posterolateral aspects of the resected proximal tibia have up to 20% more bone than the remainder of the articular surface. This observation would clearly explain why fixation can be an issue and subsidence may occur, especially anteromedially and anterolaterally, if too much tibial bone is resected or an undersized tibial component is placed without medial tibial cortex contact and support.

Malalignment

Alignment is critical to the success of UKA. Squire et al. originally reported this concept in 1999 when they noted in a series of UKA patients that 46% had loss of lateral joint space postoperatively.[37] The etiology of lateral compartment wear subsequent to medial UKA is usually secondary to overcorrecting preoperative varus alignment and placing the patient into postoperative valgus (**Fig. 24–8**). In one consecutive series of 100 patients,[16] 83% developed progressive lateral joint space collapse due to progressive wear of the lateral compartment (**Fig. 24–9**). Berger et al.,[23] however, noted that only 18%

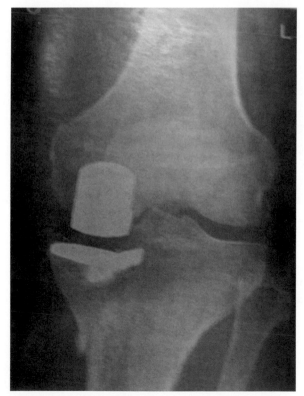

Figure 24-5 Fracture of tibia medially status post pin placement.

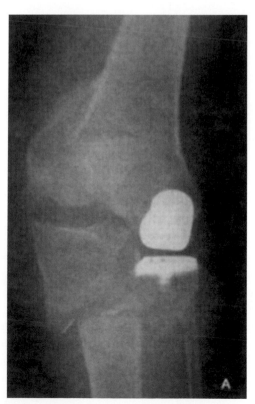

Figure 24-6 Catastrophic fracture of tibia status post lateral UKA.

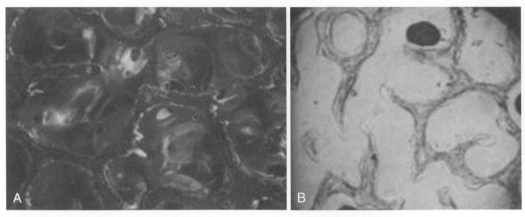

Figure 24-7 Electron microscopic polarized view **(A)** and nonpolarized view **(B)** of proximal tibia 8–11 mm below the articular surface.

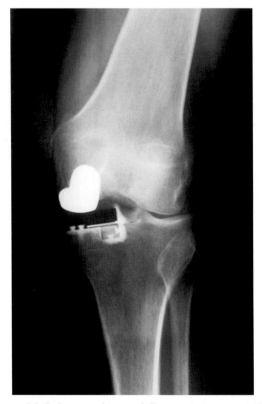

Figure 24-8 Severe valgus malalignment status post UKA.

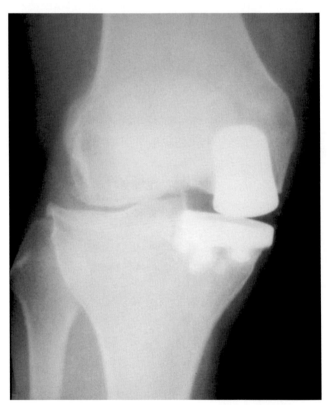

Figure 24-9 Progressive lateral joint space collapse 10 years status post medial UKA.

developed progressive joint space collapse subsequent to UKA when these patients were placed in neutral to slight mechanical varus (**Fig. 24–10**). Biopsies of the pristine surface of the lateral compartment in "normal"-appearing lateral compartment chondral surfaces has confirmed early changes of osteoarthritis histologically, indicating that preexistent degenerative arthritis may be present in asymptomatic knee compartments.[38] Medial-lateral mismatch can occur due to inappropriate placement of the components in the sagittal plane on the medial femoral condyle or the tibial plateau. In addition,

sizing of the femur and tibia is important as well since the tibial component should rest on the medial tibial cortex to avoid subsidence, which is a common failure modality if too much tibial bone is removed or the tibial component is undersized. Lateral positioning of the femoral component onto the medial femoral condyle is helpful to avoid medial-lateral mismatch.[3,25,26] Older prosthetic designs more commonly resulted in articular surface mismatch due to attempts at matching surface geometry configurations of the femoral and tibial components (**Fig. 24–11**).

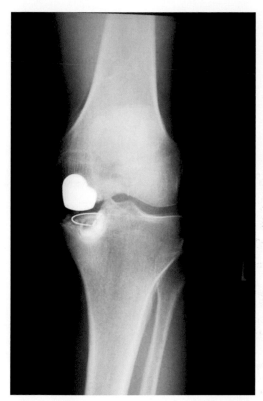

Figure 24-10 Postoperative UKA placed in neutral to slight anatomic varus.

Failure of Fixation

Failure of fixation is most commonly due to cement technique and/or component design (**Fig. 24–12**). Polyethylene wear with premature failure of the tibial insert was more common previously due to the usage of thin polyethylene inserts (**Fig. 24–13**) and sterilization issues resulting in delamination and early wear of the polyethylene tibial insert.[25] Cement removal can be compromised due to a mini-incision exposure resulting in cement retained posterior to the APT component. When implanting the tibial component, a "snowplow effect" (**Fig. 24–14A**) can occur resulting in "heaping up" of bone posteriorly (**Fig. 24–14B and 14C**), which can eventually fracture and result in loose body formation.[39] It is important to use a small curved curette or similar instrument to remove cement posteriorly when implanting the APT component.

Inappropriate Patient Selection

Inappropriate patient selection includes choosing patients with more than single-compartment disease and/or global knee pain.[3] Controversy exists, however, as to the amount of preexistent patellofemoral arthritis that can be ignored at the time of unicompartmental arthroplasty. Some authors argue that there is no contraindication to preexistent patellofemoral disease unless there is bone loss and lateral facet grooving.[40] Extremely active patients are a concern when performing this procedure since loosening and premature wear is possible.

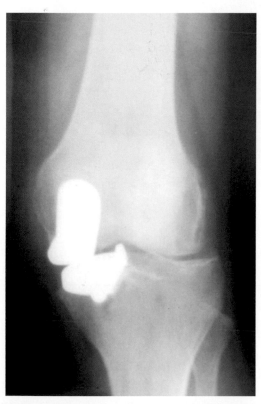

Figure 24-11 Medial-lateral mismatch of femoral and tibial components.

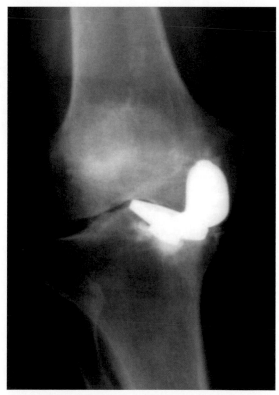

Figure 24-12 Failed fixation of UKA.

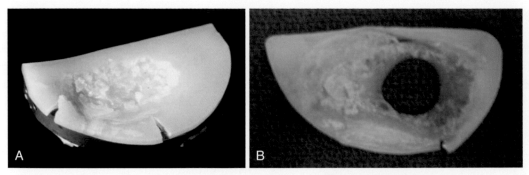

Figure 24-13 (A) Failed polyethylene insert exhibiting delamination, pitting, fracture, and wear. **(B)** Failed polyethylene insert exhibiting severe wear.

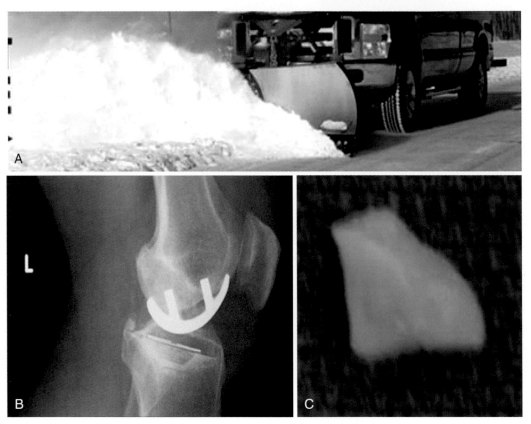

Figure 24-14 (A) Snowplow effect illustrating "heaping" of snow. **(B)** Cement buildup posterior to tibial component. **(C)** Cement "loose body" occurring 2° to fracture of built-up cement posteriorly.

Obesity has been implicated as a failure mechanism in UKA. As was noted by Behrend et al. in 2005, when other factors were excluded, obesity was a major causative factor in midterm and long-term survivorship of UKA.[41] In a retrospective review of 921 UKAs in the Healtheast Total Joint Registry,[18] a statistical analysis to compare cumulative revision rates using the Wilcoxon rank-sum test, Kaplan-Meier survival analysis, the log rank test, and the Cox proportional hazards regression test was performed. The average follow-up was 7.2 years with a range of 2 to 14 years. Obesity was defined as a body mass index (BMI) greater than 30. The results of this review confirmed no increased risk of revision for overweight or obese patients when compared to normal-BMI patients after adjustment for age and year of index procedure.[42]

CONCLUSIONS

In summary, failures of UKA are secondary to poor surgical technique resulting in tibial fracture, and medial-lateral mismatch with resultant component maltracking and loosening. Other causative factors include poor cement implantation technique as a result of ignoring the concepts of drilling, pulse lavage, and drying the bony cut surfaces prior to cementing the components. Furthermore, removal of too much tibial bone may result in component subsidence due to the significant porosity of bone occurring in the proximal tibia. Poor component design has contributed to medial-lateral mismatch, articular surface incongruity, and mobile-bearing dislocation. Component and/or limb malalignment may occur if the surgeon is not consistently monitoring alignment during the surgical procedure. Inappropriate patient selection is perhaps the most critical component resulting in prolonged survivorship for UKA. Patients with generalized knee pain tend to get incomplete relief of pain from a unicompartmental replacement. Extremely active patients tend to have earlier failure rates than those who are able to avoid significant activity levels. Obesity logically should be a contraindication to long-term survivorship for this procedure; however, midterm survivorship studies have been unable to substantiate this theory. If a well-designed UKA component system is implanted correctly in the appropriately chosen patient, UKA is a highly successful procedure in the middle-aged or older patient. As long as minimal tibial bone is removed at the time of the index procedure, revision total knee arthroplasty procedures are extremely successful for failed UKA and not difficult to perform.

REFERENCES

1. Riddle D, Jiranek W, McGlynn F. Yearly incidence of unicompartmental knee arthroplasty in the United States. J Arthroplasty 2008;23:408-412.
2. Borus T, Thornhill T. Unicompartmental knee arthroplasty. J Am Acad Orthop Surg 2008;16:9-18.
3. Bert J. Unicompartmental knee replacement. Orthop Clin North Am 2005;36:513-522.
4. Skolnick M, Coventry M, Ilstrup D. Geometric total knee arthroplasty: a two year follow-up. J Bone Joint Surg [Am] 1976;58:749-753.
5. Skolnick M, Peterson L, Combs J. Polycentric knee arthroplasty—a two year follow-up. J Bone Joint Surg [Am] 1975;57:1033-1038.
6. Bae D, Guhl J, Keane S. Unicompartmental knee arthroplasty for single compartment disease: clinical experience with an average 4 year follow-up study. Clin Orthop Relat Res 1983;(176):233-238.
7. Laskin R. Unicompartmental tibiofemoral resurfacing arthroplasty. J Bone Joint Surg [Am] 1978;60:182-185.
8. Cameron H, Hunter G, Welsh R, et al. Unicompartmental knee replacement. Clin Orthop Relat Res 1981;(160):109-113.
9. Insall J, Aglietti P. A 5 to 7 year follow up of unicondylar arthroplasty. J Bone Joint Surg [Am] 1980;62:1329-1337.
10. Marmor L. The modular knee. Clin Orthop Relat Res 1973;(94):242-248.
11. Marmor L. Unicompartmental arthroplasty of the knee with a minimum of 10 year followup. Clin Orthop Relat Res 1988;(228):171-177.
12. Scott R, Cobb A, Ewald P, et al. Unicompartmental knee arthroplasty: 8 to 12 year follow-up with survivorship analysis. Clin Orthop Relat Res 1991;(271):96-100.
13. Heck D, Marmor L, Gibson A, et al. Unicompartmental knee arthroplasty: a multicenter investigation with long term follow-up evaluation. Clin Orthop Relat Res 1993;(286):154-159.
14. Cartier A, Kozinn S, Scott R. Unicompartmental knee arthroplasty surgery. J Arthroplasty 1996;11:782-786.
15. Grelsamer RP. Unicompartmental osteoarthritis of the knee. J Bone Joint Surg [Am] 1995;77:278-292.
16. Bert J. Ten year survivorship of metal backed unicompartmental arthroplasty. J Arthroplasty 1998;13:901-905.
17. Svärd UC, Price AJ. Oxford medial unicompartmental knee arthroplasty: a survival analysis of independent series. J Bone Joint Surg [Br] 2001;83:191-194.
18. Gioe T, Bert J, Killeen K, et al. Analysis of unicompartmental arthroplasty in a community based implant registry. Clin Orthop Relat Res 2003;(416):111-119.
19. Steele R, Hutabarat S, Evans R, et al. Survivorship of the St. Georg Sled medial unicompartmental knee replacement beyond 10 years. J Bone Joint Surg [Br] 2006;88:1164-1172.
20. Repicci J. Benefits and limitations of the unicondylar knee prosthesis. J Orthop 2003;26:274-279.
21. Sah A, Springer B, Scott R. Unicompartmental knee arthroplasty in octogenerians: survival longer than the patient. Clin Orthop Relat Res 2006;(451):107-112.
22. O'Rourke M, Gardner J, Callaghan J, et al. The John Insall Award. Unicompartmental knee replacement: a minimum 21 year follow-up, end results study. Clin Orthop Relat Res 2005;(440):27-34.
23. Berger R, Meneghini R, Jacobs J, et al. Results of unicompartmental knee arthroplasy at a minimun of ten years of follow-up. J Bone Joint Surg [Am] 2005;87:999-1004.
24. Hamilton W, Collier M, Tarabee E. Incidence and reasons for reoperation after minimally invasive unicompartmental knee arthroplasty. J Arthroplasty 2006;21(6 Suppl 2):98-107.
25. Bert J, Smith R. Failures of metal-backed unicompartmental arthroplasty. Knee 1997;4:41-48.
26. Aleto TJ, Berend ME, Ritter MA, et al. Early failure of unicompartmental knee arthroplasty leading to revision. J Arthroplasty 2008;23:159-163.
27. Small S, Behrend M, Ritter M, et al. Metal backing significantly decreases tibial strains in unicompartmental knee arthroplasty. Manuscript submitted for publication, January 2010.
28. Newman J, Pydisetty R, Ackroyd C. Unicompartmental or total knee replacement: the results of a prospective randomized controlled trial. J Bone Joint Surg [Br] 2009;91:52-57.
29. Bert J. Unicompartmental arthroplasty for unicompartmental knee arthritis. Tech Knee Surg 2007;6(4):1-10.
30. Bert J, McShane M. Is it necessary to cement the tibial stem in cemented total knee arthroplasty? Clin Orthop Relat Res 1998;(356):73-78.
31. Bert J, Koeneman J. A comparison of the mechanical stability of various unicompartmental tibial components. J Orthop Arthroplasty Rounds 1994;17:559-564.
32. Rosa RA, Bert JM, Bruce W, et al. An evaluation of all-ultra-high molecular weight polyethylene unicompartmental tibial component cement fixation mechanisms. J Bone Joint Surg [Am] 2002;84(Suppl 2):102-104.
33. Yang KY, Yeo SJ, Lo NN. Stress fracture of the medial tibial plateau after minimally invasive unicompartmental knee arthroplasty: a report of 2 cases. J Arthroplasty 2003;18:801-803.

34. Brumby S, Carrington R, Zayontz S, et al. Tibial plateau stress fracture: a complication of unicompartmental knee arthroplasty using 4 guide pinholes. J Arthroplasty 2003;18:809-812.

35. Song M, Kim B, Seong J, et al. Early complications after minimally invasive mobile-bearing unicompartmental arthroplasty. J Arthroplasty 2009;24:1281-1284.

36. Bloebaum R, Bachus K, Mitchell W, et al. Analysis of the bone surface area in resected tibia. Clin Orthop Relat Res 1994;(309):2-10.

37. Squire M, Callaghan J, Goetz D, et al. Unicompartmental knee replacement: a minimum 15 year followup study. Clin Orthop Relat Res 1999;(367):61-72.

38. Bert J. Histologic appearance of pristine articular cartilage in knees with unicompartmental osteoarthritis. J Knee Surg 2007;20:15-20.

39. Hamilton W, et al. Incidence and causes of reoperation after minimally invasive unicompartmental knee arthroplasty. Presented at the AAOS 73rd Annual Meeting, Chicago, IL, March 22–24, 2006.

40. Beard DJ, Pandit H, Ostlere S, et al. Pre-operative clinical and radiological assessment of the patellofemoral joint in unicompartmental knee replacement and its influence on outcome. J Bone Joint Surg [Br] 2007;89:1602-1607.

41. Behrend K, Lombardi A, Mallory T, et al. Early failure of minimally invasive unicompartmental knee arthroplasty is associated with obesity. Clin Orthop Relat Res 2005;(440):60-66.

42. Bert J, Tatman P, Mehle S, Killeen K. The effect of body mass index on survivorship of unicompartmental knee arthroplasty. Manuscript submitted for publication, February 2010.

CHAPTER 25
The Failed Uni

Jeffrey H. DeClaire

KEY POINTS

- Despite advances in prosthetic component design, newly developed instrumentation and surgical technique, and appropriate patient selection, failure after unicompartmental knee arthroplasty can occur. As the number of unicompartmental knee arthroplasties performed continues to rise, so too will the number of failures.
- The current recommendation for management of the failed unicompartmental arthroplasty is conversion to total knee arthroplasty. In the majority of cases, the conversion of unicondylar arthroplasty to total knee arthroplasty can successfully be performed with the same approach used in primary total knee arthroplasty.
- Failure mode can be predictive of complexity of the conversion of unicompartmental arthroplasty to total knee arthroplasty. Failure modes have included polyethylene wear, progression of arthritis, patellofemoral symptoms, aseptic loosening, malpositioned implants, medial tibial collapse, poor patient selection, and technical factors.
- Polyethylene wear, with or without loosening, and progressive arthritis have been the most common failure modes reported with contemporary unicompartmental knee arthroplasty designs. When unicompartmental knees fail through these modes, the revision procedures are straightforward with minimal bone loss.
- When failure occurs in unicompartmental knee arthroplasty due to early collapse of the medial tibial plateau, there are more significant bone defects, and revisions are technically more demanding than that seen with other aseptic failure mechanisms such as polyethylene wear.
- Early failure is typically related to inappropriate patient selection, infection, medial tibial collapse, or poor surgical technique leading to ligament instability, malpositioning of the implant, or component loosening. The more common modes of failure include polyethylene wear, progression of tricompartmental arthritis, or component loosening, and will occur late after the first or second decade.
- In general, late failures are less demanding and can usually be converted using a cruciate-retained or posterior-stabilized primary total knee arthroplasty, without supplemental stabilization or constraint.
- The surgical approach follows the same principles of primary total knee arthroplasty using standard primary total knee arthroplasty instrumentation. One of the most important technical aspects of the procedure is to leave the unicompartmental arthroplasty implants intact as long as possible.
- Resection of the patella can be performed first in order to facilitate the exposure to the distal femur. This will also avoid eversion of the patella, which will minimize the soft tissue trauma to the extensor mechanism.
- There are three main critical areas of importance that must be evaluated preoperatively and attended to intraoperatively: distal femoral bone deficiency, posteromedial (or posterolateral) femoral bone deficiency, and medial (or lateral) tibial bone deficiency.

INTRODUCTION

The popularity of unicompartmental knee arthroplasty has continued to grow over the last decade and is one of the main treatment alternatives for isolated degenerative arthritis of the knee.[1–3] Since its introduction, unicondylar arthroplasty has been an alternative to total knee arthroplasty or high tibial osteotomy for the treatment of unicompartmental knee arthritis. The benefits of this procedure are attributed to the ability to provide a more rapid rehabilitation time, greater range of motion, preservation of bone stock, and more normal knee kinematics with the retention of both the anterior and posterior cruciate ligaments. With improvements in component design, surgical technique, and patient selection criteria, improved clinical outcomes have been reported in the literature. Berger et al. reported on a prospective study of 62 unicompartmental knee arthroplasties with a mean follow-up of 12 years.[3] They noted no loose components or periprosthetic osteolysis, with a 10-year survival rate of 98%. Price et al. also noted a 93% 10-year survival using the Oxford unicompartmental knee implant.[4] Because of these encouraging results, the prevalence of unicompartmental knee arthroplasty has increased significantly over the years. Between 1996 and 1997, unicondylar knee arthroplasty comprised only 1% of the U.S. total knee market.[5] This increased to 6% of all total knees performed in the United States between 2000 and 2001. Between 1998 and 2005, there has been a 10% per year increase in the number of unicompartmental knee arthroplasty procedures performed in the United States alone.[6] This growth rate is approximately three times that for total knee arthroplasty, and presently it is estimated that 12% of all total knees performed in the United States are unicompartmental knee arthroplasties.

Although early midterm studies cite a high rate of satisfactory results after unicompartmental knee arthroplasty, long-term survivorship and outcome continue to be a concern. Long-term survivorship of unicompartmental knee arthroplasty has been improving with the advancement in prosthetic component design, newly developed instrumentation and surgical technique, and appropriate patient selection. Despite advances, failure after unicompartmental knee arthroplasty can occur. When compared with total knee arthroplasty as an index arthroplasty procedure, however, the cumulative revision rate for unicompartmental knee arthroplasty tends to be higher.[7,8] Gioe et al. evaluated more than 5000 total knee arthroplasties in a community registry and noted that unicondylar arthroplasty was 7.2 times as likely to fail compared to an all-polyethylene cemented total knee arthroplasty.[9] The Norwegian Arthroplasty Registry echoed some of these same concerns, noting two times the revision rate with unicompartmental arthroplasty versus total knee arthroplasty in their evaluation of more than 2200 unicondylar knees.[10] In the Swedish Registry, Lindgren et al. found a greater than 10% cumulative revision rate at 10 years for unicondylar arthroplasty, with only a 5% cumulative revision rate for total knee arthroplasty.[11] In the Australian Registry, results were equally concerning with their 5-year revision rate of 8.9%.[12] As the number of unicompartmental knee arthroplasties performed continues to rise, so too will the number of failures. Early investigations reported technical difficulty during conversion of unicompartmental knee arthroplasty to total knee arthroplasty, citing substantial bone loss requiring bone grafting, stemmed revision components, or the need for custom implants.[8,13] More recently, with improvement in surgical technique and prosthetic designs, conversion of unicompartmental knee arthroplasty to total knee arthroplasty has been described as less technically demanding than a revision total knee arthroplasty with results comparable to the results of primary total knee arthroplasty, in terms of both function and survivorship[14] (**Figs. 25–1 and 25–2**).

CLINICAL EVALUATION AND PREOPERATIVE PLANNING

The current recommendation for management of the failed unicompartmental arthroplasty is conversion to total knee

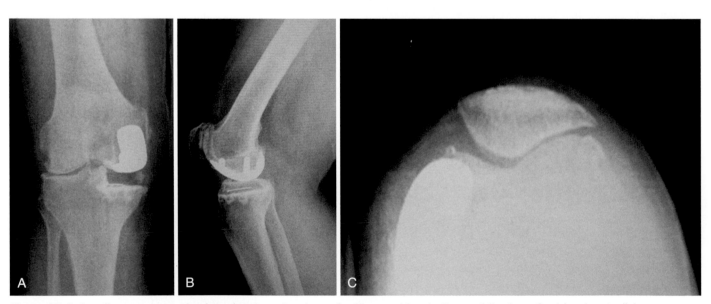

Figure 25-1 Standing anteroposterior, lateral and sunrise views of a 63-year-old male 6 years following a fixed-bearing medial unicompartmental knee arthroplasty with progressive degeneration of the lateral compartment and patellofemoral compartment requiring conversion.

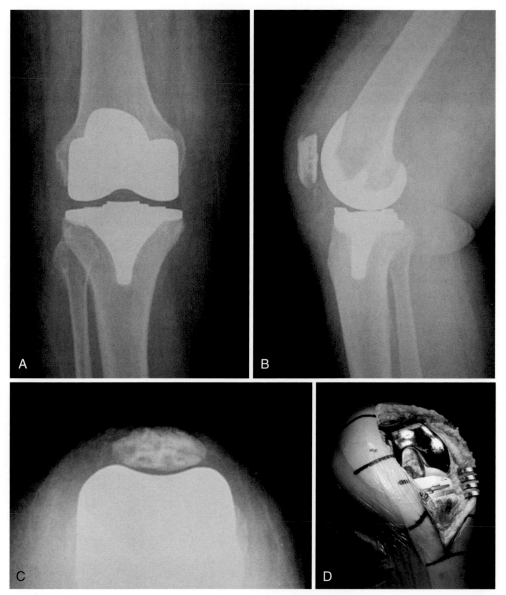

Figure 25-2 Postoperative radiographs and intra-operative photo of the same patient after conversion of the unicompartmental knee arthroplasty to a primary cruciate-retained total knee arthroplasty.

arthroplasty.[15] In the majority of cases, the conversion of uni-condylar arthroplasty to total knee arthroplasty can success-fully be performed with the same approach used in primary total knee arthroplasty. Primary total knee arthroplasty com-ponents and instrumentaion can be used. In most cases, however, it is essential to be prepared for any technical diffi-culties that may arise requiring stem fixation, metal augments, bone grafting, or a more constrained component (**Figs. 25–3 and 25–4**). Preoperative evaluation is critical in the planning process. Berend et al. have shown that the mode of failure is predictive in determining complexity of conversion and can assist in the planning for special instrumentation, or more complex reconstructive options.[15]

Factors leading to unicompartmental knee arthroplasty failure have been shown to differ based on whether failure has

occurred early or late. Early failure is typically related to inap-propriate patient selection, infection, medial tibial collapse, or poor surgical technique leading to ligament instability, mal-positioning of the implant, or component loosening. The more common modes of failure include polyethylene wear, progression of tricompartmental arthritis, or component loosening, and will occur late after the first or second decade[16] (**Fig. 25–5**). In general, late failures are less demanding and can usually be converted using a cruciate-retained or posterior-stabilized primary total knee arthroplasty, without supple-mental stabilization or constraint.[17] If failure occurs secondary to medial tibial collapse or excessive resection of tibial bone, a more complex reconstruction will typically be required. Aleto et al., in a retrospective review of 32 knees converted to total knee arthroplasty, found that the most common mode

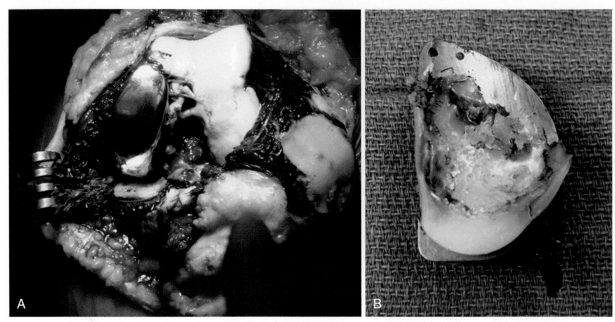

Figure 25-3 Intra-operative photos of a 68-year-old female 11 years following a fixed-bearing medial unicompartmental knee arthroplasty with extreme polyethylene wear and associated metallosis.

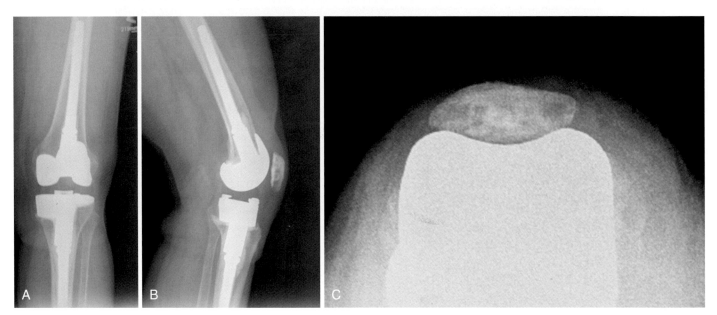

Figure 25-4 Postoperative radiographs of the same patient, which required a more constrained component with extension stems and a medial augment due to the extensive osteolysis and associated bone loss.

of failure was related to medial tibial collapse (47% of the study group)[16] (see Fig. 25–1). Of these, 87% were an all-polyethylene design, and 7 of 15 failed in less than 16 months and required a more complex reconstruction with stems, augments, and screws. In addition, they also found tibial component slope to be associated with the direction of the collapse of the implant into the tibia. Excessive posterior tibial component slope, with a mean of 12.0°, was associated with posterior failure. When failure mode is related to medial tibial

collapse, more significant bone loss can be expected, and most likely will require a more complex reconstruction (**Fig. 25–6**).

A thorough evaluation prior to surgery should be undertaken with all patients to accurately determine the cause of failure. This should include a detailed history, physical examination, radiographic evaluation, knee fluid analysis, and appropriate laboratory assessment. As in all knee arthroplasty patients, with any type of failure, it is important to consider septic arthritis until proven otherwise. Initial screening methods should be performed as in total knee arthroplasty with joint fluid analysis, including cell count, culture and sensitivity, Gram stain, and assessment for crystals. Peripheral blood evaluation should also be performed, including complete blood count, erythrocyte sedimentation rate, and C-reactive protein, as well as bone scan and sulfur colloid technetium bone scanning if indicated. A detailed physical examination should also be conducted to rule out elements of

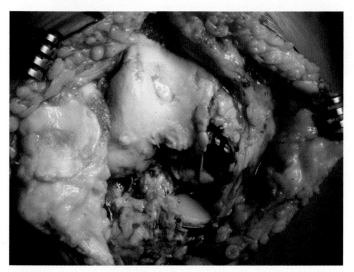

Figure 25-5 Intra-operative photo of the more common mode of failure with progressive degeneration of the patellofemoral joint and lateral compartment.

instability, with particular reference to the anterior cruciate ligament as well as the collateral ligaments. Injury or deficiency of the anterior cruciate ligament or medial collateral ligament can compromise function of the knee in the setting of unicompartmental knee arthroplasty. Lateral joint line tenderness with associated joint effusion may indicate meniscal pathology involving the opposite compartment and sometimes can be addressed with arthroscopic methods alone. Similarly, intra-articular scarring may cause impingement within the joint space, which can contribute to persistent postoperative pain and many times can be treated successfully with knee arthroscopy (**Fig. 25–7**).

It is important to note that the diagnosis of meniscal pathology, or intra-articular scarring, is based on history and clinical examination alone. It is therefore essential to first rule out all other causes for persistent pain and failure of unicompartmental arthroplasty. Standing weight-bearing radiographs are essential for evaluation of the femoral tibial joint space, which should include a standing bilateral anteroposterior view, a 45° flexion posteroanterior weight-bearing view, and lateral and skyline views. A long-leg standing weight-bearing (1.37 cm) axial alignment radiograph is also necessary to further evaluate the anatomic and mechanical axis of the knee (**Fig. 25–8**). Any progressive change of alignment may be an indication of medial tibial collapse, or possible progressive degeneration of the opposite compartment. Radiographic evaluation is also important in order to determine any evidence of radiolucent lines or concerns for component

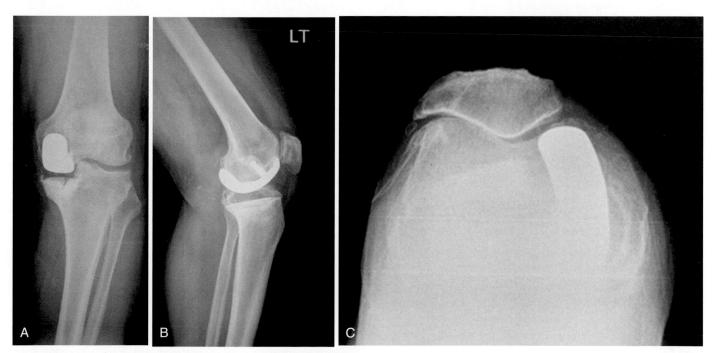

Figure 25-6 Standing anteroposterior, lateral, and sunrise radiographs of a medial unicompartmental knee arthroplasty requiring conversion to a total knee arthroplasty due to progressive degeneration of the patellofemoral joint. Note that this is an all-polyethylene tibial component with a significant posterior slope, indicating a high likelihood for a more complex reconstruction requiring augmentation and stem fixation.

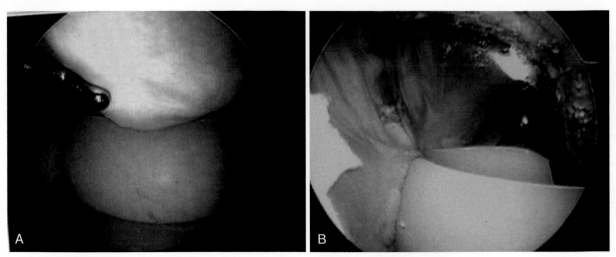

Figure 25-7 (A) Arthroscopic view of a mobile-bearing unicompartmental knee arthroplasty with medial scar impingement. **(B)** Same view after resection of scar and additional removal of bone.

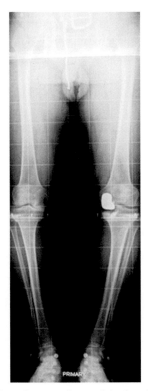

Figure 25-8 The long-leg standing weight-bearing axial alignment view is critical in evaluating the anatomic and mechanical axis of the knee. Note the varus deformity with the collapse of the medial compartment.

loosening or wear of polyethylene (**Fig. 25–9**). Serial comparison of radiographs over time is extremely helpful as changes in alignment, collapse of the tibia, or progression of arthritis can occur gradually, and sometimes can only be appreciated with prior comparison views (**Fig. 25–10**). Assessment of bone loss, on either the femoral or tibial side, is also important in planning the need for a more complex reconstruction requiring metal augments, stems, or a more constrained revision

component. Templating the level of resection on radiographs can help in this planning process to more accurately predict the need for augmentation.

SETUP AND TECHNIQUE

After confirmation of the preoperative plan, examination under anesthesia should be performed first. This will allow for further assessment of passive range of motion and collateral ligament stability, as well as the integrity of the anterior and posterior cruciate ligaments. The procedure is approached in a manner similar to that of primary total knee arthroplasty utilizing general or regional anesthesia. A short-acting spinal anesthetic with light sedation is preferable, as this will allow for a more successful approach with pain management. This has also been very beneficial in initiating early weight bearing and recovery of quadriceps muscle function within hours after the procedure. After induction of anesthesia, the patient is positioned in the supine position, with a small bolster placed at the foot of the bed to allow for knee flexion between 70° and 90° (**Fig. 25–11**). A specific leg holder is not necessary, and many times can cause further constraints of the tibia, affecting internal and external rotation during the surgical procedure.

The surgical approach follows the same principles of primary total knee arthroplasty using standard primary total knee arthroplasty instrumentation. One of the most important technical aspects of the procedure is to leave the unicompartmental arthroplasty implants intact as long as possible. This allows for a more accurate assessment of the joint line with the ability to reference the normal landmarks of the knee. Once the limb is sterilely prepped and draped, the skin incision is made utilizing the prior surgical incision, extending it proximally or distally depending on the clinical condition. A medial patellar approach is recommended to provide

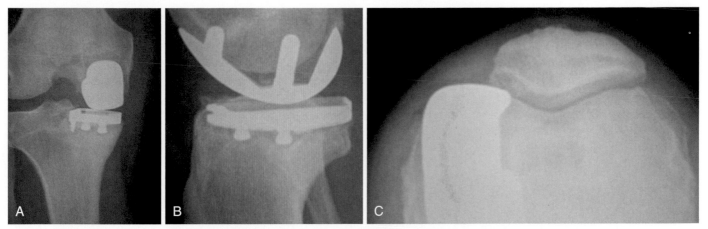

Figure 25-9 Failure of a fixed-bearing medial unicompartmental knee arthroplasty secondary to aseptic loosening of the tibial component. Note the radiolucency below the tibial component both in the anteroposterior and lateral views.

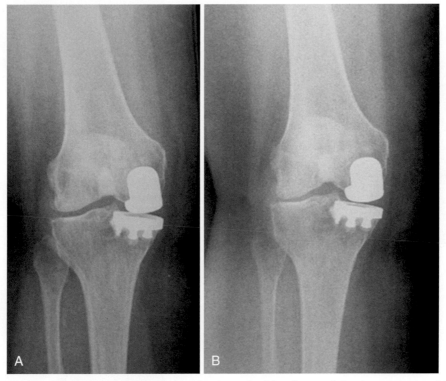

Figure 25-10 (A) Standing 45° midflexion radiograph 4 years following a fixed-bearing medial unicompartmental knee arthroplasty. **(B)** Same radiograph taken 18 months later showing progressive wear of the lateral compartment. Note: The standing midflexion 45° view is the most accurate way to assess degenerative changes of the lateral compartment.

appropriate exposure and is performed in the same manner as for a primary total knee arthroplasty. With the leg in full extension, careful dissection of the soft tissues is first carried out to develop adequate exposure. Frequently, scar may be present in the peripatellar area as well as the retropatellar fat pad. Scarring and fibrosis of the fat pad will cause obliteration of the retropatellar space with adherence of the patellar tendon to the anterior tibia. It is important for this scar to be removed and to re-create this space in order to improve patellofemoral mobility as well as facilitating exposure.

Resection of the patella can be performed first in order to facilitate the exposure to the distal femur. This will also avoid eversion of the patella, which will minimize the soft tissue trauma to the extensor mechanism. Patellar resection is performed using the same principles followed in total knee arthroplasty with a measured resection approach. Using a towel clip, the patella can be easily everted and stabilized for preparation (**Fig. 25–12**). Removing the surrounding synovial tissue from the periphery of the patella is helpful in accurately identifying the level of resection. Once the periphery of the

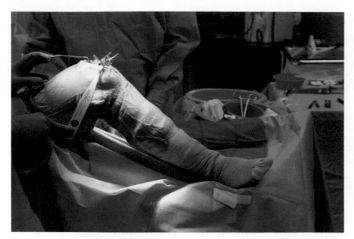

Figure 25-11 Patient positioning with knee flexion between 70° and 90°.

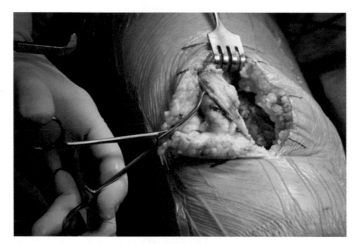

Figure 25-12 With the leg in full extension, the patella can be prepared first by using a towel clip to evert and stabilize the patella. Removal of the peripatellar synovium from the periphery of the patella can more accurately identify the appropriate level of resection.

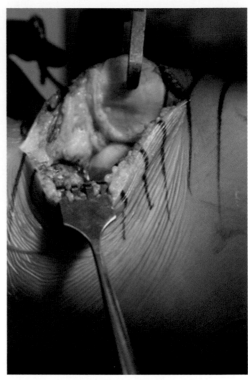

Figure 25-13 Patellar thickness is measured with the caliper, with assessment of both the medial and lateral facets.

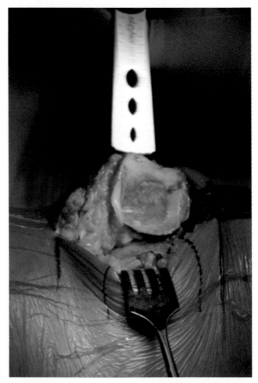

Figure 25-14 Transverse osteotomy can be performed using a freehand technique or instrumented method, depending on the surgeon's preference.

patella is cleared of synovial tissue to define its margins, a measured resection can be performed. It is important to restore the native patellar thickness to avoid overstuffing the patellofemoral joint, which can affect patellar articulation, patellar tracking, and range of motion. The patella should be measured using calipers in all four quadrants in order to retain the normal patellar height in the most accurate manner, and to avoid an oblique level of resection (**Fig. 25–13**). Transverse patellar osteotomy can be performed utilizing a freehand method or instrument method, depending on the surgeon's preference (**Fig. 25–14**). The resection level should be parallel, and once again, assessment should be made with the caliper in all four quadrants to avoid the risk of an oblique cut, and any abnormality with patellar tracking (**Fig. 25–15**). Sizing of the patella can then be performed in the usual manner, taking

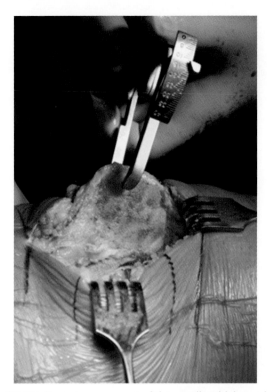

Figure 25-15 Repeat assessment of the patellar thickness is made following resection to verify appropriate thickness and symmetric resection of bone.

care to medialize the patella to prevent any overhang beyond the margins of the bone (**Fig. 25–16**). The thickness of the patella should then be reassessed following insertion of the prosthetic component trial. Ideally the goal is to have the thickness of the remaining patella and the patellar prosthesis equal to the appropriate patellar thickness.

Once the patella has been appropriately prepared, it can be easily displaced into the lateral gutter, thereby avoiding eversion of the patella with much less surgical trauma or injury to the quadriceps extensor mechanism. A custom-designed patellar retractor has been developed to facilitate the retraction of the patella, as well as protect the resected surface throughout the procedure (**Fig. 25–17**). The knee is then flexed and held in a position between 70° and 90° of flexion to provide excellent exposure of the distal femur and proximal tibia. It is important to note that hyperflexion should be avoided as this can cause greater difficulties with exposure of the distal femur due to the increased tension that is applied across the extensor mechanism the further the knee is flexed. If a modular tibial component is present, then removal of the tibial polyethylene component should be performed first. This will facilitate exposure and preparation of the distal femur. If an all-polyethylene tibial component is present, then removal should be delayed until after resection of the distal femur. Removal of an all-polyethylene tibial component can be

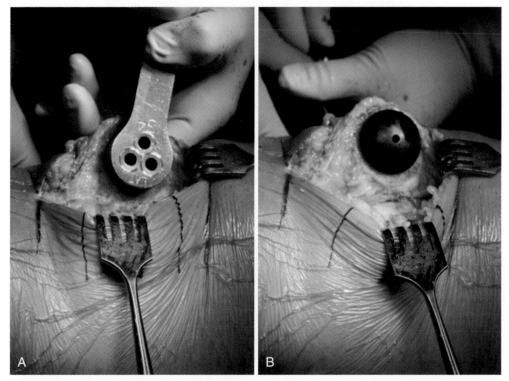

Figure 25-16 The patellar sizing guide is applied and medialized for improved patellar tracking. Three lug holes are drilled that are standardized to allow for interchangeability of the component for determining the exact size.

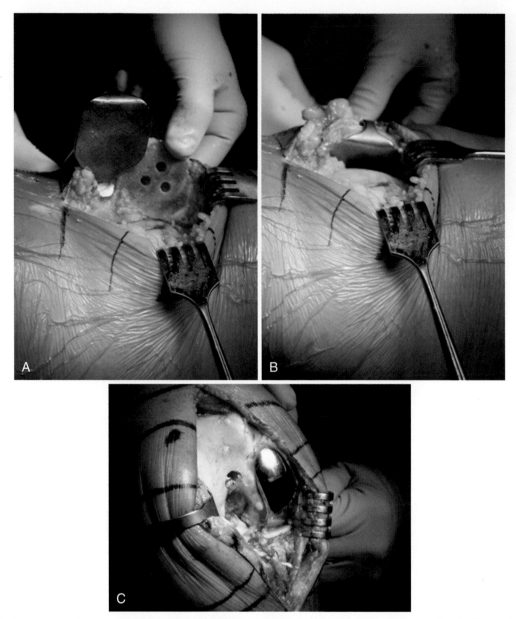

Figure 25-17 (A) A custom-designed patellar retractor is used to protect the resected patellar surface and to facilitate displacement of the patella into the lateral gutter for exposure of the distal femur. **(B)** The patellar surface is protected and displaced into the lateral gutter without eversion. **(C)** The knee is flexed between 70° and 90° to achieve excellent exposure of the distal femur. The femoral component is left intact, and the intramedullary canal can be entered for placement of the distal femoral resection guide.

achieved more easily and more accurately once the distal femoral resection is complete (**Fig. 25–18**).

Distal femoral resection is performed next. It is extremely important to leave the femoral component intact on the distal femur. This is a critical step, and will allow for more accurate assessment of the joint line for preparation of the distal femur. With the femoral component intact, the intramedullary canal can be entered for insertion of the distal resection guide, referencing off of the medial femoral condyle with the existing component in place (**Fig. 25–19**). Reference should also be made to the resection level of the lateral compartment with an angel wing to further verify the appropriate level of distal femoral resection. With the distal resection guide in place, and

the femoral component left intact, the majority of the distal resection can be performed. A small ($\frac{1}{4}$-inch) osteotome can be used next to carefully, and meticulously, disrupt the bone-cement interface of the femoral component. It is extremely important to address the entire periphery of the prosthesis as well as the posterior condylar area in order to minimize any significant bone loss during implant removal (**Fig. 25–20**). Once the femoral component has been removed, the distal resection of the femur can be completed in the usual manner (**Fig. 25–21**). Frequently this will create a resection level with minimal or no deficiencies of bone in the distal femoral condyle. Bone loss in the distal femoral condyle can usually be addressed with simple bone grafting techniques. Loss of

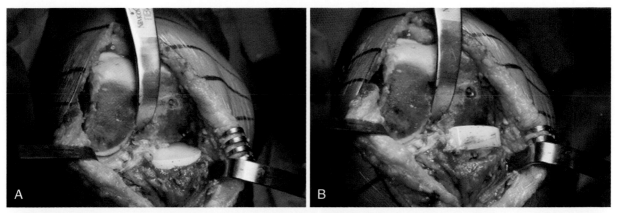

Figure 25-18 Exposure of the proximal tibia and removal of an all-polyethylene tibia can be more easily achieved after resection of the distal femur and removal of the anterior cruciate ligament. Removal of an all-polyethylene tibial component can be easily removed using the oscillating saw to disrupt the cement-implant interface first, followed by removal of the retained cement and pegs.

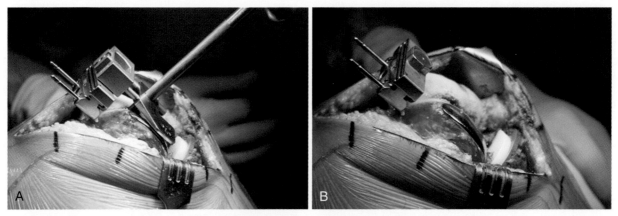

Figure 25-19 Resection of the distal femur should be performed first. The distal femoral resection guide is positioned in the same manner as a primary total knee arthroplasty leaving the femoral component intact. This is a critical step allowing for a more accurate assessment and restoration of the joint line.

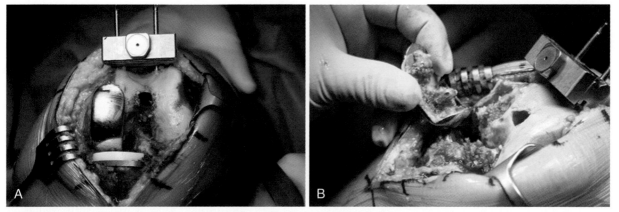

Figure 25-20 Removal of the femoral component is performed next after accurate placement of the distal femoral resection guide. This can be accomplished with a small osteotome, taking care to address the entire periphery of the component. It is important to pay special attention to the posterior condylar area to avoid excess loss of bone.

bone in the posterior condyle of the femur is common, but rarely will require bone grafting or augmentation.

Once the distal femoral resection is complete, exposure of the proximal tibia is significantly easier to achieve. If the anterior cruciate ligament is still intact, this should be incised

first to facilitate anterior displacement of the proximal tibia and improve exposure. A Hohmann retractor carefully placed into the intercondylar notch on the posterior tibia will provide excellent exposure of the proximal tibia. A Z retractor is placed behind the patellar tendon at the level of the joint line in order

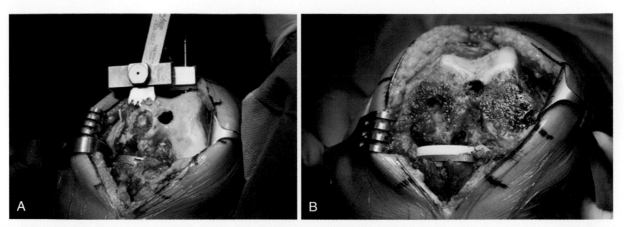

Figure 25-21 After removal of the femoral component, distal femoral resection can be completed similar to a primary total knee arthroplasty. Bone loss is rare in the distal femur, but frequently occurs posterior-medially.

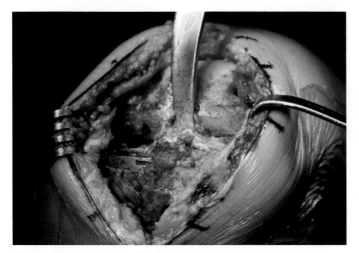

Figure 25-22 With the distal femoral resection complete, exposure of the proximal tibia can be achieved more easily. It is important to excise the anterior cruciate ligament at this time to facilitate anterior displacement of the tibia. Tibial component removal can be accomplished using the reciprocating saw and the small osteotome.

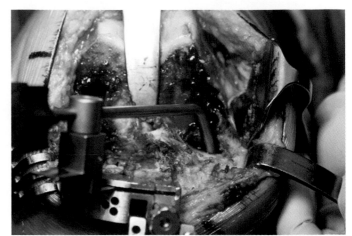

Figure 25-23 Depth of tibial resection should be referenced off the intact lateral bone in order to perform the most conservative level of resection. It is extremely important not to reference the deficient area of bone.

to protect the tendon and to further displace the patella into the lateral gutter and improve exposure (**Fig. 25–22**). A Hohmann retractor placed at the midlevel of the lateral tibial plateau may also be necessary for adequate exposure depending on the anatomy. Attention can now be directed toward removal of the tibial component. Once again, careful and meticulous disruption of the cement-mantle interface is critical in order to minimize any significant bone loss. A reciprocating saw should be used first to disrupt the bone-cement interface, followed by the use of a small osteotome. As with the femoral component removal, it is very important to carefully disrupt the bone-cement interface around the entire periphery of the prosthesis, with particular attention to the posterior aspect of the tibial component to avoid loss of bone in this area. Removal of an all-polyethylene tibial component can be easily accomplished using an oscillating saw to disrupt

the cement-implant interface first. The polyethylene pegs and retained cement can be addressed in the final preparation of the tibia.

Once the tibial component is removed, the tibial resection guide can be positioned using the same reference points used in primary total knee arthroplasty. Depth of tibial resection will be the more critical assessment to be made at this time. Reference should be made off the intact lateral bone, which will allow for the most conservative resection of bone (**Fig. 25–23**). Appropriate slope, as well as varus-valgus alignment, should also be verified. It is extremely important not to reference the deficient area of bone, as this will frequently cause over-resection of the proximal tibia. After the resection of the proximal tibia is complete, assessment of any medial bone deficiency can now be evaluated more accurately. If the defect is less than 6 mm and is contained, then bone grafting or screws and cement can be used successfully to restore the level of the medial compartment to the level of the lateral

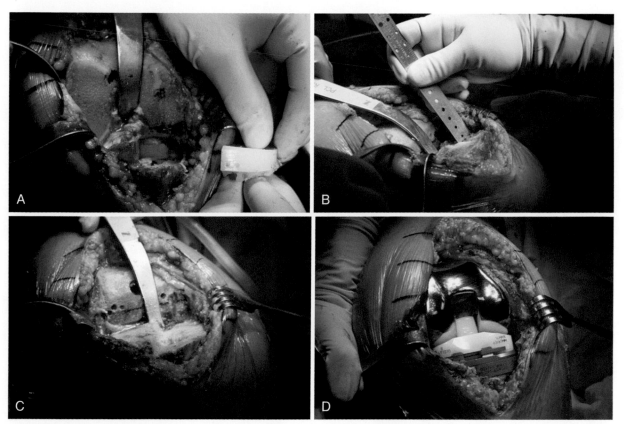

Figure 25-24 **(A)** Intra-operative view after removal of an all-polyethylene tibial component with a significant medial defect. **(B)** Initial conservative resection of tibia is performed first referencing the more normal lateral compartment. Measurement of the medial defect is found to be greater than 5 mm, therefore requiring a medial augment. **(C)** The tibia has been prepared for a medial augment and the appropriate stem fixation. **(D)** Intra-operative view of the final implant requiring a posterior cruciate stabilized femoral component, and a stemmed tibial component with a medial augment.

compartment resection. However, if there is a deficiency of 6 mm or greater, then medial augmentation with stem preparation should be carried out at this time (**Fig. 25–24**).

With the tibial resection completed, attention can be redirected toward the final preparation of the distal femur. It is essential at this time to identify and mark both Whiteside's line and the transepicondylar axis. When converting a medial unicondylar arthroplasty, bone loss from the posteromedial femoral condyle is not uncommon and will cause posterior condylar referencing for rotational alignment and sizing to be unreliable (**Fig. 25–25**). Excess external rotation of the femoral component will occur if these reference points are not identified (**Fig. 25–26**). The femoral sizing and rotation guide can now be easily applied and accurately positioned utilizing these two reference points. With the guide positioned in appropriate external rotation, two reference drill holes can be made for accurate placement of the 4-in-1 guide (**Figs. 25–27 and 25–28**). Once the femoral resection is complete, the medial posterior femoral condyle can be evaluated for bone loss, and the need for augmentation can be determined. Once again, because of improved component designs, posterior augmentation of the femur is rarely required (**Fig. 25–29**).

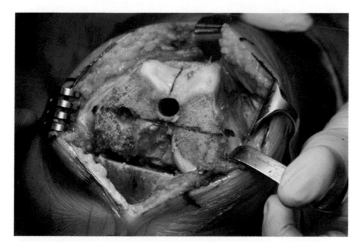

Figure 25-25 Once the tibial preparation is complete, final preparation of the femur can be achieved more easily. Because bone loss is common in the posterior medial femoral condyle, it is extremely important to identify and reference both Whiteside's line and the trans-epicondylar axis for appropriate rotational alignment of the femoral component.

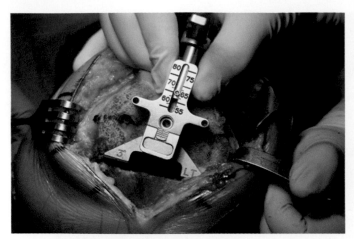

Figure 25-26 With bone loss of the posterior medial condyle, posterior condylar referencing becomes unreliable. Notice the excess external rotation of the sizing/rotation guide when reference is made using these landmarks.

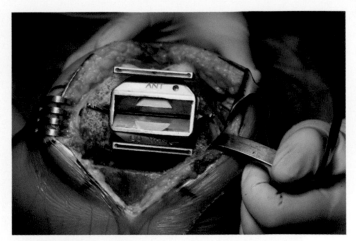

Figure 25-28 The 4-in-1 femoral resection guide can be positioned accurately for final preparation of the femur.

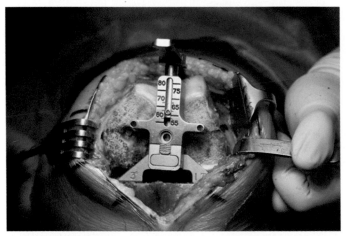

Figure 25-27 Accurate rotational alignment of the sizing/rotation guide can be achieved by using Whiteside's line and the transepicondylar axis.

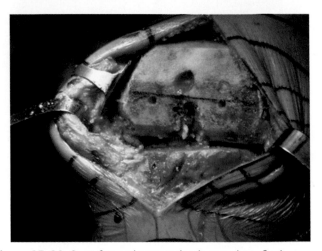

Figure 25-29 Once femoral preparation is complete, final assessment can be made for any residual bone defects in the medial femoral condyle. Because of improved femoral component designs, posterior augmentation of the femur is rarely required.

With the completion of all bone cuts, both on the femur and tibia, ligament balance as well as flexion-extension gap balance can be evaluated. Spacer block technique should then be performed, and is a critical step to verify that appropriate mechanical alignment has been restored, as well as appropriate balance and stability of the flexion and extension space (**Fig. 25–30**). Using a laminar spreader, with the knee flexed at 90°, the posterior compartment can be evaluated for any debris, meniscal remnants, or residual posterior osteophytes (**Fig. 25–31**). Trial reduction is then performed, assessing appropriate stability, range of motion, and the integrity of the posterior cruciate ligament. If there is deficiency of the posterior cruciate ligament, then a more constrained posterior-stabilized component can be utilized. Patellar tracking should be assessed utilizing a "no-thumbs technique" to assure that there is no lateral subluxation or dislocation that occurs throughout range of motion. Patellar malalignment or maltracking should be addressed, which should include a reevaluation of femoral component

rotational alignment. This should be performed before routinely performing a lateral retinacular release. The final evaluation should show central tracking of the patella, with full extension of the limb, and appropriate stability and balance of the posterior cruciate ligament in both extension and flexion. In addition, there should be appropriate stability with anterior and posterior drawer testing.

Preparation is then performed in the usual manner utilizing appropriate cement technique. The affected bone surfaces are prepared with a jet lavage system to accurately remove any blood and debris for cementation. Cement is applied first to the tibial surface with digital pressurization in order to achieve an appropriate bone-cement mantle, as well as to the undersurface of the tibial component.[18] Following application of the tibial tray, the femoral component is then cemented. Cement is applied to all surfaces with the exception of the posterior condylar surface to avoid the introduction of excess cement into the posterior compartment.[19] Cement is applied to all surfaces of the backside of the femoral component, including

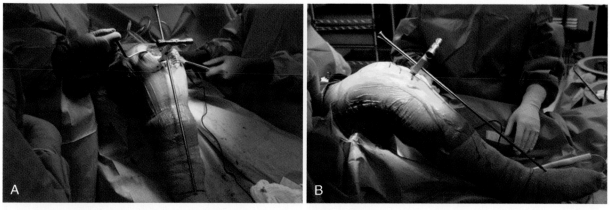

Figure 25-30 After preparation of both femur and tibia is complete, spacer block technique can be used to verify accurate restoration of mechanical alignment, as well as appropriate balance and stability of the flexion and extension space.

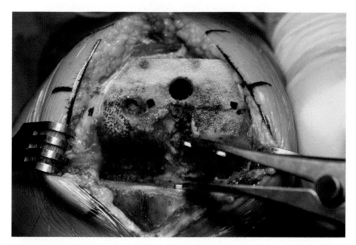

Figure 25-31 Using a laminar spreader with the knee in 90° of flexion, the flexion gap can be assessed. The posterior compartment can also be evaluated for any debris, meniscal remnants, or residual posterior osteophytes.

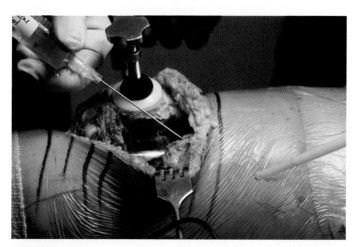

Figure 25-32 For improved postoperative pain management, the deep capsular tissues medially and laterally are injected with a "pain cocktail", as is the subcutaneous layer, prior to closure.

the posterior condylar surface. Following insertion and cement clearing of the femoral component, the tibial bearing surface is then applied and the knee is reduced and placed in full extension. The patellar component is then cemented last and pressurized with a clamp. The deep capsular tissues medially and laterally are injected with a "pain cocktail," as is the subcutaneous layer, prior to closure[20] (**Fig. 25–32**). The deep capsule is closed with an absorbable suture. Skin closure is accomplished with 4-0 absorbable running subcutaneous suture closure (**Fig. 25–33**). This can avoid the irritation and wound complications that have been identified with the use of staples.

SPECIAL CONSIDERATIONS

With a systematic approach, conversion of a unicompartmental knee arthroplasty to a total knee arthroplasty can be successfully performed using standard primary total knee arthroplasty instrumentation and components in the majority of cases. Careful preoperative planning, with particular attention to all-polyethylene tibial components and the presence of

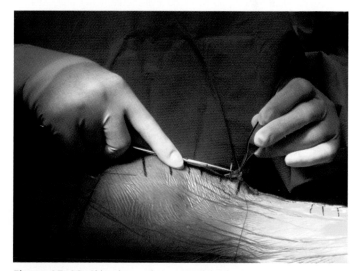

Figure 25-33 Skin closure is accomplished with a 4-0 absorbable running subcutaneous suture to avoid the irritation and wound complications that have been identified with the use of staples.

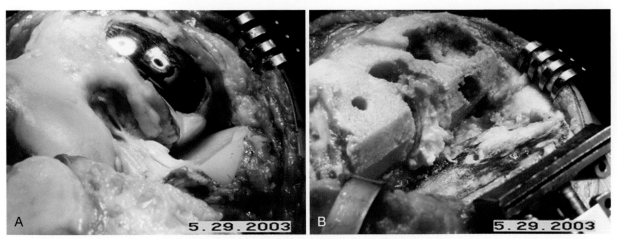

Figure 25-34 (A) Intra-operative photo of a 58-year-old female with failure of a fixed-bearing medial unicompartmental knee arthroplasty secondary to osteolysis and loosening of the femoral component. **(B)** After femoral preparation is complete, the distal femoral bone deficiency can be addressed with autogenous bone graft. Rarely is distal femoral augmentation required.

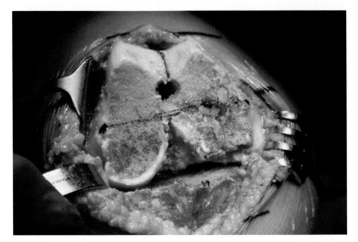

Figure 25-35 Notice the deficiency of the posterior medial femoral condyle making posterior condylar referencing unreliable. Referencing Whiteside's line and the trans-epicondylar axis is critical in establishing accurate femoral rotational alignment.

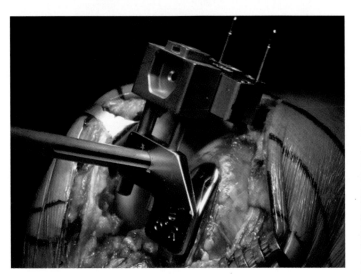

Figure 25-36 Retaining the femoral component is a critical step in the preparation of the distal femur. This will prevent overresection of the distal femur, and allow for more accurate restoration of the joint line.

medial tibial collapse, will help in predicting the complexity of the conversion. There are three main critical areas of importance that have to be evaluated preoperatively and attended to intraoperatively:

1. Distal femoral bone deficiency (**Fig. 25–34**).
2. Posteromedial (or posterolateral) femoral bone deficiency (**Fig. 25–35**).
3. Medial (or lateral) tibial bone deficiency (see Fig. 25–24).

Retaining the femoral component for preparation of the distal femur is a critical step (**Fig. 25–36**). This will allow for more accurate restoration of the joint line and also avoid overresection of the distal femur. Attention to femoral rotation is also critical. Identifying the transepicondylar axis and longitudinal axis (Whiteside's line) should be performed in all cases (see Figs. 25–24 and 25–35). The deficiency of the posteromedial femoral condyle (posterolateral for lateral

unicompartmental knee arthroplasty) will create excess external rotation (or internal rotation for lateral unicompartmental knee arthroplasty) in preparing the femur if not recognized (see Fig. 25–26). The most conservative tibial resection should be performed initially, with an assessment of flexion and extension gap in order to help determine the need for a medial (or lateral) augment. Spacer block technique, which can allow for the assessment of ligament balance as well as alignment and stability, has also been helpful (see Figs. 25–30 and 25–31). The use of a cruciate-retained or a posterior-stabilized prosthetic component can be determined at the time of surgery, depending on the integrity of the posterior cruciate ligament. Success has been reported with both types of components.[14] With attention to detail and a stepwise approach to the technical aspects of the surgical procedure, high clinical success can be achieved comparable to the success that has been achieved with primary total knee arthroplasty.

POSTSURGICAL FOLLOW-UP

Postoperative recovery is similar to that utilized for primary total knee arthroplasty. A preemptive multimodal approach to pain management is utilized in the early postoperative phase in order to restore quadriceps function and to prevent shutdown of the extensor mechanism. An intra-articular injection is performed at the time of surgery with a pain cocktail, which can significantly minimize pain in the early postoperative phase.[20] Quadriceps isometric exercises, straight leg raises, and range-of-motion exercises are started on the day of surgery. Full weight bearing is permitted immediately, and patients are encouraged to begin weight bearing on the day of surgery with the use of crutches, walker, or a cane. Ketorolac (Toradol) 15 mg intravenously has been extremely helpful in controlling the inflammatory response when given preoperatively, in addition to every 6 hours for the first 24 hours in patients without allergy to nonsteroidal anti-inflammatories. It is important that physical therapy is not too aggressive in the early phase, as this will contribute to excessive soft tissue swelling and progressive limitation of motion, quadriceps muscle weakness, increased wound drainage, and possible wound healing complications. A continuous passive motion machine during hospitalization may be used at the surgeon's discretion. Thromboembolism prophylaxis is used similar to total knee arthroplasty with coumadin (Warfarin) being utilized during the hospital stay. The majority of patients will continue with enteric-coated aspirin (325 mg, twice daily) for 4–6 weeks, unless there is an increased risk for thromboembolism or increased bleeding tendency where aspirin cannot be utilized. In these situations, coumadin is used for 2 weeks. Intravenous antibiotics are used for the first 24 hours in order to prevent infection. When quadriceps strength returns, patients are allowed to progress with unrestricted activities, with recommendation to avoid excessive loading and deep flexion, and high-impact activities.

CONCLUSION

In the past, conversion of unicompartmental knee arthroplasty to total knee arthroplasty has created some concerns for a more technically demanding procedure requiring a more complex reconstructive approach necessitating the use of bone grafting, augments, and stemmed revision components.[21] With newer prosthetic designs and more conservative surgical techniques, the conversion of unicompartmental arthroplasty to total knee arthroplasty has improved significantly, with results that are comparable to the results of primary total knee arthroplasty. Johnson et al. reported on a

series of 35 patients who had undergone conversion of unicompartmental knee replacement to total knee replacement with 91% survivorship at 10 years of follow-up.[14] This study also demonstrated that the conversion of a unicompartmental knee arthroplasty to a total knee arthroplasty is a much less demanding procedure than revision total knee arthroplasty, with results comparable to those of primary total knee arthroplasty. Only 3 of the 35 cases in this series required a stem or augmentation device. Studies on clinical outcome comparing unicompartmental knee arthroplasty conversion to primary total knee arthroplasty are rare. Miller et al. found that unicompartmental knee arthroplasty patients had a higher complication rate with inferior clinical results compared to primary total knee arthroplasty patients.[22] Jarvenpaa et al. noted that the knee scores were improved in patients who underwent conversion to a posterior cruciate ligament substituting design.[23] Saragaglia et al. evaluated the radiologic and clinical results of medial unicompartmental arthroplasty converted to total knee arthroplasty.[24] When comparing their results to the literature, they suggested that conversion of unicompartmental arthroplasty would give better results than revision total knee arthroplasty.

As previously reported, failure mode can be predictive of complexity of the conversion of unicompartmental knee arthroplasty to total knee arthroplasty.[15] Failure modes have included polyethylene wear, progression of arthritis, patellofemoral symptoms, aseptic loosening, malpositioned implants, medial tibial collapse, poor patient selection, and technical factors. Of these, polyethylene wear, with or without loosening, and progressive arthritis have been the most common failure modes reported with contemporary unicompartmental knee arthroplasty designs. Both McAuley et al. and Levine et al. demonstrated that, when unicompartmental knees fail through these modes, the revision procedures are straightforward with minimal bone loss.[25,26] In all cases, primary femoral components were used, and on the tibial side, the defects encountered were easily dealt with using autogenous nonstructural bone graft, augments, and stems, where indicated.[16] Aleto et al. found that the more significant bony defects were encountered in knees that failed by medial tibial collapse, and required increased implant requirements as compared to other failure modes.[16] In this review of 32 knees, 13 of the 15 required screws and cement and/or augments, and 10 of the 15 required stems on the tibial side. This suggests that, when failure occurs in unicompartmental knee arthroplasty due to early collapse of the medial tibial plateau, there are more significant bone defects, and revisions are technically more demanding than those seen with other aseptic failure mechanisms such as polyethylene wear. Furthermore, of the failures that occurred in this series as a result of medial tibial collapse, 87% of the 15 knees were of all-polyethylene design, which was highly significant compared to metal-backed components (**Fig. 25–37**). Using a

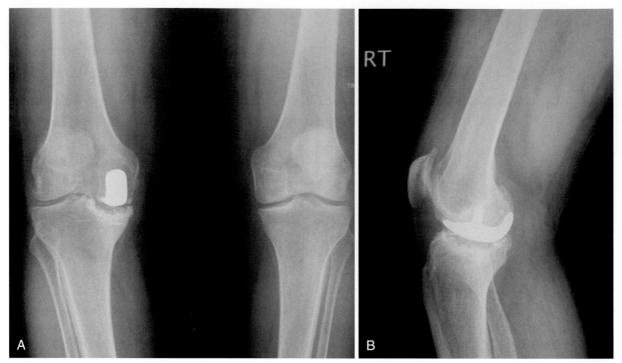

Figure 25-37 (A) Standing bilateral anteroposterior radiograph of a 63-year-old male with a fixed-bearing medial unicompartmental knee arthroplasty with an all-polyethylene tibial component. Notice the medial tibial collaspe and the increased varus alignment. **(B)** Lateral view of the same patient showing the medial tibial collaspe, and the significant increased posterior slope of the tibia. These pre-operative radiographic findings are predictive for a more complex reconstruction possibly requiring augmentation of the tibia and stem fixation.

three-dimensional finite element model to evaluate contact stresses, Morra and Greenwald found a strikingly different polyethylene loading pattern for fixed-bearing, all-polyethylene unicompartmental knee arthroplasty designs versus metal-backed designs.[27] In particular, the fixed-bearing designs showed much higher contact stresses in the polyethylene, with highly localized contact points in the anterior and medial locations. Based on the clinical data, coupled with finite element analysis estimations, it can be concluded that an all-polyethylene, fixed-bearing, low-conformity unicompartmental knee arthroplasty would be most susceptible to excessive peripheral or localized edge loading resulting in cancellous bone overload and medial tibial collapse.[16] Understanding these failure modes not only will help in the planning for conversion of the failed unicompartmental knee arthroplasty, but hopefully will also allow for improvements in understanding the technical factors required in achieving long-term clinical success. The ultimate goal in converting a unicompartmental knee arthroplasty to a total knee arthroplasty is to achieve the clinical result of a primary total knee arthroplasty, in terms of both function and survivorship.

TIPS AND PEARLS

- Preoperative evaluation is critical in determining the mode of failure of unicompartmental knee arthroplasty, which can have predictive value for the complexity of the

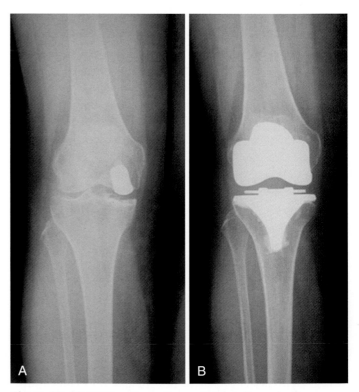

Figure 25-38 (A) Standing anteroposterior radiograph of a fixed-bearing medial unicompartmental knee without medial tibial collapse indicating a more standard conversion to a primary cruciate-retained or posterior-stabilized total knee arthroplasty. **(B)** Postoperative standing anteroposterior view of the same patient with a primary cruciate-retained total knee arthroplasty.

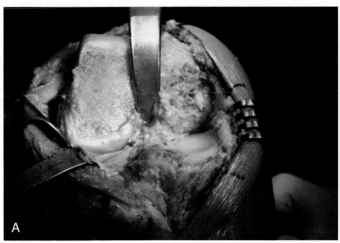 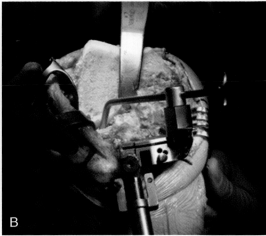

Figure 25-39 (A) When the distal femoral resection is performed first, combined with excision of the anterior cruciate ligament, a more adequate exposure of the proximal tibia can be achieved. **(B)** Depth of tibial resection should be referenced off the opposite compartment for the most conservative level of resection.

procedure and determining the need for bone grafting, metal augments, stem fixation, and more constrained revision components.

- Early failure due to medial tibial bone collapse, most frequently associated with an all-polyethylene tibial component, will typically necessitate a more complex procedure requiring bone grafting of the medial defect, or possibly screws with cement, augments, and stems (see Fig. 25–37).
- Femoral bone defects are easily addressed with simple bone grafting and rarely require augmentation or stemmed implants (see Figs. 25–34 and 25–35).
- The majority of unicompartmental knee arthroplasty–to–total knee arthroplasty conversions can be performed using primary total knee instrumentation with a standard primary cruciate-retained or posterior-stabilized total knee arthroplasty (**Fig. 25–38**).
- The distal femoral resection should be addressed first, with the existing femoral component left intact. This will allow more accurate approximation of the joint line and will avoid possible overresection of the distal femur (see Fig. 25–36).
- Tibial component removal is performed after the distal femoral resection is complete, which will allow for a more adequate exposure of the proximal tibia. An accurate level of resection should be determined by referencing the opposite compartment for a more conservative level of resection (**Fig. 25–39**).
- Removal of an all-polyethylene tibial component can be easily accomplished using the oscillating saw to disrupt the cement-implant interface first. The polyethylene peg and retained cement can be addressed in the final preparation of the tibia (see Figs. 25–18 and 25–24).
- Final preparation of the femur can be performed after the tibia preparation is complete. Bone loss of the posterior femoral condyle is common, making posterior referencing inaccurate. It is essential to identify and mark both Whiteside's line and the transepicondylar axis to assure accurate sizing and rotational alignment of the femoral component (see Figs. 25–25 through 25–27 and 25–35).
- Assessment of flexion-extension gap balance and ligament stability should be performed with every procedure using a spacer block technique (see Fig. 25–30).
- Revision components should be available with every procedure in order to address the possibility of unanticipated deficiencies requiring the need for augments, stems, or a more constrained component (see Figs. 25–3, 25–4, and 25–24).

REFERENCES

1. Kozinn SC, Marx C, Scott RD. Unicompartmental knee arthroplasty: a 4.5 to 6 year follow up study with a metal backed tibial component. J Arthroplasty 1989;4(Suppl):S1-S9.
2. Cobb AG, Kozinn SC, Scott RD. Unicondylar or total knee replacement: the patient's preference. J Bone Joint Surg [Br] 1990;72:166.
3. Berger RA, Meneghine RM, Jacobs JJ, et al. Results of unicompartmental knee arthroplasty at a minimum of ten years of follow-up. J Bone Joint Surg [Am] 2005;87: 999-1006.
4. Price AJ, Waite JC, Svärd U. Long-term clinical results of the medial Oxford unicompartmental knee arthroplasty. Clin Orthop Relat Res 2005;(435):171-180.
5. U.S. Markets for Reconstructive Devices 2001. Toronto, Ontario, Canada: Millennium Research Group, 2002.

6. U.S. Markets for Reconstructive Devices 2002. Toronto, Ontario, Canada: Millennium Research Group, 2003.

7. Goie TJ, Killeen KK, Hoeffel DP, et al. Analysis of unicompartmental knee arthroplasty in a community-based implant registry. Clin Orthop Relat Res 2003;(416):111-119.

8. Dudley TE, Goie TJ, Sinner P, Mehle S. Registry outcomes of unicompartmental knee arthroplasty revisions. Clin Orthop Relat Res 2008;(466):1666-1670.

9. Goie TJ, Killeen KK, Grimm K, et al. Why are total knee replacements revised? Analysis of early revision in a community knee implant registry. Clin Orthop Relat Res 2004;(428):100-106.

10. Furnes O, Espehaug B, Lie SA, et al. Early failures among 7,174 primary total knee replacements: a follow-up study from the Norwegian Arthroplasty Register 1994–2000. Acta Orthop Scand 2002;73:117-129.

11. Lidgren L, Knutson K, Robertsson O. Swedish Knee Arthroplasty Register: 2003 Annual Report. Lund: Swedish Knee Arthroplasty Register, 2003.

12. Australian Orthopaedic Association National Joint Registry. Annual Report. Adelaide, Australia: Australian Orthopaedic Association, 2007.

13. Bohm I, Landsiedl F. Revision surgery after failed unicompartmental knee arthroplasty: a study of 35 cases. J Arthroplasty 2000;15:982-989.

14. Johnson S, Jones P, Newman JH. The survivorship and results of total knee replacements converted from unicompartmental knee replacements. Knee 2007;14:154-157.

15. Berend K, George J, Lombardi A. Unicompartmental knee arthroplasty to total knee arthroplasty conversion: assuring a primary outcome. Orthopedics 2009;32:684.

16. Aleto TJ, Berend ME, Ritter MA, et al. Early failure of unicompartmental knee arthroplasty leading to revision. J Arthroplasty 2008;23:159-163.

17. Springer BD, Scott RD, Thornhill TS. Conversion of failed unicompartmental knee arthroplasty. Clin Orthop Relat Res 2006;(446):214-220.

18. Vanlommel J, Luyckx JP, Labey L, et al. Cementing the tibial component in total knee arthroplasty: which technique is the best? J Arthroplasty 2010;April 7. [Epub ahead of print]

19. Vaninbroukx M, Labey L, Innocenti B, Bellemans J. Cementing the femoral component in total knee arthroplasty: which technique is the best? Knee 2009;16:265-268.

20. Busch CA, Shore BJ, Bhandari R, et al. Efficacy of periarticular multimodal drug injection in total knee arthroplasty: a randomized trial. J Bone Joint Surg [Am] 2006; 88:949-963.

21. Padgett DE, Stern SH, Insall JN. Revision total knee arthroplasty for failed unicompartmental replacement. J Bone Joint Surg [Am] 1991;73:186-190.

22. Miller M, Benjamin JB, Marson B, Hollstein S. The effect of implant constraint on results of conversion of unicompartmental knee arthroplasty to total knee arthroplasty. Orthopedics 2002;25:1353-1357.

23. Jarvenpaa J, Kettunen J, Miettinen H, Kroger H. The clinical outcome of revision knee replacement after unicompartmental knee arthroplasty versus primary total knee arthroplasty: 8–17 years follow-up study of 49 patients. Presented at the International Orthopaedics (SICOT) meeting, 2009.

24. Saragaglia D, Estour G, Nener C, Colle PE. Revision of 33 unicompartmental knee prostheses using total knee arthroplasty: strategy and results. Int Orthop 2009;33:969-974.

25. McAuley JP, Engh GA, Ammeen DJ. Revision of failed unicompartmental arthroplasty. Clin Orthop Relat Res 2001;(392):279-282.

26. Levine WN, Ozuna RM, Scott RD, et al. Conversion of failed modern unicompartmental arthroplasty to total knee arthroplasty. J Arthroplasty 1996;11:797.

27. Morra EA, Greenwald AS. The effects of walking gait on UHMWPE damage in unicompartmental knee systems: a finite element study. Presented at the Annual Meeting of the American Academy of Orthopedic Surgeons, 2003.

SUGGESTED READINGS

Ansari S, Newman JH, Ackroyd CE. 10 year survivorship analysis of medial sled arthroplasty. Acta Orthop Scand 1997;68:430-434.

Barrett WP, Scott RD. Revision of failed unicondylar unicompartmental knee arthroplasty. J Bone Joint Surg [Am] 1987;69:1328.

Cartier P, Cheaib S. Unicondylar knee arthroplasty: 2–10 years of follow-up evaluation. J Arthroplasty 1987;2:157-162.

Chakrabarty G, Newman JH, Ackroyd CE. Revision of unicompartmental arthroplasty: clinical and technical considerations. J Arthroplasty 1998;13:191-196.

Fehring TK, Odum SM, Masonis JL, Springer BD. Early failures in unicondylar arthroplasty. Orthopedics 2010;33:11.

Knutson K, Lindstrand A, Lidgren L. Survival of knee arthroplasties: a nation-wide multicentre investigation of 8000 cases. J Bone Joint Surg [Br] 1986;68:795.

Kozinn SC, Scott RD. Current concepts review: unicondylar knee arthroplasty. J Bone Joint Surg [Am] 1989;71:145.

Lai C, Rand J. Revision of failed unicompartmental total knee arthroplasty. Clin Orthop Relat Res 1993;(267):193.

Laurencin CT, Zelicof SC, Scott RD, Ewald FC. Unicompartmental versus total knee arthroplasty in the same patient. Clin Orthop Relat Res 1991;(273):151-156.

Lewold S, Robertsson O, Knutson K, Lidgren L. Revision of unicompartmental knee arthroplasty: outcome in 1135 cases from the Swedish Knee Arthroplasty study. Acta Orthop Scand 1998;69:469-474.

Mackinnon J, Young S, Bailey RAJ. The St. Georg sledge for unicompartmental replacement of the knee. J Bone Joint Surg [Br] 1988;70:217.

Murray DW, Goodfellow JW, O'Connor JJ. The Oxford medial unicompartmental knee arthroplasty: a ten-year survival study. J Bone Joint Surg [Br] 1998;80:983-989.

Newman JH, Ackroyd CE, Ahmed S. The early results of prospective randomised study of unicompartmental or total knee arthroplasty. J Bone Joint Surg [Br] 1994;76(Suppl 57).

Newman JH, Ackroyd CE, Shah NA. Unicompartmental or total knee replacement? Five year results of a prospective, randomised trial of 102 osteoarthritic knees with unicompartmental arthritis. J Bone Joint Surg [Br] 1998;80:862-865.

Svärd UC, Price AJ. Oxford medial unicompartmental knee arthroplasty: a survival analysis of an independent series. J Bone Joint Surg [Br] 2001;83:191-194.

CHAPTER 26
The Painful Medial Unicompartmental Knee Arthroplasty

Michael E. Berend

KEY POINTS

- The decision to revise a painful UKA to a TKA may have a lower threshold than a painful TKA.
- Careful implant sizing in the medial-lateral position is critical to avoid overhang and possibly pain following medial mobile-bearing UKA.
- Many patients undergoing UKA have anterior knee pain; medial PFJ changes are associated with outcomes similar to those without changes, and pain resolves in most patients.
- Radiolucencies are quite common after UKA and not always indicative of a pathologic process.
- Aspirations should be performed to examine for current hemarthroses, infection, and crystalline arthropathy.
- Metal-backed tibial implants demonstrate more diffuse loading distributions while all-polyethylene tibial components have more focal loading concentrations.
- Careful revision is warranted only after appropriate time has transpired as pain resolves out to 2 years following medial UKA.

INTRODUCTION

Long-term survivorship of unicompartmental knee arthroplasty (UKA) has increased with contemporary prosthetic designs and improved patient selection and has been reported to be between 96% and 98% at 10–13 years of follow-up.[1–4] Failure leading to revision in UKA has been ascribed to progression of arthritis in retained compartments, polyethylene wear, patient selection, implant malpositioning, loosening, fracture, and *persistent pain*.[1–5] This chapter describes the evaluation and management of a painful UKA. A differential diagnosis is outlined in **Box 26–1**. Clinical and radiographic evaluations should seek to understand the diagnoses that may account for pain with well-positioned and stable implants. In addition, the assumption that the painful UKA will be solved with a conversion to a total knee arthroplasty (TKA) is discussed.

Often the evaluation of a painful UKA may lead the surgeon biased against medial UKA to believe that a TKA should have been indicated as the original arthroplasty. The reality, however, is that not all TKAs are pain free,[6] with a series by Price et al. reporting pain at midterm follow-up at 41%. In addition, patient satisfaction following TKA may not be as high as assumed by many surgeons (many of whom do not perform UKAs), as Bourne et al. reported a 19% patient dissatisfaction rate in a large cohort of TKAs.[7] Finally, the decision to revise a painful UKA to a TKA may have a lower threshold than a painful TKA and must be carefully considered. This "threshold for revision" may underscore higher revision rates in national registry data. A UKA may also have been performed prematurely without full-thickness cartilage loss and result in incomplete pain relief following the arthroplasty.[8]

CLINICAL EVALUATION

The clinical evaluation of a painful UKA begins with a history and physical examination to determine the location, time course, and inciting variables producing the pain. As with most arthroplasties about the knee (UKA, TKA, and total knee revision), complete pain resolution may take up to 12–18 months. Early weight-bearing pain after UKA may be amenable to treatment with the use of an assist device such as a cane or walker to allow the bone and soft tissues to settle over a 4- to 6-week period. Often the pain is over the anteromedial tibia and is correlated with tenderness over the pes anserine insertion. Debate continues as to whether this is soft tissue related or bony in nature and is discussed below.

The "appropriate" indications for medial UKA have long been debated.[9–12] Some have suggested a combination of patient factors and examination findings that may limit the number of appropriate candidates to 4–6% of varus knees.[9–12] Others have followed more physiologic criteria as documented by "anteromedial osteoarthritis" with intact collateral and cruciate ligaments, which may increase the percentage of varus knees that are appropriate candidates for medial UKA to as high as 30%.

Box 26–1 A Differential Diagnosis of a Painful Medial UKA

- Infection
- Implant loosening
- Stress fracture
- Ipsilateral hip disease
- Radiculopathy
- Implant impingement
  - Bearing on bone (mobile-bearing design)
  - Patella with implant (fixed-bearing design)
- Loose bodies
  - Cement
  - Bone
- Lateral meniscus tear
- Patellofemoral joint wear
- Polyethylene wear (see Fig. 26–3)
- Inappropriate indications (minimal changes on preoperative radiographs)
- Reflex sympathetic dystrophy
- Lateral joint degeneration (see Fig. 26–2)
- Implant overhang

The published long-term data support the latter approach.[4] The status of the patellofemoral joint (PFJ) as a contraindication to UKA is misunderstood, and long-term data by Beard et al.[13,14] shed important light on this subject, demonstrating that anterior knee pain resolves after medial UKA with central and medial PFJ degeneration. Further, anterior knee pain does not correlate with intraoperative or radiographic findings in patients with anteromedial osteoarthritis (OA). There are no published data to refute this approach of largely ignoring the PFJ in patients with anteromedial OA of the knee and proceeding with medial UKA.

RADIOGRAPHIC EVALUATION

Weight-bearing anteroposterior, lateral, and sunrise patellar radiographic views should be obtained and assessed. Review of the original preoperative radiographs is also quite helpful as partial-thickness cartilage loss has been associated with inconsistent pain relief following UKA.[8] This may be an indication that the early medial degenerative changes did not fully account for the preoperative knee pain leading to the UKA. Tibial implant overhang greater than 3 mm has been associated with increased pain following medial mobile-bearing UKA.[15] Correlation of pain and implant position—most notably overhang with other implant designs—is needed. Careful implant sizing in the medial-lateral position is important to avoid this scenario.

Anterior Knee Pain and Radiographic Appearance

Anterior knee pain and radiographic signs of PFJ degeneration have been considered contraindications to UKA and a possible source of pain after UKA. It is interesting to reflect on how these unnecessary contraindications developed. Kozinn and Scott[10] suggested PFJ degeneration as a contraindication to a medial UKA and therefore have no data to support that ignoring anterior knee pain and PFJ degeneration leads to persistent pain and progressive deterioration of the knee. Beard et al.,[13,14] however, reported on the outcomes of medial UKA in such patients. These data, rather than prior hypotheses and historical traditions, should dictate our clinical practice. These authors found that over half (54%) of patients undergoing UKA had anterior knee pain. Furthermore, 54% of patients had degenerative changes observed on preoperative skyline radiographs. Medial PFJ changes were associated with outcomes similar to those knees without changes. Furthermore, anterior knee pain resolved in all patients. Our historical suspicion of all anterior knee pain originating from the PFJ appears not to be supported by published evidence as it resolved following medial UKA for anteromedial OA.[13]

Pain and Radiolucencies

An important consideration is the radiographic appearance of a medial UKA. In the United States, the majority of surgeons follow their UKA patients with standard radiographs. However, radiolucent lines (RLL) often are detected only on "screened" radiographs[16] (**Fig. 26–1**). The Oxford group (Nuffield Orthopaedic Centre) has long utilized a screened or fluoroscopic imaging system to track the radiographic appearance of medial UKAs in the long term. This is a critical point as radiolucencies beneath the tibial tray are often misinterpreted to be a source of pain and result in unnecessary revision.[17] Progressive RLL with implant migration indicates implant loosening; however, a stable radiolucency often does not. Retrieval of well-functioning implants has demonstrated a partial fibrocartilage layer that may be a biologic response to loading conditions.[16] In other words, RLL are quite common and not always indicative of a pathologic process. The incidence of RLL is highly variable and is directly related to screened (fluoroscopic) versus nonscreened films. Small changes in the tilt of the x-ray beam may obscure RLL. RLL alone must be treated with great care as pain and the presence of RLL after UKA have not been clearly linked.

Additional Radiographic and Related Evaluations

The lateral compartment of the knee may show joint space collapse in the second decade and lead to revision.[18,19] It may also be an indication of unrecognized inflammatory arthritis (**Fig. 26–2**). Polymer wear is also noted (**Fig. 26–3**) on standard radiographs and is more common in fixed-bearing devices, especially in those with oxidized polyethylene and long shelf lives prior to implantation. Bone scans may be "hot" or show increased activity in the medial compartment

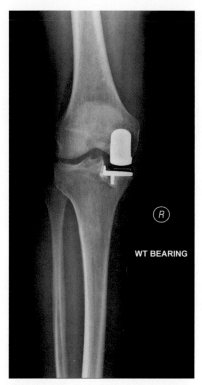

Figure 26-1 Stable radiolucencies under medial UKA tibial components. These are very common following mobile-bearing UKA and do not indicate loosening in the absence of implant migration. Careful revision should be performed as these radiographic findings are stable over time.[13]

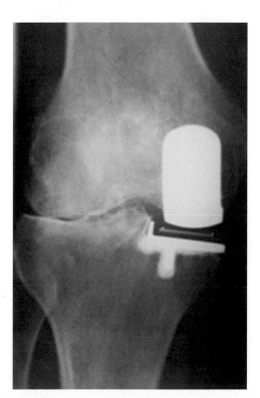

Figure 26-2 Anteroposterior radiograph demonstrating lateral compartment joint space loss from progressive lateral joint degeneration.

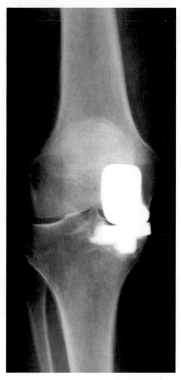

Figure 26-3 Anteroposterior radiograph demonstrating severe polyethylene wear in a fixed-bearing modular medial UKA.

for many years after UKA and must be interpreted with caution in the face of a painful UKA. Aspirations should be performed to examine for recurrent hemarthroses, infection, and crystalline arthropathy. Routine synovial fluid analysis is performed.

BIOMECHANICS OF UKA LOADING ... A POSSIBLE EXPLANATION OF PAIN?

The in vivo loading conditions of a medial UKA and the associated osseous and soft tissue adaptations are not well understood. We have hypothesized that changes in loading, as quantified by osseous stresses and strains, may at least in part explain the persistence and resolution of pain following a medial UKA. We have reported on the effects of significant overload of the tibial bone leading to implant subsidence and bony collapse in some fixed-bearing UKA designs.[5] In our study of 32 consecutive UKA revisions of both metal-backed and all-polyethylene tibial component designs, we observed medial tibia collapse in 47% of the cases studied (**Fig. 26–4**); half of these occurred early in the postoperative course, within 16 months of the surgery. We found increased tibial slope was associated with tibial collapse, with increased posterior slope in those cases that collapsed posteriorly as opposed to in anterior collapse. Hernigou et al.[20] reported similar influences of tibial slope on failure mechanisms following a UKA. While some studies have reported relatively clear-cut conversion to

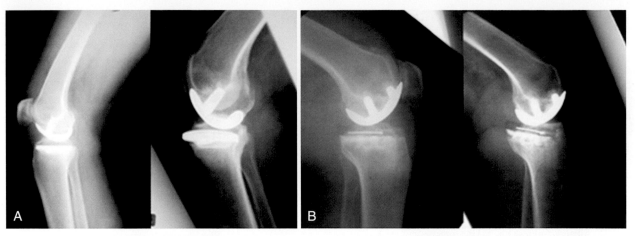

Figure 26-4 (A) UKA tibial component failure due to posterior tibial collapse. **(B)** Anterior tibial bony collapse.

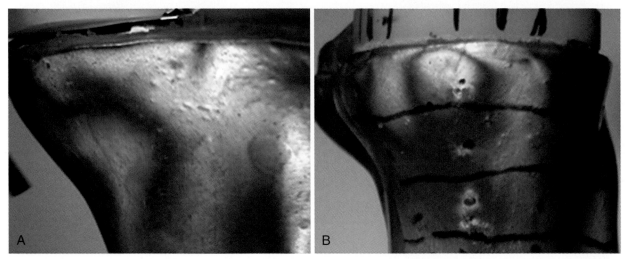

Figure 26-5 (A) Diffuse strain distribution during loading of a metal-backed UKA tibial component with the bearing in the anterior position simulating heel strike and knee extension.[21] **(B)** Localized strain distribution during loading of an all-polyethylene UKA tibial component in a posterior position simulating deep flexion and femoral roll-back.[22]

TKA for common UKA failure modes, this study noted the increased complexity of revision in cases of medial collapse as requiring screws, augments, and ancillary bone cement during revision to TKA. We have also quantified the influence of knee kinematics[21] and metal backing on the loading patterns of metal-backed mobile-bearing and all-polyethylene fixed-bearing medial UKAs.[22] We found metal-backed tibial implants demonstrated more diffuse loading distributions while all-polyethylene tibial components had more focal loading concentrations (**Fig. 26-5**). We simulated the flexion and extension of the knee experienced during gait and dynamic loading conditions and demonstrated that both component designs demonstrated significantly different loading patterns based on loading contact position. More work is needed in this area to further characterize the effects of these laboratory findings and postoperative pain in a medial UKA.

SUMMARY

The evaluation of the painful UKA is most likely best approached by a surgeon who performs medial UKAs in his or her practice. A thoughtful differential diagnostic evaluation should be undertaken. Appropriate time should transpire prior to revision as pain resolves out to 2 years following medial UKA. Careful revision is warranted only after appropriate evaluation and identification of a clear diagnosis.

REFERENCES

1. Squire MW, Callaghan JJ, Goetz DD, et al. Unicompartmental knee replacement: a minimum 15 year follow-up study. Clin Orthop Relat Res 1999;(367):61-72.

2. Berger RA, Meneghini RM, Jacobs JJ, et al. Results of unicompartmental knee arthroplasty at a minimum of ten years of follow-up. J Bone Joint Surg [Am] 2005;87:999-1006.

3. Price AJ, Waite JC, Svärd U. Long-term clinical results of the medial Oxford unicompartmental knee arthroplasty. Clin Orthop Relat Res 2005;(435):171-180.

4. Murray DW, Goodfellow JW, O'Connor JJ. The Oxford medial unicompartmental arthroplasty: a ten-year survival study. J Bone Joint Surg [Br] 1998;80:983-989.

5. Aleto TJ, Berend ME, Ritter MA, et al. Early failure of unicompartmental knee arthroplasty leading to revision. J Arthroplasty 2008;23:159-163.

6. Price AJ, Longino D, Rees J, et al. Are pain and function better measures of outcome than revision rates after TKR in the younger patient? Knee 2010;17:196-199.

7. Bourne RB, Chesworth BM, Davis AM, et al. Patient satisfaction after total knee arthroplasty: who is satisfied and who is not? Clin Orthop Relat Res 2010;(468):57-63.

8. Pandit H, Gulati A, Jenkins C, et al. Unicompartmental knee replacement for patients with partial thickness cartilage loss in the affected compartment. Knee 2010;June 1. [Epub ahead of print]

9. Stern SH, Becker MW, Insall JN. Unicondylar knee arthroplasty: an evaluation of selection criteria. Clin Orthop Relat Res 1993;(286):143-148.

10. Kozinn SC, Scott R. Unicondylar knee arthroplasty. J Bone Joint Surg [Am] 1989;71:145-150.

11. Kozinn SC, Marx C, Scott RD. Unicompartmental knee arthroplasty: a 4.5–6-year follow-up study with a metal-backed tibial component. J Arthroplasty 1989;4(Suppl):S1-S10.

12. Kozinn SC, Scott RD. Surgical treatment of unicompartmental degenerative arthritis of the knee. Rheum Dis Clin North Am 1988;14:545-564.

13. Beard DJ, Pandit H, Ostlere S, et al. Pre-operative clinical and radiological assessment of the patellofemoral joint in unicompartmental knee replacement and its influence on outcome. J Bone Joint Surg [Br] 2007;89:1602-1607.

14. Beard DJ, Pandit H, Gill HS, et al. The influence of the presence and severity of pre-existing patellofemoral degenerative changes on the outcome of the Oxford medial unicompartmental knee replacement. J Bone Joint Surg [Br] 2007;89:1597-1601.

15. Chau R, Gulati A, Pandit H, et al. Tibial component overhang following unicompartmental knee replacement—does it matter? Knee 2009;16:310-313.

16. Tibrewal SB, Grant KA, Goodfellow JW. The radiolucent line beneath the tibial components of the Oxford meniscal knee. J Bone Joint Surg [Br] 1984;66:523-528.

17. Gulati A, Chau R, Pandit HG, et al. The incidence of physiological radiolucency following Oxford unicompartmental knee replacement and its relationship to outcome. J Bone Joint Surg [Br] 2009;91:896-902.

18. Emerson RH Jr, Higgins LL. Unicompartmental knee arthroplasty with the Oxford prosthesis in patients with medial compartment arthritis. J Bone Joint Surg [Am] 2008;90:118-122.

19. Collier MB, Eickmann TH, Anbari KK, Engh GA. Lateral tibiofemoral compartment narrowing after medial unicondylar arthroplasty. Clin Orthop Relat Res 2007;(464):43-52.

20. Hernigou P, Deschamps G. Posterior slope of the tibial implant and the outcome of unicompartmental knee arthroplasty. Bone Joint Surg [Am] 2004;86:506-511.

21. Small SR, Berend ME, Ritter MA, Buckley CA. Bearing mobility affects tibial strain in mobile-bearing unicompartmental knee arthroplasty. Surg Technol Int 2010;19:185-190.

22. Small SR, Berend ME, Ritter MA, et al. Metal backing significantly decreases tibial strain in medial unicompartmental knee arthroplasty model. J Arthoplasty 2010;September 14. [Epub ahead of print]

SECTION 7
Putting It All Together

CHAPTER 27
Practical Issues in Unicompartmental Knee Arthroplasty—The Secrets for Success

David F. Dalury

KEY POINTS

- Careful surgical technique is important.
- UKA is more technically challenging than a TKR.
- Patient selection is paramount.
- There has been a cautious expansion of indications from traditional criteria.

INTRODUCTION

Unicompartmental knee arthroplasty (UKA) is an attractive alternative to tibial osteotomy and total knee replacement (TKR) in certain patients. Advantages of UKA include more retained native bone and soft tissues, including both cruciate ligaments in most cases, and less bone resection on both the femur and the tibia. Smaller incisions, less pain, and earlier return of function are also associated with UKAs. The fact that the conversion from a failed UKA to a TKR is usually easier than a conversion of a failed osteotomy to a TKR is another reason that surgeons find UKA an appealing option in the patient with isolated femoral-tibial compartment disease. It is generally agreed that the UKAs are more challenging than TKRs. With that in mind, there are several important considerations when planning a UKA.

The single most important determinant in a good outcome following a UKA is patient selection (**Fig. 27–1**). Most authors refer to the traditional selection criteria originally written by Kozinn and Scott.[1] These criteria say that UKAs should not be used in patients with more than a 10° fixed flexion contracture or varus or valgus deformity, and they should be used predominantly in thin, elderly, low-demand patients. Flexion deformity is usually considered the most important of these exclusions. More recently, there has been a cautious expansion of the indications to include younger[2,3] and heavier[4–6] patients. While the data are still relatively short term, there are increasing reports of the successful use of this concept in young (less than 60 years of age) patients at midterm follow-up. If this

procedure can provide reasonable outcomes at 10 years, the thinking goes, then this relatively less involved procedure will have served as a "time buyer" until a further conversion to a TKR is performed. There is a growing appeal of thinking of a UKA as a patient's first arthroplasty for the younger patient and a last arthroplasty for an elderly patient. Another reason for the increased use of UKA in younger patients is that the concept is an appealing one to these patients and, with the increased use of the Internet and direct-to-patient marketing, patients in this age category are increasingly aware of these surgical options and frequently seek out these procedures. Weight has been a concern with UKA procedures but, like use in younger patients, there are reports showing that excess weight, in and of itself, is not a contraindication. These reports are still in the midterm, but the traditional criterion of an 85- to 90-kg limit is being challenged.

There are several other important aspects to patient selection. These include the status of the anterior cruciate ligament (ACL), the amount of disease present in the other compartments, the presence of crystalline disease and other inflammatory arthropathies, and location of a patient's pain. Most surgeons feel that a functioning ACL is important, particularly with mobile-bearing devices. The amount of disease in other compartments is controversial. Most surgeons will accept up to Grade 3 Outerbridge damage but not Grade 4, but some surgeons ignore cartilage damage in the patellofemoral joint entirely. The damage often seen on the medial aspect of the lateral femoral compartment due to irritation of the tibial spine is usually ignored (**Fig. 27–2**). The presence of calcium pyrophosphate dihydrate crystals on radiographs or at surgery or the finding of an inflammatory synovium at the time of arthrotomy would be considered by most to be a contraindication to proceeding with a UKA. Some surgeons feel that, for a patient to be a UKA candidate, he or she should be able to point with one finger to the area of pain (medial femoral-tibial joint for medial UKA). Patients with more anterior knee pain or those who complain of pain while going up or down stairs are, in their minds, less ideal candidates for this type of surgery. This idea, however, is also being challenged and now many surgeons are not as concerned with the location of the pain as

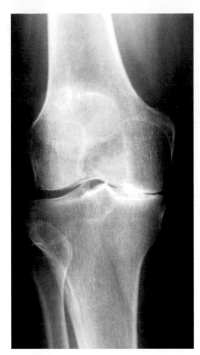

Figure 27-1 Radiograph showing isolated disease in AP view of the knee.

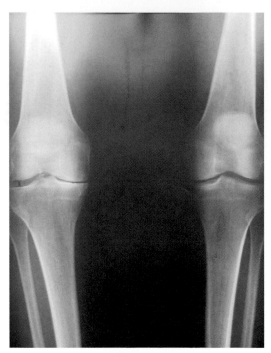

Figure 27-3 AP view of the knee. The surgeon should aim for perpendicular or slight undercorrection of the knee.

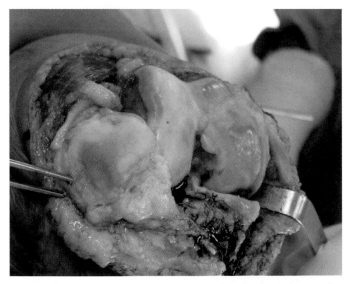

Figure 27-2 Open arthrotomy demonstrating Grade IV changes in the patellofemoral joint: not an ideal candidate for a UKA.

they are with the preoperative radiographs and examination. Another important factor in patient selection is the patient's understanding of the concept and the procedure. Patients looking for the most predictable surgical management of their knee disease are probably best served by having a TKR despite the isolated nature of their disease. On the other hand, many patients find the idea of a less invasive procedure, where only the diseased part of the knee is replaced, an appealing one even if it does not have as good long-term follow up as a TKR. It is

important that the patient understand the differences and the pros and cons of both approaches.

Once appropriate patient selection has occurred, UKA preoperative planning is important. A UKA should be thought of as replacing what has worn away. It should not be used to correct a significant malalignment or deformity. A general sense of the patient's knee is important. Has the patient always had a varus knee? If so, it is important not to overcorrect the joint line. Using the anteroposterior (AP) radiograph, the surgeon should plan the level of tibial resection to be essentially perpendicular to the long axis of the tibia, although slight undercorrection is acceptable (**Fig. 27–3**). Because only one part of the joint is being replaced, it is imperative that the lateral radiograph be evaluated so the UKA will reproduce the preexisting posterior tibial slope. Failure to do so will lead to loosening and implant failure. The range of posterior tibial slope has been measured to be anywhere from 0° to 22° (**Fig. 27–4**).

TECHNIQUE

There are several surgical techniques for UKA implantation that can be utilized with various devices. An extramedullary, tibia-first approach is described here as it is the most commonly used technique. The sequence for this procedure is as follows:

- Appropriate exposure
- Conservative tibia resection

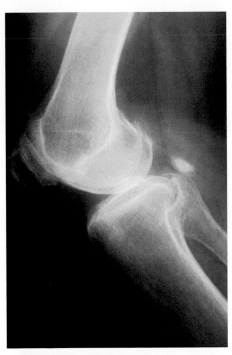

Figure 27-4 Lateral view of the knee. Beware of variability of the posterior tibial slope.

- Assessment of the flexion and extension gaps
- Mating the femoral cut to the tibial cut in extension
- Sizing and orienting the femoral component relative to the tibial surface at 90°
- Preparing the femur
- Removing the remaining meniscus and osteophytes posteriorly
- Sizing and preparing the tibia
- Final soft tissue balancing
- Cementation and removal of debris
- Appropriate closure and repair

At each step of the procedure there are several keys to success.

Appropriate Exposure

Most UKAs are now performed via a "minimally invasive" approach (**Fig. 27–5**). In the strictest sense, this does not describe the length of the incision; rather, it means that the extensor mechanism is not displaced from the trochlear groove. With the patella in place, the femoral-tibial alignment and orientation are easier to gauge and evaluate. Incisions should extend approximately from the top of the patella to the joint line. An adequate synovectomy at the arthrotomy enhances visualization and allows for further inspection of the remaining joint, ligaments, and synovium. As opposed to a TKR, where most of the surgery is done either at full extension or at 90° of flexion, a UKA is performed at a variety of flexion positions, and therefore the incision should be large enough to

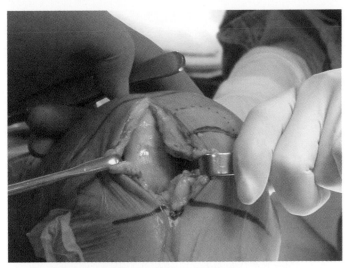

Figure 27-5 "Minimally invasive" exposure. Note that the extensor mechanism is not displaced.

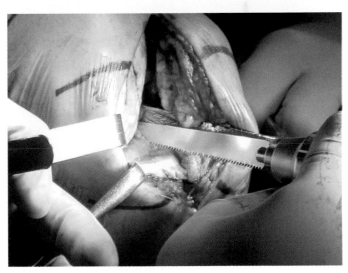

Figure 27-6 Using the lateral border of the medial femoral condyle is a good guide for the sagittal saw cut.

allow an adequate view of the joint. Soft tissues are at risk in these small incisions, so retractor placement is important, particularly along the medial joint line to protect damage to the medial collateral ligament. Extending the length of the incision should always be done if visualization is compromised.

Conservative Tibial Resection

Following the idea that a UKA should be replacing what is worn, based on the preoperative planning radiographs, a minimal amount of tibial bone should be removed—a few millimeters at most off the medial plateau for a medial UKA. Both the vertical and horizontal cuts are important. It can be helpful to use the lateral border of the medial femoral condyle as a cutting guide for the L or vertical cut of the tibial bone resection (**Fig. 27–6**). Placing the reciprocating saw along the

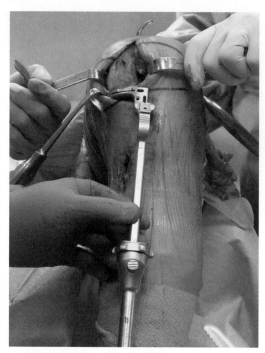

Figure 27-7 External tibial cutting guide for planning tibial resection.

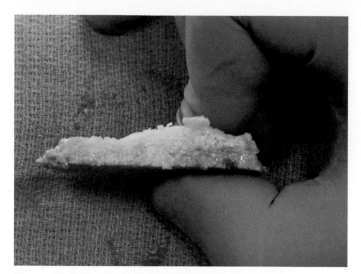

Figure 27-8 Resected tibial bone. Note the equal anterior and posterior bone thickness, which means resection has matched the patient's native slope.

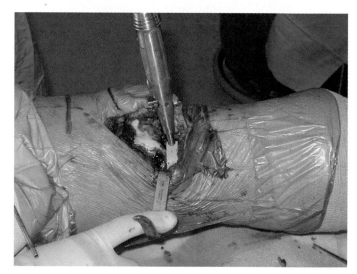

Figure 27-9 Various sizes and thicknesses of spacers are used to assess the flexion and extension gaps.

lateral aspect of the medial condylar bone and medial to the ACL is a remarkably consistent landmark for the vertical cut for the tibia. The horizontal cut should be approximately at 90° to the long axis of the tibia and at 90° to the "L" cut. Various cutting guides can be helpful for planning this cut (**Fig. 27–7**). The amount of posterior slope must match the native knee and should be carefully planned on the preoperative radiographs. In many cases, because the majority of bone loss in UKA knees is anterior, when the knee is flexed there is a normal amount of residual cartilage between the femur and tibia. Placement of a thin guide in this position is an intraoperative check to ensure appropriate slope to the tibial cut. Because this is a tibia-first sequence, this cut is extremely important. Care must be taken to avoid lifting the hand when making the vertical cut as the tibial bone becomes quite soft posteriorly. Because there is almost never any bone or cartilage loss in the notch, inspection of the medial aspect of the removed tibial bone should show that the anterior and posterior parts of the cut surface are the same thickness. This confirms that the appropriate slope has been applied to the tibial cut (**Fig. 27–8**).

Assessing the Flexion and Extension Gaps

At this point the resected tibial bone can be used to get an approximate size of the tibia to be replaced. Spacers of various thicknesses can be used to assess the flexion and extension gaps (**Fig. 27–9**). For proper balance in extension, the knee should fully extend and have about 1–2 mm of laxity in full

extension. To test the flexion gap, the knee should be flexed and the same spacer should be placed into the flexion gap. Most UKA patients have extension gap loss (anterior tibia and weight-bearing femur cartilage loss) and the posterior femoral cartilage is often of normal thickness. If the knee is too tight in flexion but stable in extension, one option is to use the oscillating saw to resect 1–2 mm of cartilage off the posterior aspect of the femur; this will usually equalize the gaps.

Mating the Distal Femoral Cut to the Tibial Cut

To ensure stability in stance and fixation of implants, the femoral cut should be mated to the tibial cut in extension. As was previously mentioned, the tibial cut can be placed in anywhere from 0° to 22° of posterior slope. This slope is

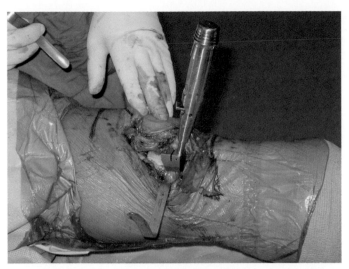

Figure 27-10 Distal femoral cut in extension mated to the tibial cut surface.

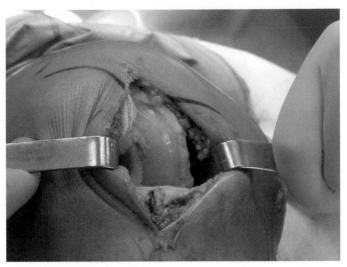

Figure 27-11 The so-called tidemark is the area where cartilage loss ends on the femur, and it can be a landmark for placement of the femoral component.

usually approximately 5° but it needs to be considered in the planning of the femoral cut. This cut can be planned with either intra- or extramedullary guides. Use of a cutting guide that sits on the cut tibial surface ensures that the distal femur cut matches the tibial cut. If the tibial cut has been made in posterior flexion (as is usually the case), the knee should be held in slight flexion while the guide is pinned to the femur. This will make the femoral cut in slight extension and this will help mate the femoral and tibial cuts (**Fig. 27–10**). It is important that enough bone has been resected off the distal femur so that the femoral implant will sit on a large enough bed that is not overly sclerotic, this will allow the cement to interdigitate with the bone and allow more durable fixation of the femoral component.

Sizing and Orienting the Femoral Trial

There is great variability in the shape and size of the distal femoral condyles. The femoral sizing in most modern UKA systems is independent of the tibial size. In many cases the so-called tidemark (**Fig. 27–11**) where the cartilage loss ends on the distal femur is a good landmark for placement of the femoral trial. In general, the femoral trial is measured in the AP plane while the knee is in flexion. Often a wedge can be used to anteriorize the femoral trial. This ensures that the femur is placed in an appropriately anterior position. From this starting point, the goal is to stay within about 10–15° of varus-valgus angulation of the tibial surface so as to not edge load the final construct. The femoral trial can be moved medial or lateral depending upon coverage so long as the nose of the trial does not point into the trochlear groove, as this could cause patellar impingement. Avoiding excessive internal rotation is important as this will bring the posterior aspect of the femoral component too medial in extension (**Fig. 27–12**). Most surgeons

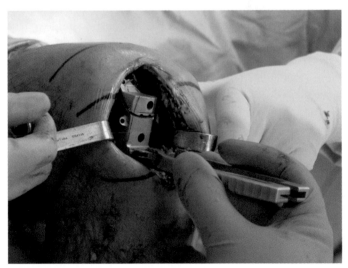

Figure 27-12 Correct rotation of the femoral cutting guides is critical.

aim for slight external rotation of the femur relative to the tibial cut in flexion. The actual rotation of the femoral component is dependent upon the type of implant used. If the system is a round-on-flat design, as most are, there is some forgiveness in the orientation of the femur. If, on the other hand, the system is a fully congruent one, this orientation is critically important. Most UKA systems have trials to ensure appropriate femoral-tibial alignment, tracking and balance.

Final Femoral Preparation

Most systems utilize a single block for cutting the distal femur. These blocks allow the anterior and posterior chamfers and the posterior cut. In many instances, the sequence should be as follows: anterior chamfer, which is usually quite small, then

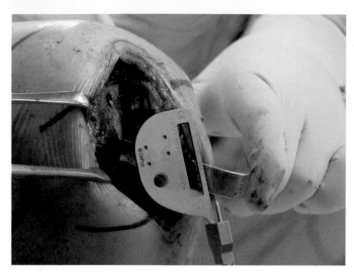

Figure 27-13 After all bone cuts have been made, it is easier to size and prepare the tibia.

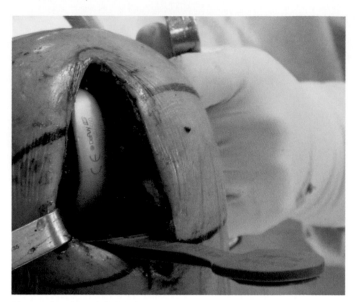

Figure 27-14 Trials in place allow testing of soft tissue balance and implant alignment.

the posterior cut, and lastly the posterior chamfer cut. The reason to do the posterior chamfer cut last is that occasionally, when this bone is removed, it allows the cutting guide to slip into a flexed position. Oftentimes the posterior chamfer is very sclerotic and, with the smaller guides, the smaller blades in these smaller guides can be less accurate, so greater care is needed on this cut. Several guides incorporate the drill holes for the lugs for the femur into the one guide. Until the lugs have been drilled, there is still the possibility to translate the femur more laterally if necessary. Femoral rotation obviously can no longer be changed. The lug holes should be drilled last for this reason.

Removal of the Meniscal Remnant

The smaller incisions that are commonly used today make visualization of the meniscal remnant difficult. Moving the leg into various degrees of flexion can be helpful in delivering the meniscus into view. It is important not to damage the medial collateral ligament during excision—an event that happens more frequently than one would think. This is also an opportune time to remove osteophytes from behind the femur. This is an important step to allow better range of motion.

Tibial Sizing and Preparation

With the meniscal fragment removed and the femoral cuts done, the tibial plateau can be more easily visualized (**Fig. 27–13**). For an all-poly tibial component, it is more important to have good AP coverage than medial-lateral coverage. This gives the tibial insert the best support. If necessary, it is possible to cut more into the medial aspect of the tibial spine, which in effect lateralizes the tibial component and allows for a larger size if needed. Slight overhang medially is tolerated on the tibia, and this is preferable to cutting too far into the tibial spine, which could potentially destabilize the

insertion of the ACL. For an inlay tibial component, leaving a rim of bone for cement containment is important and leaving a base of sclerotic bone is helpful for tibial support.

Depending upon the type of undersurface preparation needed for tibial fixation, a combination of saws, burrs, and hand tools can safely prepare the bone. There is great variability in the density of the medial tibial bone, and therefore it is important to be careful in removing it to accomodate various tibial component undersurfaces. In particular, it is easy to violate the posterior aspect of the tibia while preparing for a keel-type fixation, and this could theoretically diminish tibial cement penetration and fixation.

Final Balance Check and Trial Reduction

Once all bone preparation is complete, this is the time to perform a trial reduction (**Fig. 27–14**). Most systems have adequate trials for insertion, but if not, the real components can be used; however, it is important to remove them carefully after the trialing so as to not scratch their surfaces. A trial reduction will be helpful in determining the amount of flexion necessary to seat the components and also allows for final soft tissue balancing. It is possible to do slight adjustments to the medial soft tissues if the knee is too tight in both flexion and extension, although it is not recommended to perform a large medial release in the UKA knee.

Cementation

Retained cement is a relatively common cause for early reoperations in UKA. Removal of all cement fragments is very important. Smaller incisions limit visibility, and insertion of the tibial component in particular has the tendency to push cement out the back of the knee. This is particularly a problem

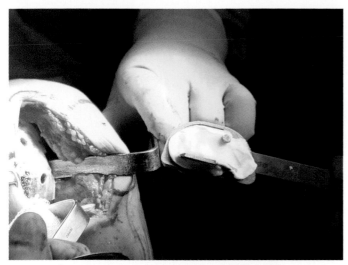

Figure 27-15 Cement on the undersurface of the tibia. Avoid placing too much cement.

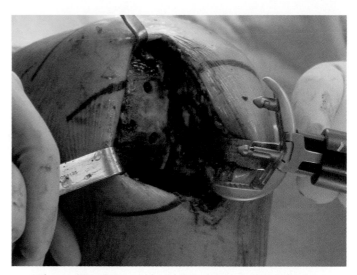

Figure 27-16 Femoral position of the implant in flexion.

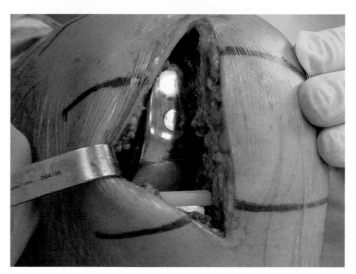

Figure 27-17 Final position of the implant in flexion.

with all-poly tibial components. Placement of a sponge behind the knee during cementation is one way to help prevent this from occurring (**Fig. 27–15**). Avoiding too much cement on the posterior aspect of the tibia is another. It is important to recognize that it is possible to have the front of the tibia in contact on the anterior tibial bone at the same time that the posterior part of the component is actually extended and not seated. The best way to prevent this is to insert the tibia in a hyperflexed position and to engage the back of the tibial implant on the tibia and to then bring the anterior edge of the tibia down. This can have the effect of pushing the cement anteriorly rather than out the back of the joint. It is important to inspect along the medial aspect of the knee to see that the posterior aspect is, in fact, in contact with the tibia. On the femoral side, good cement penetration onto the femoral surface is imperative. If sclerotic bone persists after bony prep, small drill holes can be helpful in improving the interdigitation. Most femoral components have lugs, and good cement compression into these lugs is also important to prevent femoral loosening (**Figs. 27–16, 27–17, and 27–18**).

Closure

A good capsular closure is particularly important in the UKA knee. Many of these patients have little pain and experience a relatively quick return to function. This can put an abnormal amount of stress on a fresh wound. To help prevent wound breakdown, meticulous repair of the soft tissues is needed.

LATERAL UKA

Lateral UKA represents less than 10% of UKAs. Historically the literature shows a comparable or even slightly higher longevity when compared to medial UKA. However, this may be

due to more careful patient selection and the fact that the majority of these procedures tend to be done by more high-volume UKA surgeons. There are a few technical tips related to the lateral UKA. The incision can be done either through a full medial arthrotomy or, more commonly, via a lateral incision where the patella is not displaced from the groove. If a lateral incision is made and a conversion to a TKR needs to be performed, the surgeon should be familiar with the lateral approach to the knee. The lateral incision tends to be more vertical and slightly shorter when compared to the medial one.

The lateral knee joint is laxer than the medial side, and it is therefore important to not overstuff the lateral joint with the implant. As opposed to the medial side, there frequently will be retained cartilage on the distal femoral surface as compared with the posterior femoral region; therefore, with a lateral UKA, the surgeon often has to remove cartilage off the

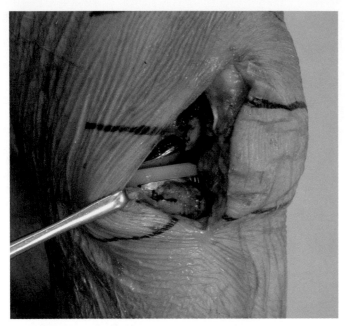

Figure 27-18 Final position of the implant in extension.

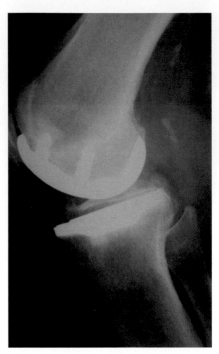

Figure 27-19 Lateral radiograph of UKA.

distal femur to balance the flexion and extension gap. The lateral knee joint is usually smaller than the medial one, so it is important to have available the smaller components of the particular system that will be used. The femoral size is even often downsized to avoid patellar impingement. The lateral femoral condyle is also generally more vertical than the medial side, so the femoral placement is usually more vertical than one is used to on the medial side. Internal rotation (10–20°) of the tibial component is desirable in the lateral UKA as it better accommodates the "screw-home" mechanism of the knee.

CONCLUSION

UKA is generally thought to be a more technically difficult surgery. In particular, in comparison to a TKR, the smaller incision usually used in UKA and the fact that the surgeon must mate the replaced compartment to the remaining tibial plateau are two reasons for the increased technical difficulty. However, if the surgeon is careful in patient selection, follows a meticulous surgical technique, and utilizes a well-designed implant, UKA can provide an excellent option for the patient with isolated compartment disease (**Fig. 27–19**).

REFERENCES

1. Kozinn SC, Scott R. Unicondylar knee arthroplasty. J Bone Joint Surg [Am] 1989;71:145-150.
2. Pennington DW, Swienckowski JJ, Lutes WB, Drake GN. Unicompartmental knee arthroplasty in patients sixty years of age or younger. J Bone Joint Surg [Am] 2003;85:1968-1973.
3. Parratte S, Argenson JN, Pearce O, et al. Medial unicompartmental knee replacement in the under-50s. J Bone Joint Surg [Br] 2009; 91:351-356.
4. Deshmukh RV, Scott RD. Unicompartmental knee arthroplasty: long-term results. Clin Orthop Relat Res 2001;(392):272-278.
5. Naal FD, Neuerburg C, Salzmann GM, et al. Association of body mass index and clinical outcome 2 years after unicompartmental knee arthroplasty. Arch Orthop Trauma Surg 2009;129:463-468.
6. Tabor OB Jr, Tabor OB, Bernard M, Wan JY. Unicompartmental knee arthroplasty: long-term success in middle-age and obese patients. J Surg Orthop Adv 2005;14:59-63.

CHAPTER **28**

Anesthesia, Pain Management, and Early Discharge for Partial Knee Arthroplasty

Richard A. Berger

KEY POINTS

- The implementation of specialized clinical pathways in joint replacement has simultaneously decreased the length of hospital stay while significantly decreasing complications.
- We have developed newer perioperative anesthesia and rehabilitation protocols and combined them with a minimally invasive approach to partial knee replacement in order to hasten recovery and perform outpatient partial knee replacement.
- Using these newer protocols with a minimally invasive approach to partial knee replacement, we have found that patients recover faster and outpatient partial knee replacement is not only possible, but has become routine for our patients.
- Furthermore, this combined surgery and clinical pathway has been proven safe and effective and decreases the postoperative complication rate.

HISTORICAL PERSPECTIVE

Unicompartmental knee arthroplasty was originally popularized in the 1970s, promising minimal bone sacrifice and the potential ease of future revision to a total knee arthroplasty, if required. Unfortunately, an incomplete understanding of appropriate indications and surgical techniques, combined with flawed early prosthetic designs, resulted in a high rate of failure. Subsequently, unicompartmental knee arthroplasty was all but abandoned in the United States by the late 1980s. Fortunately, renewed interest in the concept was initiated by Repicci and colleagues,[1,2] who in the 1990s described a minimally invasive technique for unicompartmental knee arthroplasty. Subsequently, unicompartmental knee arthroplasty has increased in usage secondary to a combination of interest in less invasive knee arthroplasty[1-3] and reports from multiple centers of survivorship that rivals that of total knee arthroplasty in appropriately selected patients.[4]

In the past decade, efforts have been made to improve the short-term outcomes of both total knee arthroplasty and unicompartmental knee arthroplasty with respect to pain control and early functional recovery with the implementation of minimally invasive surgical techniques.[5-10] The evolution of many orthopedic procedures has had this progression. Anterior cruciate ligament reconstruction has evolved from an inpatient to an outpatient procedure. In addition, spinal diskectomy has also had similar changes over the past decade. As in these procedures, minimizing soft tissue trauma is one part of a greater protocol that has led to decreased inpatient needs and, at our institution, the now commonplace outpatient unicompartmental knee arthroplasty. A comprehensive perioperative approach is essential to allow same-day discharge of unicompartmental knee arthroplasty patients. This paradigm shift involves not only the patient and surgeon, but also the patient's family, the hospital, anesthesia team, therapists, and nursing staff. A successful protocol and pathway includes pain management, decreasing medication side effects, and accelerated therapy that is delivered in a timely fashion.

INDICATIONS/CONTRAINDICATIONS

Outpatient unicompartmental knee arthroplasty continues to evolve, and the indications and contraindications are continuing to evolve as well. Furthermore, patient expectations are expanding from pure pain relief to include high functional demands. The great success and rapid recovery of unicompartmental knee arthroplasty surgery has allowed both surgeons and patients to undertake the procedure in an expanded age group, and now include younger patients. While it is easy to imagine our younger patients motivated to return to work and life as soon as possible, it is evident that older patients desire the same early functional recovery to travel, golf, and time spent with family and friends. Subsequently, fewer patients are willing to spend multiple days in the hospital, and fewer still want to spend time in a rehabilitation center or recovering slowly at home. Outpatient unicompartmental knee arthroplasty surgery represents a new style of patient care, and some patients, surgeons, and institutions simply are not yet ready for this dramatic change. However, we have found that with a few exceptions, if a patient is independent and functional at home prior to surgery, a carefully planned outpatient unicompartmental knee arthroplasty can allow resumption of the patient's preoperative status the same evening of the day of surgery.

PREOPERATIVE PLANNING

Preoperative planning occurs in many stages and is the most important part of the process. It begins long before the day of surgery and includes much more than the historic medical clearance and implant choice that we have become accustomed to. The main components are planning, perioperative education, teamwork, and follow-through. The entire plan is customized for each individual patient and is created in the office at the time the patient decides to have surgery. After choosing the surgery date, the patient's medical history is carefully scrutinized to identify relevant problems such as cardiac, pulmonary, thromboembolic, anticoagulation, and any other issues that may require more thorough preoperative investigation or an altered postoperative management. All patients attend a comprehensive educational class prior to surgery. During the same visit to our medical center for the teaching class, the patient's medical clearance appointments and laboratory tests are scheduled, as well as an appointment to donate a unit of autologous blood. Each patient is given a complete packet of information in the office when they sign up for surgery. The contents follow a clear and logical format—these are summarized in **Box 28–1**.

Comprehensive patient education is required for partial knee arthroplasty to be successfully performed on an outpatient basis. The first step in this process begins in the office by helping patients set appropriate goals and realistic expectations. To achieve these goals and expectations, we have

---

Box 28-1 Summary of Patient Information Packet

- **Contact information for support staff:** clinical nurses, physical therapists, administrative assistants, billing coordinator, discharge planners
- **Preoperative plan summary:** surgical date, preoperative appointments (to include laboratory testing, electrocardiogram, chest radiograph)
- **Medication section:** what medications to stop before surgery, what medications to take after surgery
- **Partial knee arthroplasty information:** risks, benefits, implant images
- **Physical therapy information:** includes a postdated prescription, outline of goals to achieve, range-of-motion graph
- **Frequently asked questions:** day of surgery, procedure, discharge, recovery
- **Hospital information:** parking, hospital layout, all relevant telephone numbers

---

established a mandatory preoperative group class that patients and their spouses (or caregivers) attend 2–3 weeks prior to their surgery. This class gives patients the chance to review the educational packet prior to the class and generate further questions. Our clinical support staff teaches each class, and the curriculum outlines the perioperative experience from start to finish; from the initial office visit to routine annual follow-up. At the mandatory class, the risks and benefits of total knee arthroplasty are again reviewed. The preoperative requirements are reviewed, including preoperative testing, medical clearance, and medication prior to surgery. Furthermore, the surgical day is outlined in detail from arrival to check-in, anesthesia, positioning, postanesthesia care unit, physical therapy, and finally discharge. Lastly, strong emphasis is placed on postoperative strategies that will allow same-day discharge by meeting functional, nutritional, and symptomatic goals efficiently during the immediate postoperative period.

The most significant hurdle to outpatient partial knee arthroplasty is effective pain management. Much of the difficulty stems from patient fears and beliefs. A significant portion of the preoperative class therefore focuses on pain control strategies. The patients receive their postoperative pain medications from the hospital pharmacy at the time of the class to avoid any unnecessary delays the day of surgery. We employ a long-acting narcotic for baseline pain control, a short-acting breakthrough narcotic, and a nonsteroidal anti-inflammatory. In addition, we proactively reduce side effects such as nausea and constipation. The postoperative medication strategy is outlined in **Tables 28–1 and 28–2**. Table 28–1 is the routine table we use for our patients, while Table 28–2 is for the elderly patient or the patient who cannot or will not take oxycodone (OxyContin). Furthermore, it is difficult to predict the most appropriate dose of oral narcotic pain medication, even when considering the patient's weight and age. Therefore, all patients are asked to take one dose of the strongest pain medication they will take the week before surgery and to report any side effects. The postoperative dose can then be modified appropriately. The stool softener and antinausea medication are initiated prior to surgery and continued as shown in Tables 28–1 and 28–2. Finally, the patients are given two additional sheets that give an overview (**Table 28–3**) and a detailed view (**Box 28–2**) of their medications so that they understand what to take, when, and why.

Physical therapy and rehabilitation are also a large focus of the teaching class. The goals of therapy, both preoperative and postoperative, are discussed. Patients are given a cane, and the techniques for bed transfer, gait training, and assisted walking are reviewed. Rarely is crutch training or walker training anticipated or taught. A handout is provided with diagrams that detail the exercises and therapy regimen for preoperative training and postoperative rehabilitation. Finally,

Table 28-1   Postoperative Medication Sheet for the Routine Patient

	Day 1		Day 2		Day 3		Day 4		Day 5		Day 6		Day 7	
	AM	*PM*	*AM*	*PM*	*AM*	*PM*	*AM*	*PM*	*AM*	*PM*	*AM*	*PM*	*AM*	*PM*
	OxyContin 1 pill*	OxyContin 1 pill	OxyContin 1 pill	OxyContin 1 pill	OxyContin 1 pill		OxyContin 1 pill		OxyContin 1 pill	You are now finished with OxyContin				
	Celebrex	Celebrex	Celebrex	Celebrex	Celebrex	Celebrex	Celebrex	Celebrex	Celebrex	Celebrex	Celebrex	Celebrex	Celebrex	Celebrex
	Lyrica	Lyrica	Lyrica	Lyrica	Lyrica	Lyrica	Lyrica	Lyrica	Lyrica	Lyrica	Lyrica	Lyrica	Lyrica	Lyrica
	Senokot	Senokot	Senokot	Senokot	Senokot	Senokot	Senokot	Senokot	Senokot	Senokot	Senokot	Senokot	Senokot	Senokot
	Aspirin	Aspirin	Aspirin	Aspirin	Aspirin	Aspirin	Aspirin	Aspirin	Aspirin	Aspirin	Aspirin	Aspirin	Aspirin	Aspirin
					Scopolamine patch						Scopolamine patch			

	Day 8		Day 9		Day 10		Day 11		Day 12		Day 13		Day 14	
	AM	*PM*	*AM*	*PM*	*AM*	*PM*	*AM*	*PM*	*AM*	*PM*	*AM*	*PM*	*AM*	*PM*
	Celebrex	Celebrex	Celebrex	Celebrex	Celebrex	Celebrex	Celebrex	Celebrex	Celebrex	Celebrex	Celebrex	Celebrex	Celebrex	Celebrex
	Lyrica	Lyrica	Lyrica	Lyrica	Lyrica	Lyrica	Lyrica	Lyrica	Lyrica	Lyrica	Lyrica	Lyrica	Lyrica	Lyrica
	Senokot	Senokot	Senokot	Senokot	Senokot	Senokot	Senokot	Senokot	Senokot	Senokot	Senokot	Senokot	Senokot	Senokot
	Aspirin	Aspirin	Aspirin	Aspirin	Aspirin	Aspirin	Aspirin	Aspirin	Aspirin	Aspirin	Aspirin	Aspirin	Aspirin	Aspirin

	Day 15		Day 16		Day 17		Day 18		Day 19		Day 20		Day 21	
	AM	*PM*	*AM*	*PM*	*AM*	*PM*	*AM*	*PM*	*AM*	*PM*	*AM*	*PM*	*AM*	*PM*
	Celebrex	Celebrex	Celebrex	Celebrex	Celebrex	Celebrex	Celebrex	Celebrex	Celebrex	Celebrex	Celebrex	Celebrex	Celebrex	Celebrex†
	Senokot	Senokot	Senokot	Senokot	Senokot	Senokot	Senokot	Senokot	Senokot	Senokot	Senokot	Senokot	Senokot	Senokot
	Aspirin	Aspirin	Aspirin	Aspirin	Aspirin	Aspirin	Aspirin	Aspirin	Aspirin	Aspirin	Aspirin	Aspirin	Aspirin	Aspirin

*You may take Norco (hydrocodone) as needed for pain while you are taking OxyContin.
†The Celebrex will be continued for a total of 3 months after surgery.

Table 28-2 Postoperative Medication Sheet for Elderly Patients or Patients Who Cannot Take Oxycontin

	Day 1		Day 2		Day 3		Day 4		Day 5		Day 6		Day 7	
	AM	PM	AM	PM	AM	PM	AM	PM	AM	PM	AM	PM	AM	PM
	Celebrex Lyrica Senokot Aspirin	Celebrex Lyrica Senokot Aspirin	Celebrex Senokot Aspirin	Celebrex Lyrica Senokot Aspirin	Celebrex Lyrica Senokot Aspirin	Celebrex Lyrica Senokot Aspirin	Celebrex Lyrica Senokot Aspirin	Celebrex Lyrica Senokot Aspirin	Celebrex Lyrica Senokot Aspirin	Celebrex Lyrica Senokot Aspirin	Celebrex Lyrica Senokot Aspirin	Celebrex Lyrica Senokot Aspirin	Celebrex Lyrica Senokot Aspirin	Celebrex Lyrica Senokot Aspirin

Darvon or Ultram as needed for pain. Every 4–6 hours as needed. Alternate the doses. Maximum of 12 tablets in 24 hours.*

	Day 8		Day 9		Day 10		Day 11		Day 12		Day 13		Day 14	
	PM	AM	PM	AM	PM	AM	PM	AM	PM	AM	PM	AM	PM	AM
	Celebrex Lyrica Senokot Aspirin	Celebrex Lyrica Senokot Aspirin	Celebrex Lyrica Senokot Aspirin	Celebrex Lyrica Senokot Aspirin	Celebrex Lyrica Senokot Aspirin	Celebrex Lyrica Senokot Aspirin	Celebrex Lyrica Senokot Aspirin	Celebrex Lyrica Senokot Aspirin	Celebrex Lyrica Senokot Aspirin	Celebrex Lyrica Senokot Aspirin	Celebrex Lyrica Senokot Aspirin	Celebrex Lyrica Senokot Aspirin	Celebrex Lyrica Senokot Aspirin	Celebrex Lyrica Senokot Aspirin

Darvon or Ultram as needed for pain. Every 4–6 hours as needed. Alternate the doses. Maximum of 12 tablets in 24 hours.*

	Day 15		Day 16		Day 17		Day 18		Day 19		Day 20		Day 21	
	AM	PM	AM	PM	AM	PM	AM	PM	AM	PM	AM	PM	AM	PM
	Celebrex Senokot Aspirin	Celebrex Senokot Aspirin	Celebrex Senokot Aspirin	Celebrex Senokot Aspirin	Celebrex Senokot Aspirin	Celebrex Senokot Aspirin	Celebrex Senokot Aspirin	Celebrex Senokot Aspirin	Celebrex Senokot Aspirin	Celebrex Senokot Aspirin	Celebrex Senokot Aspirin	Celebrex Senokot Aspirin	Celebrex Senokot Aspirin	Celebrex† Senokot Aspirin

Darvon or Ultram as needed for pain. Every 4–6 hours as needed. Alternate the doses. Maximum of 12 tablets in 24 hours.*

*You may take Darvon and/or Ultram as needed for pain. Maximum of 12 tablets in 24 hours.
†The Celebrex will be continued for a total of 3 months after surgery.

Table 28-3 Overview of Postoperative Medication Protocol

Long-acting narcotic	OxyContin (oxycodone HCl, controlled release; Purdue Pharma L.P., Stanford, CT)
Short-acting narcotic	Norco (hydrocodone/acetaminophen)
COX II anti-inflammatory	Celebrex (celecoxib; Pharmacia/Pfizer, Chicago, IL)
Antinausea agent	Scopolamine patch
Stool softener	Senokot S (to start 2 days prior to surgery)

Box 28-2 Medication Explanation for Patients

Daily Medications

- **OxyContin** (oxycodone): Take as directed according to the attached graph. OxyContin IS NOT an as-needed medication.
- **Celebrex** (celecoxib): Anti-inflammatory to be taken twice daily for a total of 3 months after surgery. Make sure you take with food every time you take it.
- **Aspirin**: Used as a mild blood thinner after surgery, to be taken twice daily for 3 weeks. If you normally take aspirin, you may resume your usual dosing after you finish the 3-week postoperative regimen.
- **Lyrica** (pregabalin): To help with nerve pain and tingling sensations; take twice daily for 2 weeks.
- **Senokot (Senna Plus)** (docusate plus senna): Stool softener to be taken the whole time you are on narcotics (including Norco and OxyContin).
- **Scopolamine patch**: Used to control nausea for the first week after surgery. Change it every 3 days (72 hours). Only use if you are taking narcotics.

As-Needed Medications

- **Pain**: Norco (hydrocodone/acetaminophen):
  - Use as needed for pain control.
  - Can be taken while on OxyContin.
  - Limit in a 24-hour period is 12 tablets total. Take 1–2 tablets every 4–6 hours.
  - We recommend taking Norco approximately 30 minutes prior to physical therapy sessions.
- **Nausea**: Reglan (metoclopramide): As needed for nausea not controlled by the scopolamine.
- **Sleep**: Ambien (zolpidem): As needed for insomnia. (**Do Not Take While On OxyContin.**)

the importance of motion is stressed, and patients are made aware they must achieve at least 100° of flexion by 1 week after surgery. The final part of the teaching class reviews the postoperative period. Patients are given a copy of the discharge sheet, medication protocol, and postoperative directions. The normal postoperative course is reviewed so that patients may feel comfortable recognizing symptoms and situations that are unusual and need to be reported. An understanding of the perioperative protocols and the roles of both patient and provider facilitate early recovery after surgery.

Successful outpatient partial knee surgery not only requires careful planning and preparation, but also requires cooperation between the patient and surgical team. This team includes the surgeon, office staff, anesthesia team, and the hospital team of nurses and therapists. For patients to be discharged the day of surgery, the patient must meet specific goals. To meet these requirements in a timely fashion requires an early surgical start time for patients who are planning to go home the same day. A strategy is utilized for prophylactic prevention of and treatment of pain, hypovolemia, and nausea. This approach is necessary in minimizing any symptoms or problems that would otherwise delay recovery. Preoperative medication protocols are employed to establish baseline blood levels of both narcotic and anti-inflammatory medication. Most patients take 10 mg of OxyContin and 400 mg of celecoxib (Celebrex) with a sip of water the morning of surgery. Most patients are placed on the standard postoperative protocol (see Table 28–1). Patients who are unable to take narcotics, had an adverse reaction to the trial dose of medication, or are extremely elderly are placed on an alternative pathway (see Table 28–2) and therefore just take 400 mg of Celebrex with a sip of water the morning of surgery.

Cooperation between the surgical team and the anesthesia team is a very important aspect of successful outpatient partial knee surgery. The anesthetic goal is appropriate intraoperative pain relief that minimizes postoperative symptoms.[11,12] While there are many anesthetic choices that allow outpatient partial knee replacement, our patients receive a straight bupivacaine epidural in the holding area prior to entering the operating room. A small dose of midazolam (Versed) is administered in conjunction with epidural placement. Intraoperative sedation is accomplished with propofol, which is titrated as needed for the individual patient. Narcotic use is avoided, or at least minimized as much as possible, to avoid unwanted side effects, which typically include increased nausea and sedation. Another important strategy that includes the anesthesia team is the prevention of nausea and hypovolemia. A big part of the technique begins by restricting narcotic use intraoperatively. To prevent nausea, the anesthesiologist administers 20 mg famotidine (Pepcid) IV, 4 mg ondansetron (Zofran) IV, and 10 mg metoclopramide (Reglan) IV during the surgery. This combination helps to prevent nausea postoperatively. The anesthesiologist is encouraged to aggressively manage fluid balance. To aid in this cause, if the patient has donated autologous blood, it is transfused intraoperatively to prevent anemia and hypovolemia. If the patient has not donated autologous blood, patients are typically given a fluid bolus of hetastarch in sodium chloride (Hespan) at the conclusion of the surgery. Alternatively, as another method to prevent fluid loss, a re-transfusion device can be utilized.

The surgical technique itself plays a pivotal role in our outpatient partial knee protocol. Multiple minimally invasive techniques have been described for partial and total knee arthroplasty.[1–3,5,6,8,10,13] These surgical techniques all share the common goal of limiting soft tissue injury in order to limit pain and allow early function after surgery. These strategies include making in situ bone cuts, not dislocating the knee or the patella, and preserving the quadriceps mechanism.

POSTOPERATIVE MANAGEMENT

The patient's knee is infused with 0.25% bupivacaine (Marcaine) at the conclusion of the surgery to cover pain control prior to the oral agent initiation but after the epidural being discontinued. After completion of the surgery, the patient is transferred to the recovery room. There, after verification of neurologic status of the operative extremity, an epidural drip is started with bupivacaine 0.1% and fentanyl 5 mcg/ml. The drip is run with a continuous infusion of 6 ml/hr in addition to a patient-controlled bolus of 1 ml/15 min with a 40-ml total infusion per hour maximum. The patient can be discharged from the recovery room or can be transferred to the inpatient ward and discharged from there. At the preoperative teaching class, patients are taught to expect a well-planned and rapid progression aimed at discharge in approximately 6 hours. Timing is critical, and we employ strict order sets to facilitate drain removal, dressing change, transition to oral pain medication, diet advancement, and physical therapy.

The patient's diet is advanced almost immediately, and patients typically receive lunch in the early afternoon. The epidural catheter and urinary catheter are removed 6 hours after surgery. A 10-mg dose of OxyContin is administered 2 hours prior to epidural removal as a bridge for pain management. Patients who experience significant postoperative pain may receive 30 mg ketorolac intramuscularly. This pain management protocol minimizes narcotic use and side effects while effectively controlling pain. Patients are required to pass physical therapy prior to discharge. Therapy sessions typically begin in the early afternoon, depending on when the patient reaches the floor. It is imperative that patients are not experiencing hypotension or nausea when therapy is initiated. If they are experiencing either of these symptoms, we temporarily hold therapy until we correct the problem (**Table 28–4**). Therapy starts by sitting the patient on the side of the bed and progressing if he or she is symptom free. Ambulatory aids are used as needed as determined by the therapist. Physical therapy goals include walking 150 feet and managing a single flight of stairs. Achieving these goals takes approximately 30 minutes.

Discharge is dependent not only on physical therapy, but also upon pain and nausea control. The discharge instructions are reviewed and patients are instructed not to operate a motor vehicle if they are using any narcotic medication. The patients must have a family member or friend to drive them home and

Table 28-4	Summary of Remedies for Potential Problems	
	Preemptive	*Treatment*
Nausea	Minimize or avoid opioids	Metoclopramide
	Ondansetron (Zofran) or scopolamine patch	(Reglan)
	Keep adequate hydration	Hydration
	Steroids	(Zofran does not work well for treatment)
Hypotension (orthostatic)	Adequate hydration	Hydration
		Ephedrine
Hypotension (drug induced)	Avoid opioids	Reverse drug
		Wait
		Hydration
Pain	Anti-inflammatories and opioids prior to surgery	Opioids for breakthrough
	Local injection for bridge	Ketorolac (Toradol)
	Start oral medications in recovery room	
	Avoid PRN dosing	

stay with them during the immediate postoperative period. The patient's postdischarge care plan is clearly delineated at the teaching class and outlined on written materials that the patients take home. Patients are encouraged to work on range of motion on their own and are weight bearing as tolerated. They already have their postoperative long-acting and short-acting pain medications. The 1-week follow-up appointment is prearranged and they are seen again at 3 and 6 weeks. A wide variety of anticoagulation protocols exist, and any of them may be utilized in conjunction with rapid rehabilitation techniques. We choose to use 325 mg of aspirin twice a day for 3 weeks after surgery. We also use graded compression stockings for the first 3 weeks. Several other aspects of the overall protocol also decrease the rate of thrombosis.[14] The minimally invasive techniques themselves do not require patellar eversion, hyperflexion, or tibial dislocation. Autologous blood donation and epidural anesthesia contribute as well.

Patients begin therapy in their homes with a visiting therapist three times per week. The therapy prescription at home is identical to our outpatient protocol. The protocol focuses on motion, extension when at rest, and flexion to a minimum of 100° by 1 week. The patient and therapist determine when the patient progresses to a cane and then no walking aid. Patients are encouraged to bike, golf, and engage in aqua therapy as soon as they feel ready. A wound check is performed at 1 week after the surgery. Most patients are ready to transition to outpatient therapy by this visit. This often depends on their ability to drive, which is prohibited if they are still using narcotic pain medication. Patients arrange their outpatient therapy at a convenient location and typically attend sessions 3 days per week for 6 weeks. The actual length of time in therapy depends on progress and success in achieving functional goals.

This entire protocol is outlined in **Box 28–3**.

Box 28-3	Summary of Anesthesia, Pain Management, and Early Discharge Protocol

Preoperative

- Internist appointment for medical clearance
- Teaching class
  - Go through risks and benefits of surgery
  - Explain rapid discharge protocol
  - Session of physical therapy

Morning of Surgery

- Celebrex 400 mg orally
- OxyContin 10 mg orally

Intraoperative

- Epidural anesthesia with fentanyl 5 mcg/ml and Marcaine 0.1%
- Preventative measures for side effects include:
  - Reglan 10 mg
  - Zofran 4 mg
  - Pepcid 20 mg
- Twilight sedation with propofol drip titrated to mcg/kg (per body weight)
- Local infiltration of surgical area with Marcaine 0.25% (per body weight)

Postoperative

- Give postoperative dose as soon as patient is in postanesthesia recovery
  - Norco 5 mg for patients over 70 years old
  - OxyContin 10 mg for patients under 70 years old
- Patients are given a fluid bolus of 500 ml of lactated Ringer s solution
- Remove epidural—2 hours after surgery
- Change surgical dressing and remove drain—3 hours after surgery
- Physical therapy session with weight bearing as tolerated—4 hours after surgery

Discharge patient, if medically stable, comfortable on oral analgesia, and patient agrees.

Start oral program of Celebrex, asprin, and oral analgesia (10 mg OxyContin for most patients, with a wean schedule).

RESULTS

We have previously reported results with outpatient partial and total knee arthroplasty.[5,6,13] The successes of our initially conservative selection criteria have led us to expand the indication to all patients. In fact, in our most recent report,[13] we found that 94% of the partial and total knee arthroplasties performed before noon were done on an outpatient basis. In this study of all comers, we assessed the feasibility and perioperative complications following outpatient total knee and unicompartmental knee replacement where no patient was excluded. To accomplish these goals, a minimally invasive surgical technique, improved perioperative anesthesia, and an expedited rehabilitation protocol were developed. One hundred twenty-one consecutive patients who had primary partial or total knee replacement completed by noon were prospectively studied.[13] While no patient was excluded by the investigator, 10 patients refused participation. The remaining 25 unicompartmental knee arthroplasty and 86 total knee arthroplasty patients (111 total) followed the comprehensive perioperative clinical pathway described above (see Box 28–3), which included preoperative teaching, regional anesthesia, preemptive oral analgesia, and preemptive antiemetics. In addition, a rapid rehabilitation pathway with full weight bearing and range of motion was implemented within a few hours after surgery. Only if standard discharge criteria were met did the patient have the option of discharge to home the day of surgery.

Twenty-four of the 25 unicompartmental knee replacement patients (96%) and 80 of the 86 total knee replacement patients were discharged directly to home on the day of surgery.[13] The remaining seven patients were hospitalized overnight and discharged the next day. The only unicompartmental knee arthroplasty patient who required overnight stays experienced nausea that could not be adequately controlled on the day of surgery. Four patients who had undergone total knee replacement remained hospitalized due to difficulty with pain control; all had their surgeries completed between 11:00 AM and noon. One total knee patient had chest pain that required a workup for myocardial infarction, which was negative, and another total knee patient chose not to leave the hospital due to apprehension and fear of discharge. All of these seven patients successfully and easily met discharge criteria by the morning of postoperative day 1 and were discharged to home at that time. There were no statistically significant differences with regard to average age ($p = .46$), body weight ($p = .47$), or body mass index ($p = .17$) between the 104 patients who were successfully treated as outpatients and the seven patients who required an overnight stay. There were no readmissions or emergency room visits within the 3 months following surgery for any of the unicompartmental patients. There were no deaths, cardiac events, or pulmonary complications during this study. This study has shown that the comprehensive perioperative clinical pathway that we have developed and described above not only is effective for allowing early discharge and rehabilitation for unicompartmental knee surgery patients, but also is safe.[13]

In 2009, we started a study of patients undergoing partial knee replacements using the anesthesia, pain management, and early discharge protocol. In this prospective study, 56 consecutive patients who had primary partial knee replacements completed by noon were invited to participate in this study evaluating the above-described protocol. While we excluded no patients, 6 patients declined participation. Among the remaining 50 partial knee replacement patients, 34 had medial unicompartmental replacements, 10 had lateral unicompartmental replacements, and 6 had patellofemoral replacements. The average age was 71 (range 57–81), the average weight was 180 lbs (range 120–320 lbs), 21 were females and 29 were males. This group of 50 partial knee replacement patients followed the comprehensive perioperative clinical pathway described above, which included preoperative teaching, regional anesthesia, preemptive oral analgesia, and preemptive antiemetics. In addition, a rapid rehabilitation pathway with full weight bearing and range of motion was implemented within a few hours after surgery. Only if standard discharge criteria were met did the patient have the option of discharge to home the day of surgery. We found that, in this group of 50 consecutive patients who agreed to be in this study, all 50 were discharged home the day of surgery. There were no readmissions following surgery for any of these 50 patients. There were no deaths, cardiac events, or pulmonary complications during this study. This study has again demonstrated that the comprehensive perioperative clinical pathway that we have developed and described above is effective for allowing early discharge and is safe.

POSSIBLE CONCERNS, FUTURE OF THE TECHNIQUE

Through the use of minimally invasive surgical techniques for partial and total knee arthroplasty, rapid rehabilitation,

and comprehensive pain management, we have successfully instituted a protocol for outpatient partial and total knee arthroplasty at our institution. The techniques and protocols are evolving. A great deal of planning must be done prior to embarking upon such a pathway to ensure patient safety and success. The high rate of discharge to home the day of surgery was in part due to our team's responsiveness to early signs of nausea and hypotension, which were swiftly acted upon. Continuing work in this arena may make it possible to perform outpatient minimally invasive partial knee arthroplasty in specialized surgical centers in the future. Future developments in technique that require even less soft tissue disruption may broaden the scope of outpatient partial and total knee arthroplasty. Improved fluid management, pain control, and side effect reduction will also allow more patients and surgeons to explore this pathway. The same financial pressures and patient demands that have led to successful outpatient anterior cruciate ligament reconstruction and diskectomy apply to partial and total knee replacement patients, and a response by the orthopaedic community has the potential to meet patient, surgeon, and health-care system goals.

REFERENCES

1. Repicci JA, Eberle RW. Minimally invasive surgical technique for unicondylar knee arthroplasty. J South Orthop Assoc 1999;8:20-27 [discussion appears in J South Orthop Assoc 1999;8:27].
2. Romanowski MR, Repicci JA. Minimally invasive unicondylar arthroplasty: eight year follow-up. J Knee Surg 2002;15:17-22.
3. Gesell MW, Tria AJ. MIS unicondylar knee arthroplasty: surgical approach and early results. Clin Orthop Relat Res 2004;(428):53-60.
4. Berger RA, Menghini RM, Jacobs JJ, et al. Results of unicompartmental knee arthroplasty at a minimum of ten years of follow-up. J Bone Joint Surg [Am] 2005;87:999-1006.
5. Berger RA, Sanders S, Gerlinger T, et al. Outpatient total knee arthroplasty with a minimally invasive technique. J Arthroplasty 2005;20(3 Suppl):33-38.
6. Berger RA, Sanders S, D'Ambrogio E, et al. Minimally invasive quadriceps-sparing TKA: results of a comprehensive pathway for outpatient TKA. J Knee Surg 2006;19:145-148.
7. Rosenberg AG. Anesthesia and analgesia protocols for total knee arthroplasty. Am J Orthop 2006;35(7 Suppl):23-26.
8. Scuderi GR. Minimally invasive total knee arthroplasty: surgical technique. Am J Orthop 2006;35(7 Suppl):7-11.
9. Scuderi GR. Preoperative planning and perioperative management for minimally invasive total knee arthroplasty. Am J Orthop 2006;35(7 Suppl):4-6.
10. Goble EM, Justin DF. Minimally invasive total knee replacement: principles and technique. Orthop Clin North Am 2004;35:235-245.
11. McGuire DA, Sanders K, Hendricks SD. Comparison of ketorolac and opioid analgesics in postoperative ACL reconstruction outpatient pain control. Arthroscopy 1993;9:653-661.
12. White PF. Management of postoperative pain and emesis. Can J Anaesth 1995;42:1053-1055.
13. Berger RA, Kusuma SK, Sanders SA, et al. The feasibility and perioperative complications of outpatient knee arthroplasty. Clin Orthop Relat Res 2009;(467):1424-1430.
14. Berend KR, Lombardi AV Jr. Multimodal venous thromboembolic disease prevention for patients undergoing primary or revision total joint arthroplasty: the role of aspirin. Am J Orthop 2006;35:24-29.

CHAPTER 29

Deep Vein Thrombosis Prophylaxis following Unicompartmental Knee Arthroplasty

Adolph V. Lombardi, Jr. and Vincent Y. Ng

KEY POINTS

- Modernization of all aspects of total joint arthroplasty have significantly reduced many surgery-related risk factors for venous thromboembolic disease (VTED).
- There are many different pharmaceutical options, adjunctive measures, and expert or evidence-based recommendations for reducing the risk of VTED.
- Unicompartmental knee arthroplasty may impose a lower risk of VTED than total knee or hip arthroplasty.
- Risk stratification, multimodal prophylaxis, hypotensive epidural anesthesia, and rapid mobilization appear to be effective in reducing the incidence of both symptomatic VTED and clinically important bleeding.
- Despite significant advances relevant to VTED, the arthroplasty community should remain vigilant in staying ahead of this potentially devastating complication.

INTRODUCTION

Venous thromboembolic disease (VTED) represents a spectrum of pathology ranging from asymptomatic deep vein thrombosis (DVT) to fatal pulmonary embolism (PE). Historically, VTED was one of the most feared complications of lower extremity total joint arthroplasty (TJA), with rates of fatal PE as high as 3.4%.[1] General surgical studies demonstrated that, before 1990, PE accounted for approximately 10% of in-hospital deaths.[2,3] However, modern orthopaedic surgical techniques, anesthetic care, and rehabilitation protocols have vastly improved the incidence of VTED and death after TJA. The Global Orthopaedic Registry found that only 0.3% of total knee arthroplasty (TKA) patients died within 3 months after TKA.[4] The National Registry for England and Wales demonstrated that the overall mortality rates at 1 year were actually 66% lower than age- and gender-matched controls from the general population.[5,6] Nevertheless, VTED remains a significant concern for patients and surgeons alike. DVT is still the most frequent in-hospital complication after TKA[4] and the most common reason for emergency readmission.[7]

ETIOPATHOGENESIS OF VTED

The etiopathogenesis of VTED is multifactorial. Known as Virchow's triad,[8] the combination of venous stasis, endothelial injury, and hypercoagulability are predispositions for VTED. Undergoing TJA exposes patients to all three of these states. Venous stasis can occur intraoperatively with manipulation of the limb, kinking of the vessels, and use of the tourniquet, and postoperatively during recuperation. A certain degree of endothelial injury inevitably happens from the physical nature of surgery and the hypoxic, hypothermic conditions during tourniquet inflation.[9–11] The cause of intraoperative hypercoagulability is not certain, but the 10–15% venographic incidence of DVT in the upper or contralateral limbs clearly demonstrates an iatrogenic systemic diathesis for clotting.[7] Further evidence is that over 80% of DVTs after TKA are already present by the first postoperative day.[12] In addition to the numerous surgery-related components of VTED, there are many patient-based risk factors as well (**Box 29–1**).

SEQUELAE OF VTED

While fatal PE is the most devastating consequence of VTED, it is relatively rare. The 90-day rate after TKA was 0.22% after almost 27,000 patients in the Scottish Registry,[13] and that for symptomatic, nonfatal PE was 0.41% in over 200,000 patients in a California database.[14] Approximately 25–30% of untreated symptomatic distal DVTs can propagate to proximal veins[15] and are associated with a greater embolic risk.[16,17] Asymptomatic VTED may not pose an immediate clinical problem, but at least three well-recognized sequelae can cause significant morbidity. Characterized by chronic venous insufficiency, pain, swelling, and recurrent ulcers, postphlebitic or postthrombotic syndrome (PTS) can develop in 25% of patients within 3 years after a DVT.[18,19] Although there is no gold standard for diagnosing PTS,[20] there is evidence that the incidence

Box 29-1 Commonly Cited Patient-Related Risk Factors for VTED after TJA

- History of VTED
- History of malignancy
- Family history of VTED
- Preexisting medical condition requiring use of chemical thromboprophylaxis
- Postoperative ileus[89]
- Long-term steroid use
- Oral contraceptive use
- Heritable thrombophilia or hypercoagulable state (protein C or S deficiency)
- Expected prolonged postoperative immobility
- Marked venous stasis
- Morbid obesity
- Age > 75 years (controversial)
- ASA (American Society of Anesthesiologists) Physical Classification[90,91] > 2
- High Charlson Comorbidity Index[57,92]
- History of cardiovascular disease[57]

of developing PTS may not necessarily be significantly elevated in patients who experience DVT after TKA,[21,22] and the use of thromboprophylaxis may not be effective in allaying that risk.[23,24] A second concern is recurrent VTED. An initial DVT has been shown to be an independent risk factor for subsequent DVTs.[25,26] Third, chronic pulmonary hypertension leading to right ventricular hypertrophy and right heart failure is a serious condition that can develop in 3.8% of patients at 2 years after an acute episode of PE.[27]

MODERNIZATION OF THROMBOPROPHYLAXIS

Modern developments have significantly mitigated the surgery-related risk factors for VTED after TJA. Forty years ago, the average patient underwent 2.4 hours of operation, 1650 ml of blood loss, 3 units of transfusion, 1 week of bed rest, and 3 weeks of hospitalization.[1,7] Warfarin was typically started 5 days postoperatively. Without thromboprophylaxis, the rates of DVT after TKA are exceedingly high, with proximal clots occurring in as many as 22% of patients at 14 days.[28] The last randomized, placebo-controlled study was over 20 years ago, and it is unlikely that another would ever be ethically approved. Although the need for some form of thromboprophylaxis is rarely questioned, there is considerable debate between two main governing bodies, the American College of Chest Physicians (ACCP) and the American Academy of Orthopaedic Surgeons (AAOS), regarding the type and extent of prevention necessary after TJA.

ACCP Guidelines

The eighth edition of the Clinical Practice Guidelines on antithrombotic agents was published in 2008 by the ACCP, an organization formed by practitioners in multiple fields such as pulmonology, critical care medicine, and cardiology.[29] In their analysis, the ACCP used objectively diagnosed DVT or PE as end points and examined only randomized controlled trials (RCTs) or meta-analyses of RCTs.[30] Some of their stronger recommendations for TKA were: against using aspirin (acetylsalicylic acid; ASA) or low-dose unfractionated heparin as the only means of prophylaxis (Grade 1A); continuing thromboprophylaxis for at least 10 days (Grade 1A) and extending it to 35 days (Grade 2B); using a high-risk dose of low-molecular-weight heparin (LMWH) started preoperatively or postoperatively, or fondaparinux started 6–24 hours postoperatively, or warfarin started preoperatively with a target international normalized ratio (INR) of 2.5 (range, 2–3) (Grade 1A); and using intermittent pneumatic compression devices (IPCDs) in patients with a high risk of bleeding (Grade 1A).[31] Because there are no prospective RCTs comparing multimodal prophylaxis to single modalities, the ACCP did not make any recommendations for or against it. Although the ACCP accepts that DVT is not a perfect surrogate for PE and that PE is the most important outcome for patients, it believes that DVT is a valid surrogate for PE based on a consistent correlation on imaging studies and parallel reduction of both entities with antithrombotic agents.[30,32] In addition, because of the relative rarity of PE and death after TJA, the sample size necessary to prove a statistical difference in either entity with thromboprophylaxis would near 30,000 patients for each arm of an RCT.[6,33]

Risks of Bleeding

Pharmaceutical thromboprophylaxis is not without risk of bleeding. The ACCP recommendations were based on studies with no date criterion, including those published far before the introduction of modern surgical and rehabilitation protocols. Many orthopaedists feel that the ACCP unduly focused on the prevention of all VTED at the expense of iatrogenic hemorrhage.[34] The challenge in achieving the appropriate balance was aptly put by Freedman et al.[33] "The decision regarding prophylaxis against thromboembolic disease depends primarily on which events one is attempting to prevent: all DVTs, proximal DVTs, all PEs, fatal PEs, death, or all of the above. When considering the issue of safety, one must determine which adverse consequences are important: minor wound-bleeding, major wound-bleeding, or major nonwound bleeding (gastrointestinal or intracerebral hemorrhage)."

AAOS Guidelines

In 2008, the AAOS published their own clinical guidelines addressing specific concerns with the ACCP recommendations.[35] First, only studies with patient recruitment since 1996 were included to better reflect the true underlying risk of VTED with modern protocols. Second, in addition to RCTs, large prospective cohort studies (>100 patients) were included. Third, instead of relying on the incidence of DVT as the primary efficacy outcome, prevention of symptomatic PE was used as the main goal of thromboprophylaxis. The AAOS challenged the validity and appropriateness of DVT, especially asymptomatic cases, as a proxy for PE or representative of clinical benefit.[36] Fourth, a formal consideration of the benefits *and harms* of potent thromboprophylaxis was made in the context of TJA. Patients who return to the operating room within 30 days after TKA have a significantly increased risk for deep infection or for requiring other major surgery.[37] Each day of prolonged wound drainage is associated with a 42% increased risk of infection.[38] Fifth, in order to choose the appropriate aggressiveness of prophylaxis, the AAOS emphasized the need to risk-stratify each patient in terms of PE and hemorrhage. The ACCP, in contrast, considered all TJA patients to be high-risk candidates for VTED. The most important distinctions of the AAOS guidelines are the allowance of ASA as the sole chemoprophylaxis except in patients with elevated risk for PE, a lower target INR with warfarin of ≤2.0, and the avoidance of LMWH in patients with elevated risk of bleeding. In addition, mechanical prophylaxis and early mobilization are recommended in all patients.[35]

Warfarin

Warfarin (Coumadin; Bristol-Myers Squibb, Princeton, NJ) acts at multiple sites in the clotting cascade, inhibiting the synthesis of vitamin K–dependent factors II, VII, IX, and X. It is a time-honored method of anticoagulation, but has several drawbacks. Because of its effect on endogenous anticoagulants protein C and protein S, warfarin is initially prothrombotic, and even with early administration, the INR does not usually reach its target range until 36 hours. Unlike most other anticoagulants, warfarin requires frequent INR monitoring and close titration of doses in order to prevent catastrophic bleeding. This can be challenging in the presence of numerous diet and drug interactions. Contemporary rates of hemorrhage while on warfarin range from 1.2% to 3.7%,[39–41] and at-risk medical patients have a 0.3% risk of bleeding for each additional month while on therapy.[42,43] A meta-analysis of warfarin prophylaxis found a 45% incidence of DVT, 8.2% of asymptomatic PE, and 0.4% of symptomatic PE after TKA.[44]

Low-Molecular-Weight Heparin

Enoxaparin (Lovenox; Sanofi-Aventis, Bridgewater, NJ) and the less commonly used dalteparin (Fragmin; Pfizer, Brooklyn, NY) are LMWHs. Unlike commercial unfractionated heparin (molecular weight 12–15 kDa), enoxaparin is smaller and more uniform in weight (molecular weight 5 kDa).[7] Its anticoagulant effect is mediated by enhanced inactivation of factor Xa and, to a lesser extent, factor IIa.[45] Enoxaparin has many advantages, including a more predictable dose response, a

dose-independent mechanism of clearance, a longer plasma half-life, and lower incidence of heparin-induced thrombocytopenia than unfractionated heparin.[46] Unlike warfarin, no regular laboratory monitoring is necessary other than a baseline and an early platelet count to rule out heparin-induced thrombocytopenia. Several disadvantages are high cost (~$40 per dose) and painful route of administration (subcutaneous injection). Enoxaparin is associated with lower DVT and hemorrhage rates than unfractionated heparin.[7,47] Compared to warfarin, enoxaparin is generally more efficacious after TKA in preventing distal DVT (24% vs. 34%), proximal DVT (2% vs. 11%), and pulmonary embolism (0% vs. 0.6%),[48] but multiple studies[4,7] have demonstrated a significantly higher incidence of major hemorrhage (5.2% vs. 2.3%) and clinically important operative site bleeding (6.9% vs. 3.4%).[48]

Aspirin

Aspirin is inexpensive and easy to administer, does not need monitoring, and has undergone a recent resurgence secondary to increased attention to bleeding complications from other agents. By inhibiting the production of thromboxane, ASA exerts an antiplatelet effect and is often used to prevent arterial tree embolism. For patients intolerant of ASA, dipyridamole (Persantine; Boehringer Ingelheim Pharmaceuticals, Ridgefield, CT) or clopidogrel bisulfate (Plavix; Bristol-Myers Squibb, Princeton, NJ) is typically substituted. To reduce the risk of gastrointestinal ulcer, a histamine$_2$ antagonist (e.g., ranitidine) or proton pump inhibitor (e.g., omeprazole) is administered. The Antiplatelet Trialists' Collaboration[49] and Pulmonary Embolism Prevention Trial[50] provided some evidence that aspirin may be effective in reducing VTED, but the data were somewhat confounded by multiple factors, including nonorthopaedic patients and concomitant anticoagulants.[7] Although there are no recent well-controlled studies examining the relative effectiveness and efficacy of ASA,[51] it is increasingly being used as one facet of a multimodal regimen. However, several large cohort studies have demonstrated its efficacy and safety in this context. When ASA (325 mg twice a day for 6 weeks) is combined with early mobilization, mechanical prophylaxis, and hypotensive epidural or regional anesthesia, rates of VTED and bleeding are exceedingly low, with 2.5–10.2% DVT, 0–0.1% fatal PE, and 0.2–0.5% hematoma or minor distant bleeding.[51–53] A recent review of multiple studies presented debatable evidence that the rate of all-cause mortality and incidence of nonfatal PE were significantly lower with multimodal prophylaxis and ASA compared to patients receiving LMWH and other heparin derivatives.[54,55]

New Pharmaceutical Agents

There are several newer anticoagulants that have received recent press. Fondaparinux (Arixtra; GlaxoSmithKline,

London, UK) is a synthetic pentasaccharide analog of the antithrombin binding site of heparin.[7] By triggering a conformational change in antithrombin, fondaparinux indirectly enhances inactivation of factor Xa, but unlike enoxaparin, does not affect factor IIa.[45] Although associated with lower rates of VTED after TKA than enoxaparin, it is also associated with a higher incidence of major bleeding.[56] Thrombin, an enzyme that converts soluble fibrinogen to insoluble fibrin and enhances clot formation, is the target of several oral medications such as ximelagatran (Exanta; AstraZeneca, London, UK) and dabigatran (Pradaxa; Boehringer Ingelheim Pharmaceuticals). Apixaban (Pfizer; Bristol-Myers Squibb) and rivaroxaban (Xarelto; Ortho-McNeil Pharmaceutical, Raritan, NJ) are direct factor Xa inhibitors, but data from clinical trials are only emerging and, along with dabigatran, they are not currently approved within the United States.[45] Ximelagatran has been discontinued secondary to hepatotoxicity during clinical trials.

Duration of Thromboprophylaxis

The appropriate postoperative duration of pharmaceutical thromboprophylaxis is debatable. Like the ACCP, the AAOS does not provide a strong or high-grade recommendation beyond providing a range between 2 and 6 weeks for warfarin and ASA.[35] Regarding LMWH and fondaparinux in TKA, the ACCP recommends a 35-day extended course while the AAOS feels that they have not been sufficiently evaluated for periods longer than 12 days.[31,35] Although the risk for VTED is highest within the first several days after surgery, the ongoing process of clot formation and lysis persists[7] and the risk remains elevated for at least 90 days.[57] Several studies have shown that, while short-duration anticoagulant therapy significantly decreases the risk of VTED, approximately 1 in 32 of these patients will have a symptomatic nonfatal VTED-related event and 1 in 1000 will have a fatal PE within the following 3 months.[46,58,59] A cost-utility analysis of enoxaparin showed that prolonged therapy led to increased health benefits through reduction of VTED, but at a significantly increased overall monetary cost.[60] This study, however, did not consider the ramifications of bleeding complications from additional anticoagulation. There is little evidence in this regard, but one study found that the additional enoxaparin did not increase the risk of major hemorrhage and only increased minor bleeding slightly from 2.5% to 3.7%.[59]

MECHANICAL THROMBOPROPHYLAXIS

The concept behind mechanical thromboprophylaxis is the replication of normal skeletal muscular contractions enhancing venous return. The most commonly used methods are graduated compression stockings (GCSs) and intermittent pneumatic compression devices (IPCD). GCSs statically provide a gradient of pressure ranging from 18 mm Hg at the ankle to 8 mm Hg at the thigh and prevent venous distention and pooling of blood.[7,61] Achieving the correct fit and maintaining the stocking in position are not only sometimes difficult, but also essential to its function. A recent study demonstrated that about half of all applied GCSs produced a "reversed" gradient of pressure and the incidence of DVT was greater than four times higher than in patients with correctly fitted stockings.[62] Intermittent pneumatic compression devices actively squeeze the lower extremity to 40 mm Hg for 12 seconds each minute (calf and thigh IPCDs) or 130 mm Hg for 3 seconds every 20 seconds (foot pumps).[7] Although smaller and quieter IPCDs have been developed, their main disadvantage is patient discomfort. Nevertheless, they have been found to be highly effective compared to placebo (62% risk reduction) and GCSs (47% risk reduction),[63] and even comparable to LMWH.[33,44] There is evidence that mechanical thromboprophylaxis is protective by both enhancing fibrinolysis and decreasing procoagulation activation.[7] Concomitant use of GCSs with IPCDs may reduce the hematogenous preload and emptying velocity of the veins, but there is little evidence to judge the merit of simultaneous mechanical modalities.[7] Because thrombogenesis often occurs during surgery and because of the beneficial systemic effect of mechanical thromboprophylaxis, IPCDs should be started intraoperatively on the nonsurgical limb.

INFERIOR VENA CAVA FILTERS

Inferior vena cava (IVC) filters are used in approximately 0.5% of TJA patients for either treatment or prophylaxis of VTED.[64] The most common indications are contraindication to anticoagulation, failure of anticoagulation, cessation of anticoagulation secondary to bleeding, and saddle embolus.[64] Although multiple studies have demonstrated strong efficacy of IVC filters in preventing PE in high-risk patients (0–3.1% incidence),[64-67] they should not be used without careful consideration. There is evidence that IVC filters may not affect overall mortality rates, and their presence is associated with an increased risk of primary or recurrent DVT.[68-70] While removal can theoretically reduce the long-term risk of an indwelling filter, actual retrieval rates are low secondary to filter site thrombosis and incorporation into the vessel wall, and range from only 13% to 64%.[64,71] Complications associated with filter insertion are low, but can occur in up to 11% of cases during retrieval.[64,65]

HYPOTENSIVE REGIONAL ANESTHESIA

Regional anesthesia, most commonly a spinal (subarachnoid) or epidural injection before TKA, when combined with hypotensive protocols, is thought to enhance lower extremity blood flow in the immediate postoperative period.[72] Epidural anesthesia causes a blockade of the sympathetic cardioaccelerator fibers originating from the upper thoracic spinal segments.[73] Although there appears to be no significant change in either thrombin generation or fibrinolytic activity during tourniquet elevation intraoperatively,[74] several studies have found that neuraxial anesthesia compared to general anesthesia decreased rates of proximal DVT from 9% to 4% after TKA,[75] and the odds of DVT by 44% and PE by 55%.[76] A review of 2500 total hip arthroplasties (THAs) performed with hypotensive epidural anesthesia reported rates of symptomatic and fatal PE at 0.42% and 0.04%.[77] Although the intraoperative hematologic impact of hypotensive anesthesia may be blunted for TKA with the use of a tourniquet, deliberate hypotension has been shown to decrease blood loss and transfusion requirements in orthopaedic procedures.[78] The exact definition of hypotension varies between institutions from a mean arterial pressure of 50 mm Hg to 70 mm Hg.[78] A combination of an opioid and local anesthetic typically provides adequate analgesia and neural blockade for patient comfort and surgery, yet allows early recovery of sensory and motor function in the early postoperative period to start rehabilitation.[79] Nevertheless, epidurals can fail in up to 20% of cases, and adjuvant pain control protocols should be in place to smooth the transition if an infusion catheter is removed at 24 hours.[79]

The timing of anticoagulation is critical when patients have received or are receiving neuraxial anesthesia. To reduce the risk of spinal or epidural hematoma and potential paraplegia, needle placement should be at least 10–12 hours apart from the nearest dose of LMWH and infusion catheters should not be placed or removed if the patient has an elevated INR.[51] Contraindications to hypotensive anesthesia include severe aortic or mitral stenosis and occlusion of the carotid artery, and extreme care should be taken in patients with congestive heart failure, uncontrolled hypertension, or severe atherosclerosis. Cerebral hypoperfusion, myocardial infarction, and renal failure are all potential risks.[80]

ROUTINE SCREENING AND RISK STRATIFICATION

Although routine screening in asymptomatic patients for VTED, specifically DVT, prior to hospital discharge to tailor levels of thromboprophylaxis may be intuitively appealing, both the AAOS and ACCP recommend against it.[33,35] Early surveillance imaging for DVT is a poor predictor of overall VTED risk and should not be used as a guide to decide whether extended thromboprophylaxis is necessary.[77,81,82] Risk stratification, in contrast, is likely more effective at protecting both high- and low-risk patients, and at the same time minimizing

their risk for bleeding. In a study of 1179 TJA patients, individuals were stratified according to their risk factors.[83] The low-risk group received ASA for 1 month while the high-risk group received LMWH for 10 days, then ASA for 1 month, or warfarin (INR 2–2.5) for 6 weeks or otherwise prescribed for a preexisting condition. All patients received IPCDs and early mobilization, and 82% had epidural anesthesia plus supplemental general sedation. Mean length of stay was 5 days, and all patients underwent Doppler ultrasound 24 hours prior to discharge. Low-risk patients and high-risk patients on LMWH who were found to have a proximal DVT or experienced a PE were switched to warfarin for 3–6 months. The overall rates were 5.2% asymptomatic DVT, 0.4% symptomatic DVT, 0.25% symptomatic PE, 0% fatal PE, 0.4% wound hematoma, and 0.17% nonfatal GI bleeding. Of note, this study differed from many RCTs by including "all comers" and not excluding high-risk individuals. Particularly interesting was that the incidence of hemorrhage and hematoma was 35 times higher in the patients who received non-ASA drug therapy either as thromboprophylaxis (high-risk group) or for treatment of VTED.[83]

DIFFERENCES BETWEEN UNICOMPARTMENTAL KNEE ARTHROPLASTY AND TKA AND THA

There are many important differences between THA, TKA, and unicompartmental knee arthroplasty (UKA) germane to thromboprophylaxis and VTED. First, intravasation and embolization of bone marrow fat during medullary canal preparation are commonly implicated as the sentinel event in activation of the clotting cascade.[84,85] With traditional instrumentation, violation of the canal is significantly less during UKA than THA and TKA. Second, because patients eligible for a UKA typically have smaller deformities than those undergoing TKA, they require lesser soft tissue releases for balancing the knee. In addition, the exposure necessary to perform a UKA is less invasive than a TKA. These factors reduce the risk of hematoma formation postoperatively. One must remember, however, that the knee has less soft tissue coverage and is much less forgiving than the hip in regard to wound healing. Third, there is generally less blood loss and a more rapid recovery period after a UKA than a TKA. The traditional perception that TKA is the highest VTED risk orthopaedic procedure has been challenged by new evidence,[58] and additional research may demonstrate that UKA incurs a significantly lower risk than TKA. Fourth, the generation and nature of DVT vary between TKA and THA, and may be distinct in UKA as well. Routine thromboprophylaxis in THA has changed the distribution of DVT from primarily proximal (50–60%) to nearly all distal (>90%). In TKA, however, 90% of all DVTs begin distally with or without prophylaxis. When proximal thrombi are present, in TKA they are usually contiguous with distal clots and do not extend beyond the popliteal vein, but in THA they are separate from distal clots and occur near the lesser trochanter.[7]

OUR PROTOCOL AND EXPERIENCE

At our institution, UKA is utilized in approximately 16% of knee arthroplasty patients. In a review of 1000 UKA cases, within 90 days postoperatively, there was only one (0.1%) symptomatic DVT, three (0.3%) hematomas requiring reoperation, and five (0.5%) blood transfusions for anemia.[86] Our thromboprophylaxis protocol for UKA is oral ASA 325 mg twice daily for 6 weeks (low risk); LMWH subcutaneous injection 30 mg twice daily or 40 mg once daily for 2 weeks, then ASA for an additional 4 weeks (moderate risk); and dose-adjusted warfarin (target INR 2.0) for 6–12 weeks (high risk). Clopidogrel bisulfate is used in ASA-intolerant patients. A general medical consultant assists in risk stratification. All patients receive IPCDs intraoperatively on the opposite limb and both IPCDs and GCSs are started bilaterally in the recovery room. Rehabilitation, including full weight-bearing and range-of-motion exercises, is initiated on the day of surgery. The average hospitalization is 1.4 days. We do not perform routine screening ultrasounds in asymptomatic patients. When it can be safely utilized, hypotensive epidural anesthesia is preferred. If neuraxial anesthesia is contraindicated, a femoral nerve block is used instead.[81,86,87] We also use perioperative cyclooxygenase-2 inhibitors; aggressive antiemetic medications; periarticular soft tissue injections with ketorolac, epinephrine, and ropivacaine prior to wound closure; long-acting oral narcotics for 24 hours; and short-acting oral narcotics for breakthrough pain.[88] These measures facilitate rapid recovery, early mobilization, consistent pain relief, and early discharge, leading to very low rates of both VTED and bleeding.

CONCLUSIONS

With modern advances in surgical technique and perioperative management, the threat of VTED after TJA has been greatly reduced. Nevertheless, symptomatic PE and the sequelae of DVT remain valid and important concerns for patients and surgeons alike. Equally important are the risks of bleeding associated with pharmaceutical prophylaxis. While the merits of multimodal therapy and risk stratification are rarely debated in the arthroplasty community, a consensus on appropriate anticoagulation is lacking. Recent evidence may support a shift in philosophy that no longer emphasizes medication as the lone main pillar in preventing VTED. Performing a UKA requires a related, but unique set of techniques compared to TKA. Similarly, it may require adjustments in the management of VTED.

REFERENCES

1. Coventry M, Beckenbaugh R, Nolan D, Ilstrup D. 2,012 total hip arthroplasties: a study of postoperative course and early complications. J Bone Joint Surg [Am] 1974;56:273-284.
2. Lindblad B, Eriksson A, Bergqvist D. Autopsy-verified pulmonary embolism in a surgical department: analysis of the period from 1951 to 1988. Br J Surg 1991;78:849-852.
3. Sandler D, Martin J. Autopsy proven pulmonary embolism in hospital patients: are we detecting enough deep vein thrombosis? J R Soc Med 1989;82:203-205.
4. Cushner F, Agnelli G, Fitzgerald G, Warwick D. Complications and functional outcomes after total hip arthroplasty and total knee arthroplasty: results from the Global Orthopaedic Registry (GLORY). Am J Orthop 2010;39:22-28.
5. National Joint Registry 4th Annual Report. Available at www.njrcentre.org.uk (accessed September 20, 2008).
6. Cusick L, Beverland D. The incidence of fatal pulmonary embolism after primary hip and knee replacement in a consecutive series of 4253 patients. J Bone Joint Surg [Br] 2009;91:645-648.
7. Pellegrini V, Sharrock N, Paiement G, et al. Venous thromboembolic disease after total hip and knee arthroplasty: current perspectives in a regulated environment. Instr Course Lect 2008;57:637-661.
8. Virchow R. Thrombose und Embolie: Gefassentzundung und septische Infektion. Frankfurt: Von Meidinger & Sohn, 1856.
9. Malone P, Morris C. The sequestration and margination of platelets and leucocytes in veins during conditions of hypokinetic and anaemic hypoxia: potential significance in clinical postoperative venous thrombosis. J Pathol 1978;125:119-129.
10. Naesh O, Haljamae H, Skielboe M, et al. Purine metabolite washout and platelet aggregation at reflow after tourniquet ischaemia: effect of intravenous regional lidocaine. Acta Anaesthesiol Scand 1995;39:1053-1058.
11. Ogawa S, Gerlach H, Esposito C, et al. Hypoxia modulates the barrier and coagulant function of cultured bovine endothelium. J Clin Invest 1990;85:1090-1098.
12. Maynard M, Sculco T, Ghelman B. Progression and regression of deep vein thrombosis after total knee arthroplasty. Clin Orthop Relat Res 1991;(273):125-130.
13. Howie C, Hughes H, Watts A. Venous thromboembolism associated with hip and knee replacement over a ten-year period: a population-based study. J Bone Joint Surg [Br] 2005;87:1675-1680.
14. SooHoo N, Lieberman J, Ko C, Zingmond D. Factors predicting complication rates following total knee replacement. J Bone Joint Surg [Am] 2006;88:480-485.
15. Kearon C. Natural history of venous thromboembolism. Circulation 2003;107:122-130.
16. Moser K, Le Moine J. Is embolic risk conditioned by location of deep venous thrombosis? Ann Intern Med 1981;94:439-444.
17. Pellegrini VJ, Clement D, Lush-Ehmann C, et al. The John Charnley Award. Natural history of thromboembolic disease after total hip arthroplasty. Clin Orthop Relat Res 1996;(333):27-40.
18. Kahn S, Ginsberg J. Relationship between deep venous thrombosis and the postthrombotic syndrome. Arch Intern Med 2004;164:17-26.
19. Prandoni P, Lensing A, Cogo A, et al. The long-term clinical course of acute deep venous thrombosis. Ann Intern Med 1996;125:1-7.

20. Kahn S, Solymoss S, Lamping D, Abenhaim L. Long-term outcomes after deep vein thrombosis: postphlebitic syndrome and quality of life. J Gen Intern Med 2000;15:425-429.

21. Ginsberg J, Gent M, Turkstra F, et al. Postthrombotic syndrome after hip or knee arthroplasty: a cross-sectional study. Arch Intern Med 2000;160:669-672.

22. McAndrew C, Fitzgerald S, Kraay M, Goldberg V. Incidence of post-thrombotic syndrome in patients undergoing primary total knee arthroplasty for osteoarthritis. Clin Orthop Relat Res 2010;(468):178-181.

23. Khuangsirikul S, Sampatchalit S, Foojareonyos T, Chotanaphuti T. Lower extremities' postthrombotic syndrome after total knee arthroplasty. J Med Assoc Thai 2009;92:S39-S44.

24. Schindler O, Dalziel R. Post-thrombotic syndrome after total hip or knee arthroplasty: incidence in patients with asymptomatic deep venous thrombosis. J Orthop Surg 2005;13:113-119.

25. Laporte S, Tardy B, Quenet S, et al.; PREPIC Study Group. The location of deep-vein thrombosis as a predictive factor for recurrence and cancer discovery after proximal deep-vein thrombosis [letter]. Haematologica 2003;88:ELT08.

26. Heit J, Mohr D, Silverstein M, et al. Predictors of recurrence after deep vein thrombosis and pulmonary embolism. Arch Intern Med 2000;160:761-768.

27. Pengo V, Lensing A, Prins M, et al. Incidence of chronic thromboembolic pulmonary hypertension after pulmonary embolism. N Engl J Med 2004;350:2257-2264.

28. Cushner F, Nett M. Unanswered questions, unmet needs in venous thromboprophylaxis. Orthopedics 2009;32:62-66.

29. Guyatt G, Cook D, Jaeschke R, et al. Grades of recommendation for antithrombotic agents: American College of Chest Physicians Evidence-Based Clinical Practice Guidelines (8th Edition). Chest 2008;133(6 Suppl):123S-131S.

30. Eikelboom J, Karthikeyan G, Fagel N, Hirsh J. American Association of Orthopedic Surgeons and American College of Chest Physicians guidelines for venous thromboembolism prevention in hip and knee arthroplasty differ. Chest 2009;135:513-520.

31. Geerts W, Bergqvist D, Pineo G, et al.; American College of Chest Physicians. Prevention of venous thromboembolism: American College of Chest Physicians Evidence-Based Clinical Practice Guidelines (8th Edition). Chest 2008;133(6 Suppl):381S-453S.

32. Eikelboom J, Hirsh J. Response. Chest 2009;136:1700-1701.

33. Freedman K, Brookenthal K, Fitzgerald RJ, et al. A meta-analysis of thromboembolic prophylaxis following elective total hip arthroplasty. J Bone Joint Surg [Am] 2000;82:929-938.

34. Johanson N, Lachiewicz P, Lieberman J, et al. Prevention of symptomatic pulmonary embolism in patients undergoing total hip or knee arthroplasty. J Am Acad Orthop Surg 2009;17:183-196.

35. Lachiewicz P. Comparison of ACCP and AAOS guidelines for VTE prophylaxis after total hip and total knee arthroplasty. Orthopedics 2009;32:74-78.

36. Weber K, Zuckerman J, Watters W, Turkelson C. Deep vein thrombosis prophylaxis. Chest 2009;136:1699-1700.

37. Galat D, McGovern S, Hanssen A, et al. Early return to surgery for evacuation of a postoperative hematoma after primary total knee arthroplasty. J Bone Joint Surg [Am] 2008;90:2331-2336.

38. Patel V, Walsh M, Sehgal B, et al. Factors associated with prolonged wound drainage after primary total hip and knee arthroplasty. J Bone Joint Surg [Am] 2007;89:33-38.

39. Amstutz HA, Friscia D, Dorey F, Carney B. Warfarin prophylaxis to prevent mortality from pulmonary embolism after total hip replacement. J Bone Joint Surg [Am] 1989;71:321-326.

40. Paiement G, Wessinger S, Hughes R, Harris W. Routine use of adjusted low-dose warfarin to prevent venous thromboembolism after total hip replacement. J Bone Joint Surg [Am] 1993;75:893-898.

41. Pellegrini VJ, Clement D, Lush-Ehmann C, et al. The natural history of thromboembolic disease following hospital discharge after total hip arthroplasty. Clin Orthop Relat Res 1996;(333):27-40.

42. Landefeld C, Cook E, Flatley M, et al. Identification and preliminary validation of predictors of major bleeding in hospitalized patients starting anticoagulation therapy. Am J Med 1987;82:703-713.

43. Landefeld C, Goldman L. Major bleeding in outpatients treated with warfarin: incidence and prediction by factors known at the start of outpatient therapy. Am J Med 1989;87:144-152.

44. Westrich G, Haas S, Mosca P, Peterson M. Meta-analysis of thromboembolic prophylaxis after total knee arthroplasty. J Bone Joint Surg [Br] 2000;82:795-800.

45. Friedman R. New oral anticoagulants for thromboprophylaxis after total hip or knee arthroplasty. Orthopedics 2009;32:79-84.

46. Colwell C. The ACCP guidelines for thromboprophylaxis in total hip and knee arthroplasty. Orthopedics 2009;32:67-73.

47. Geerts W, Jay R, Code K, et al. A comparison of low-dose heparin with low-molecular-weight heparin as prophylaxis against venous thromboembolism after major trauma. N Engl J Med 1996;335:701-707.

48. Fitzgerald R, Spiro T, Trowbridge A, et al. Prevention of venous thromboembolic disease following primary total knee arthroplasty. J Bone Joint Surg [Am] 2001;83:900-906.

49. Collaborative overview of randomized trials of antiplatelet therapy: III. Reduction in venous thrombosis and pulmonary embolism by antiplatelet prophylaxis among surgical and medical patients: Antiplatelet Trialists' Collaboration. BMJ 1994;308:235-246.

50. Prevention of pulmonary embolism and deep venous thrombosis with low dose aspirin: Pulmonary Embolism Prevention (PEP) Trial. Lancet 2000;355:1295-1302.

51. Daniel J, Pradhan A, Pradhan C, et al. Multimodal thromboprophylaxis following primary hip arthroplasty: the role of adjuvant intermittent pneumatic calf compression. J Bone Joint Surg [Br] 2008;90:562-569.

52. Della Valle A, Serota A, Go G, et al. Venous thromboembolism is rare with a multimodal prophylaxis protocol after total hip arthroplasty. Clin Orthop Relat Res 2006;(444):146-153.

53. Lotke P, Lonner J. The benefit of aspirin chemoprophylaxis for thromboembolism after total knee arthroplasty. Clin Orthop Relat Res 2006;(452):175-180.

54. Eriksson B, Friedman R, Cushner F, Lassen M. Letter to the Editor. Potent anticoagulants are associated with a higher all-cause mortality rate after hip and knee arthroplasty. Clin Orthop Relat Res 2008;(466):2009-2011.

55. Sharrock N, Della Valle A, Go G, Salvati E. Potent anticoagulants are associated with a higher all-cause mortality rate after hip and knee arthroplasty. Clin Orthop Relat Res 2008;(466):714-721.

56. Bauer K, Eriksson B, Lassen M, Turpie A; Steering Committee of the Pentasaccharide in Major Knee Surgery Study. Fondaparinux compared with enoxaparin for the prevention of venous thromboembolism after elective major knee surgery. N Engl J Med 2001;345:1305-1310.

57. Pederson A, Sorensen H, Mehnert F, et al. Risk factors for venous thromboembolism in patients undergoing total hip replacement and receiving routine thromboprophylaxis. J Bone Joint Surg [Am] 2010;92:2156-2164.

58. Douketis J, Eikelboom J, Quinlan D, et al. Short-duration prophylaxis against venous thromboembolism after total hip or knee replacement. Arch Intern Med 2002;162:1465-1471.

59. Eikelboom J, Quinlan D, Douketis J. Extended-duration prophylaxis against venous thromboembolism after total hip or knee replacement: a meta-analysis of the randomised trials. Lancet 2001;358:9-15.

60. Haentjens P, De Groote K, Annemans L. Prolonged enoxaparin therapy to prevent venous thromboembolism after primary hip or knee embolism: a cost-utility analysis. Arch Orthop Trauma Surg 2004;124:507-517.

61. Coleridge-Smith P, Hasty J, Scurr J. Deep vein thrombosis: effect of graduated compression stockings on distension of the deep veins of the calf. Br J Surg 1991;78:724-726.

62. Best A, Williams S, Crozier A, et al. Graded compression stockings in elective orthopaedic surgery: an assessment of the in vivo performance of commercially available stockings in patients having hip and knee arthroplasty. J Bone Joint Surg [Br] 2000;82:116-118.

63. Vanek V. Meta-analysis of effectiveness of intermittent pneumatic compression devices with a comparison of thigh-high to knee-high sleeves. Am Surg 1998;64:1050-1058.

64. Bass A, Mattern C, Voos J, et al. Inferior vena cava filter placement in orthopedic surgery. Am J Orthop 2010;39:435-439.

65. Emerson RJ, Cross R, Head W. Prophylactic and early therapeutic use of the Greenfield filter in hip and knee joint arthroplasty. J Arthroplasty 1991;6:129-135.

66. Golueke P, Garrett W, Thompson J, et al. Interruption of the vena cava by means of the Greenfield filter: expanding the indications. Surgery 1988;103:111-117.

67. Vaughn BK, Knezevich S, Lombardi AV Jr, Mallory TH. Use of the Greenfield filter to prevent fatal pulmonary embolism associated with total hip and knee arthroplasty. J Bone Joint Surg [Am] 1989;71:1542-1548.

68. PREPIC Study Group. Eight-year follow-up of patients with permanent vena cava filters in the prevention of pulmonary embolism: The PREPIC (Prevention du Risque d'Embolie Pulmonaire par Interruption Cave) randomized study. Circulation 2005;112:416-422.

69. Decousus H, Leizorovicz A, Parent F, et al. A clinical trial of vena caval filters in the prevention of pulmonary embolism in patients with proximal deep-vein thrombosis. N Engl J Med 1998;338:409-415.

70. Gorman P, Qadri S, Rao-Patel A. Prophylactic inferior vena cava (IVC) filter placement may increase the relative risk of deep venous thrombosis after acute spinal cord injury. J Trauma 2009;66:707-712.

71. Strauss E, Egol K, Alaia M, et al. The use of retrievable inferior vena cava filters in orthopaedic patients. J Bone Joint Surg [Br] 2008;90:662-667.

72. Davis F, Laurenson V, Gillespie W, et al. Leg blood flow during total hip replacement under spinal or general anesthesia. Anaesth Intensive Care 1989;17:136-143.

73. Kleinert K, Theusinger O, Nuernberg J, Werner C. Alternative procedures for reducing allogeneic blood transfusion in elective orthopedic surgery. Hosp Special Surg J 2010;6:190-198.

74. Sharrock N, Go G, Williams-Russo P, et al. Comparison of extradural and general anaesthesia on the fibrinolytic response to total knee arthroplasty. Br J Anaesth 1997;79:29-34.

75. Sharrock N, Haas S, Hargett M, et al. Effects of epidural anesthesia on the incidence of deep-vein thrombosis after total knee arthroplasty. J Bone Joint Surg [Am] 1991;73:502-506.

76. Rodgers A, Walker N, Schug S, et al. Reduction of postoperative mortality and morbidity with epidural or spinal anaesthesia: results from overview of randomised trials. BMJ 2000;321:1493-1497.

77. Westrich G, Farrell C, Bono J, et al. The incidence of venous thromboembolism after total hip arthroplasty: a specific hypotensive epidural anesthesia protocol. J Arthroplasty 1999;14:456-463.

78. Paul J, Ling E, Lalonde C, Thabane L. Deliberate hypotension in orthopedic surgery reduces blood loss and transfusion requirements: a meta-analysis of randomized controlled trials. Can J Anesth 2007;54:799-810.

79. Maheshwari A, Blum Y, Shekhar L, et al. Multimodal pain management after total hip and knee arthroplasty at the Ranawat Orthopaedic Center. Clin Orthop Relat Res 2009;(467):1418-1423.

80. Lieberman J, Huo M, Hanway J, et al. The prevalence of deep venous thrombosis after total hip arthroplasty with hypotensive epidural anesthesia. J Bone Joint Surg [Am] 1994;76:341-348.

81. Berend KR, Lombardi AV Jr. Multimodal venous thromboembolic disease prevention for patients undergoing primary or revision total joint arthroplasty: the role of aspirin. Am J Orthop 2006;35:24-29.

82. Pellegrini VJ, Donaldson C, Farber D, et al. The Mark Coventry award: prevention of readmission for venous thromboembolism after total knee arthroplasty. Clin Orthop Relat Res 2006;(452):21-27.

83. Dorr L, Gendelman V, Maheshwari A, et al. Multimodal thromboprophylaxis for total hip and knee arthroplasty based on risk assessment. J Bone Joint Surg [Am] 2007;89:2648-2657.

84. Mohanty K, Powell J, Musso D, et al. The effect of a venous filter on the embolic load during medullary canal pressurization: a canine study. J Bone Joint Surg [Am] 2005;87:1332-1337.

85. Sharrock N, Go G, Harpel P, et al. Thrombogenesis during total hip replacement. Clin Orthop Relat Res 1995;(319):16-27.

86. Lombardi AV Jr, Berend KR, Tucker TL. The incidence and prevention of symptomatic thromboembolic disease following unicompartmental knee arthroplasty. Orthopedics 2007;30:41-43.

87. Berend KR, Morris MJ, Lombardi AV Jr. Unicompartmental knee arthroplasty: incidence of transfusion and symptomatic thromboembolic disease. Orthopedics 2010;33:1-3.

88. Lombardi AV Jr, Berend K, Adams J. A rapid recovery program: early home and pain free. Orthopedics 2010;33:656.

89. Berend KR, Lombardi AV Jr, Mallory TH, et al. Ileus following total hip or knee arthroplasty is associated with increased risk of deep venous thrombosis and pulmonary embolism. J Arthroplasty 2004;19:82-86.

90. Mantilla C, Horlocker T, Schroeder D, et al. Risk factors for clinically relevant pulmonary embolism and deep venous thrombosis in patients undergoing primary hip or knee arthroplasty. Anesthesiology 2003;99:552-560.

91. Rozner M. The American Society of Anesthesiologists physical status score and risk of perioperative infection. JAMA 1996;275:1544.

92. Charlson M, Pompei P, Ales K, MacKenzie C. A new method of classifying prognostic comorbidity in longitudinal studies: development and validation. J Chron Dis 1987;40:373-383.

CHAPTER 30

A Multimodal Approach to Transfusion Avoidance and Blood Loss Management in Partial Knee Arthroplasty

Michael P. Nett

KEY POINTS

- Historic rates of blood transfusion following joint arthroplasty are unacceptably high.
- Preoperative hemoglobin is the best predictor of postoperative blood transfusion.
- Bloodless surgery is achievable with a multimodal approach to transfusion avoidance.

INTRODUCTION

Modern surgical techniques have reduced the amount of blood loss during total knee arthroplasty (TKA) procedures. Despite numerous advances, allogeneic transfusion rates still remain high. Transfusion rates following unilateral TKA range from 4% to 46%, while bilateral TKA results in transfusion rates between 31% and 72%.[1,2] Acute postoperative anemia, risks of allogeneic transfusion, and wound complications remain of great concern to the patient and surgeon. Allogeneic transfusions traditionally have been used to ameliorate the occurrence of anemia, but complications following allogeneic transfusion remain. Incorrect blood component transfusion, disease transmission, allergic reactions, fluid overload, transfusion reactions, and immunosuppression from allogeneic transfusions are well described.[3–8] Few data currently exist with regard to blood loss and transfusion rates in patients undergoing partial knee arthroplasty (PKA). In available studies regarding unicompartmental arthroplasty, average blood loss ranges from less than 200 to 240 ml, transfusion rates appear low, and postoperative hemoglobin drop ranges from 1.8 to 2.73 g/dl.[9–12] While patient risks for transfusion are lower with PKA, our practice follows a similar protocol with TKA and PKA with regard to minimizing perioperative blood loss and transfusion avoidance. The protocol focuses on a multimodal approach. This approach needs to be utilized in the preoperative, intraoperative, and postoperative periods to optimize the patient prior to surgery and minimize blood loss during and following arthroplasty. Conservation techniques for the preoperative, intraoperative, and postoperative periods are reviewed, and blood management protocols are presented.

WHY WE SHOULD TRY TO AVOID TRANSFUSIONS

Historically, 50% of patients undergoing total joint arthroplasty receive an allogeneic blood transfusion. The risks of allogeneic transfusions are well described in the literature for TKA, but data following PKA are sparse.[9,13–19] The main risks for direct transfusion-related morbidity and mortality include incorrect blood component transfusion (70%) and immunologic risks (28%), while transfusion-transmissible infection (2%) is of less significance.[20] With regard to transmissible infection, West Nile, TT, parvovirus B19, and SEN virus transmission has been discussed as a potential source of infection after allogeneic transfusions.[20,21] On a global scale, protozoa infections, including malaria and toxoplasmosis, remain some of the most common transfusion-transmitted infections.[20] In addition, some cases of the blood-borne transmission of prions have been described.[20]

Perhaps more concerning to the surgeon, allogeneic transfusions have been implicated in the increased incidence of infection after surgery. Tang et al.[22] performed a prospective series of 2809 consecutive colon resections. In this report, transfusion was the single most powerful risk factor for postoperative infection, with an odds ratio greater than 5. Kendall et al.[23] described immunosuppression secondary to allogeneic transfusions in 34 patients undergoing total hip arthroplasty (THA). According to Kendall et al., the lymphocyte function is impaired, which may be the etiology of the increased risk of deep prosthesis infection.[23] The effect of allogeneic transfusion on the immune system is now well documented in the literature.[20] Authors believe that the immunomodulating effect of red blood cell transfusion may be responsible for the better outcome in transplantation patients receiving transfusion, the higher risk of recurrence following malignancy resection in patients receiving transfusion, and the higher risk of postoperative infection following transfusion.[20] The incriminated pathomechanism of these effects of blood transfusion is called transfusion-related immunomodulation.[20]

The increased risk of infection following allogeneic transfusion is fairly well established in the joint arthroplasty literature. Pulido et al.[24] looked at predisposing factors for developing periprosthetic infection in a series of 9245 arthroplasty patients. They demonstrated a 2.1-fold increase in the rate of periprosthetic infection following allogeneic transfusion. Similarly, Shaunder et al.[25] demonstrated a 3.6 times greater relative risk for developing postoperative infection after cardiac and orthopaedic surgery following allogeneic blood transfusion. Similarly, Murphy et al.[26] showed an increased rate of confirmed or suspected infections in a series of 84 patients undergoing THA. They compared patients receiving autologous blood transfusion with those receiving allogeneic blood. Although the numbers were small in this series, the infection rate in the group receiving allogeneic transfusion was 32% compared to 3% in the autologous group. Other complications have also been linked to transfusion. In a recent population-based review of 28,087 THA patients, Pedersen et al.[27] compared 2254 patients receiving allogeneic transfusion with 2254 nontransfused, matched patients. In this series, transfused patients demonstrated a higher 90-day mortality and increased odds of pneumonia (odds ratio 2.2 and 2.1, respectively). Bierbaum et al.[1] evaluated 9482 patients undergoing major orthopedic surgery. This study demonstrated an increase in overall complication rate in patients requiring transfusion. Complications associated with transfusion in this series included an increase in infection, fluid overload, and a longer hospital stay.

While disease transmission may be the main concern for patients, other complications associated with allogeneic transfusion are more common and perhaps more concerning. The increase in mortality, pneumonia, and postoperative infection related to immunosuppression following transfusion is a major concern. These risks of transfusion need to be understood by the clinician when determining the risk-benefit ratio of transfusion during the postoperative period.

RISK FACTORS FOR TRANSFUSION

Preoperative blood values remain the best way to predict which patients will require perioperative allogeneic transfusion.[28–31]

Checking the hemoglobin and hematocrit before scheduling the indicated procedure identifies those patients at risk for requiring transfusion. In one of Cushner et al.'s original papers, they described factors that influence transfusion rates following TKA.[32] In this study, they found preoperative hematocrit values were the best predictor for transfusion needs. Nuttall et al.[33] as well as Boettnner et al.[28] had similar findings, also noting the importance of preoperative hemoglobin. To minimize postoperative transfusion requirements, the patient's hemoglobin must be maximized during the preoperative period. Patients average a 10% hematocrit loss routinely after total joint arthroplasty. Therefore, those who begin with higher preoperative hemoglobin concentrations are better able to tolerate the loss. Patients who are anemic preoperatively will be anemic during the postoperative period and may require transfusion. Guerin et al.[34] performed a prospective review of 162 consecutive hip and knee arthroplasties. In this series, patients with preoperative hemoglobin levels less than 13 g/dl were four times more likely to receive a transfusion than patients with preoperative hemoglobin levels greater than 15 g/dl.

Nuttall et al.[33] evaluated 299 patients who underwent primary or revision THA in an attempt to predict the risk factors for allogeneic transfusion. In this study, risk factors for transfusion included preoperative hemoglobin, weight, age, anticipated blood loss, and aspirin use. Interestingly, they noted that predonated blood was often not transfused, leading to blood wastage and an increase in cost. Nuttall and colleagues[33] concluded that identifying patients who were unlikely to require transfusion could avoid the unnecessary autologous predonation. Similar results were recently published by Boettner et al.[28] In their study of 283 patients undergoing THA, not only was preoperative autologous donation (PAD) not beneficial in nonanemic patients, but PAD increased the overall transfusion rate, as our practice has demonstrated previously.

The preoperative hemoglobin concentrate has been shown to be the best predictor for postoperative transfusion in several other studies as well. Cabibbo et al.[35] recently reviewed their autologous blood donation program in 1198 orthopaedic patients over the past 10 years. In this series, a preoperative hemoglobin level greater than 14 g/dl was a strong predictor for not requiring postoperative transfusion. Sculco and Gallina[36] evaluated 1405 patients who underwent total joint arthroplasty. Again, preoperative hemoglobin level was inversely related to the frequency of perioperative allogeneic transfusions. In a large multicenter study, Bierbaum et al.[1] evaluated 9482 patients undergoing major orthopaedic surgery. An increased transfusion rate for patients with a preoperative hemoglobin value of less than 13 g/dl was demonstrated. These studies suggest that the patient's hemoglobin should be checked and optimized prior to surgery to minimize postoperative transfusion and complication rates. In our practice, we feel that preoperative optimization of the patient's hemoglobin/hematocrit is the most valuable step in reducing perioperative transfusion rates.

PREOPERATIVE BLOOD MANAGEMENT

Preoperative Autologous Donations

In the late 1980s, the standard of care for a patient undergoing TKA was the preoperative donation of autologous blood. Although commonplace in the United States, PAD is uncommon in other areas of the world. PAD has several limitations. As discussed previously, patients who are most anemic in the preoperative period are at greatest risk for postoperative transfusion. These same patients are often excluded from PAD due to the preoperative anemia. This alone inhibits the ability of a PAD program to helping those patients with the greatest need. In addition, PAD may actually increase the risk of transfusion in the remaining patients by reducing their preoperative hemoglobin level, making a previously low-risk patient now at higher risk for transfusion.[32,33,37] The assumption cannot be made that, after donating blood, the patients return to their predonation status. Several studies have shown that PAD will lower the patient's preoperative blood levels.[28,38–40] The patient donates the blood, does not return to baseline, and arrives for the surgery in an anemic state. The patient is now more at risk for allogeneic transfusion because of the autologous donation.

In our experience, too many patients donated blood too close in time to the scheduled surgery to recover the blood lost with PAD. In addition, a 1- to 2-unit PAD program does not cause a significant erythropoietic response. Because no erythropoietic response occurs, patients do not return to their baseline level. This is demonstrated by the literature. For example, Hatzidakis and coworkers[41] performed a retrospective analysis of 489 consecutive patients undergoing total joint arthroplasty. A decrease in hemoglobin concentration from the time of the donation to the time of surgery was reported; the average decrease was 1.22 g/dl. The authors did not recommend PAD for patients with predonation status greater than 13 g/dl. We evaluated our PAD program previously with regard to preoperative hemoglobin levels. Between 1993 and 1995, 2 units of PAD were obtained on average compared with 1 unit of PAD obtained in the years between 1995 and 1997. Our studies showed a 3% decrease in hematocrit values for every unit donated before surgery.[42] When 1 unit was donated, a 3% decrease in hematocrit was noted before surgery. When 2 units were donated, a 6% decrease from baseline was noted; 2 units of PAD resulted in more anemia before the surgical procedure.[39]

Our practice tried to address the issue of wastage with automatic infusion of the autologous blood. We reviewed our results of a 1-unit PAD program with automatic infusion of the donated blood. All patients were given their PAD immediately after surgery, resulting in 0% wastage. No numerical transfusion triggers were utilized and subsequent allogeneic transfusion was based on symptoms. Despite ordering the PAD unit 1 month before surgery, significant preoperative anemia was noted. In this retrospective review of 148 patients undergoing unilateral TKA, a 1.3-g/dl decrease in hemoglobin was noted between predonation and presurgical testing.[43] We refer to this occurrence as "orthopaedic-induced anemia." Whereas only 26.2% of patients were in the high-transfusion-risk group (hemoglobin >10 g/dl and ≤13 g/dl) before surgery, 55.7% of patients were in this high-risk category after PAD. The patients did not recover from the autologous donations that occurred 4 weeks before surgery. A mean hemoglobin level of 14.0 g/dl was seen before donation, whereas the mean preoperative hemoglobin level decreased to 12.6 g/dl. As documented by others, the use of PAD resulted in anemia, and the patients did not return to the predonation hemoglobin and hematocrit values. Although the allogeneic infusion rate was low in this series, we believe this reflects our lower trigger point for transfusion in the immediate postoperative period. Had historical transfusion triggers been followed (hemoglobin concentration < 10 g/dl), a transfusion rate of 30% would have been found. Fifty percent of our patients were discharged with hemoglobin concentrations less than 9 g/dl.

The low allogeneic transfusion rate should not be misconstrued as efficacy of a 1-unit PAD program, but rather a change in our transfusion practice. PAD programs are limited by significant wastage if automatic transfusion is not followed. In a review of 1198 patients enrolled in an autologous blood donation program, Cabibbo et al.[35] demonstrated a high degree of autologous blood wastage in patients with an optimized preoperative hemoglobin. In this series, a preoperative hemoglobin level greater than 14 g/dl was a strong predictor for not requiring postoperative transfusion. In this subgroup of patients, autologous blood wastage was over 90%. Even in the subgroup of patients with preoperative hemoglobin levels between 13 and 14 g/dl, autologous blood wastage was still over 50%. Even in a recent study that concluded autologous blood donation was a cost-effective measure in reducing allogeneic transfusion rates following arthroplasty, Green et al.[44] demonstrated overall autologous blood wastage of 38% in 356 patients. When looking at TKA alone, the autologous blood wastage was 51%. These findings are similar to those of Bierbaum et al.[1] In their large prospective series including 9482 patients, the autologous blood wastage was 45%. Our institution has abandoned the aforementioned protocol based on the apparent lack of efficacy. In addition, this type of protocol places patients at an additional risk. A protocol with a 100% autologous rate exposes patients to the added risk of donation error. Goldman et al. reviewed autologous error rates in Canada and found an error rate of 6 in 149.[45] The majority of these errors were related to labeling error (48%) or error in component preparation (25%). One patient received the wrong unit of donated blood, which is not an uncommon occurrence. According to the College of American Pathologists,[46] 0.9% of the 3852 institutions studied had at least 1 unit of PAD given to the wrong patient.

Cost is the final issue of PAD, for this is not an inexpensive process. The costs of a PAD program are related to procurement and the cost connected with giving the blood. Billote et al.[38] evaluated PAD in patients who were receiving THA and found no benefit in PAD for nonanemic patients undergoing primary hip replacement. Each patient donated 2 units of autologous blood, with an additional cost of $758 per patient despite frequent blood wastage. Etchason et al.[42] studied the cost of the PAD program and concluded that increased protection afforded by autologous blood is limited and may not justify the increased cost. However, a more recent study comparing the cost of erythropoietin versus autologous and allogenic blood donation in total joint arthroplasty showed that autologous blood donation might be cost effective.[44] In 356 unilateral total joint arthroplasties performed during an 11-month period, a combination of autologous blood donation and allogeneic blood was the least costly approach at $856 and $892 per patient for THA and TKA, respectively. The most costly strategy was allogeneic blood only at $1769 and $1352 per THA and TKA patient, respectively.

Use of Erythropoietins

The importance of preoperative hemoglobin concentrations was discussed earlier. The surgeon is often limited in his or her ability to maximize the patient's predonation hemoglobin values. In the past, we participated in a PAD program. Unhappy with the anemia caused by donations, we put our patients on a new protocol. We began incorporating a patient-specific protocol to utilize epoetin alfa (EPO) (Procrit; Ortho Biotech, PA) into our busy knee practice.[39] We obtain a preoperative hemoglobin and hematocrit prior to surgical booking. Patients with a hemoglobin level greater than 10 and less than 13 g/dl are indicated to receive EPO injections prior to surgery. Patients receive 40,000 units at 3 weeks, 2 weeks, and 1 week prior to surgery, with an average rise in hemoglobin of 1.5 g.[39] We compared 50 patients who received EPO injections with 50 patients participating in the autologous program with automatic reinfusion.[43] The patients receiving EPO had higher blood parameters preoperatively, postoperatively, and on discharge than the patients who participated in the autologous program. Additionally, our overall cost was reduced because the autologous program was used in 25% of the patients with

EPO compared with 100% in previous protocols. Due to the success of this protocol, our indications have expanded. We now employ the same protocol for all arthroplasty patients, including those undergoing PKA, unilateral arthroplasty, bilateral arthroplasty, revision arthroplasty, and two-stage revisions for infections.

The success of this protocol is best demonstrated with discussion of our more complicated cases. By utilizing EPO between stages during the two-stage treatment of an infected total joint arthroplasty, our allogeneic transfusion rates were decreased from a high of 88% to 33%.[47] On evaluation of blood loss and transfusion rates following revision TKA, we found that 75% of female patients scheduled for revision were in the high-risk group (hemoglobin > 10 and <13 g/dl).[48] In our practice, approximately 25–30% of patients fall into the high-risk group and require EPO injections. This means that 75% required no preoperative intervention. This saves our office the time and inconvenience of routinely scheduling autologous blood donations for all patients, for many of whom it would be unnecessary. Treating 25% of patients with EPO injections is significantly less costly than using an autologous donation program for 100% of the patients, especially in light of potential risks with an automatic reinfusion protocol. A similar protocol was recently studied by Moonen et al.[49] and compared to re-transfusion of autologous shed blood. All patients in this study had a preoperative hemoglobin level between 10 and 13 g/dl. In 100 arthroplasty patients randomized to preoperative erythropoietin injection or re-transfusion of autologous shed blood, the allogeneic transfusion rate for the group receiving preoperative injections of erythropoietin was 4% compared to 28% for the group with a reinfusion drain. A second recent study compared the use of erythropoietin to a PAD program.[50] In this series, 121 arthroplasty patients with a preoperative hemoglobin between 11 and 14 g/dl either received weekly EPO injections or underwent PAD. The EPO group demonstrated higher hemoglobin levels, lower transfusion rates, and a significant increase in postoperative vigor.[50]

Insall-Scott Institute Protocol

We check hemoglobin values before surgery and identify patients at increased risk; approximately 25% of patients receive the EPO injections (**Fig. 30–1**). The other patients, with a preoperative hemoglobin greater than 13 g/dl, are scheduled for surgery without any PAD or recombinant human EPO prescriptions. The patients with a hemoglobin between 10 and 13 g/dl receive their EPO injections before surgery from our office. Patients with a hemoglobin less than 10 g/dl should be referred to a hematologist for thorough evaluation. This approach maximizes the hemoglobin and hematocrit levels for the high-risk patients and saves cost by allowing low-risk patients to proceed without intervention.

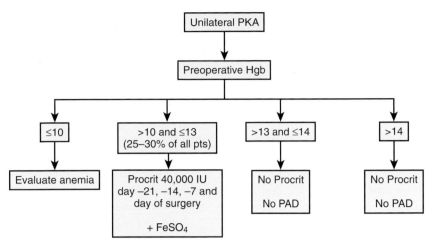

Figure 30-1 The Insall-Scott Kelly Institute protocol for preoperative risk stratification and preoperative hemoglobin (Hgb) optimization.

INTRAOPERATIVE BLOOD MANAGEMENT

Several options exist for intraoperative blood management of the arthroplasty patient. The preoperative measures work by attempting to maximize the ability of patients to tolerate the intraoperative blood loss. To avoid transfusions, the amount of intraoperative blood loss must also be addressed. In this section, hypotensive anesthesia, blood salvage, hemodilution, topical hemostatic agents, and specialized cautery are reviewed.

Acute Normovolemic Hemodilution

Acute normovolemic hemodilution involves simultaneous removal of whole blood from a patient immediately before surgery and replacement with acellular fluids (crystalloid or colloid) to maintain normal blood volume. This technique is recommended when the potential for blood loss may exceed 20% in patients with hemoglobin greater than 10 g/dl. It has a cost and preoperative time commitment similar to PAD, with the possibility of clerical error or bacterial contamination. It is often impractical in most total joint programs because of the relatively short duration of the procedure and lesser blood loss.[51] Acute normovolemic hemodilution is not necessary when blood loss is expected to be less than 500–1000 ml and therefore has little role in PKA.

Intraoperative Blood Salvage

Blood salvage requires a return of the patient's autologous blood loss during surgery. Often the indicated TKA is performed under tourniquet control. Blood salvage devices are therefore used during the postoperative period as a reinfusion drain, when most of the blood loss occurs. The use of reinfusion drains is discussed in depth in the section on postoperative blood loss management. Intraoperative blood salvage has more utility in total and revision hip arthroplasty or in patients undergoing knee arthroplasty with a contraindication to the use of a tourniquet. Intraoperative blood salvage likely plays little role in partial knee replacement.

Hypotensive Anesthesia

Hypotensive anesthesia is a technique for reducing intraoperative blood loss by significantly lowering the mean arterial pressure during surgery. Hypotensive anesthesia may reduce intraoperative blood loss, but it depends on the relative decrease in pressure and the type of anesthesia.[52–54] The reduction in blood loss does not seem to be related to cardiac output.[55] Hypotensive anesthesia is associated with tissue hypoperfusion, and complications can occur, including death. Patients with underlying cardiac, renal, cerebral, or peripheral vessel disease are at increased risk. Two recent studies have shown hypotensive anesthesia during total joint arthroplasty to be safe in patients with aortic stenosis and chronic renal dysfunction, but these series are severely limited by the number of patients evaluated (22 and 54 patients, respectively).[54,56] The possibility of increased deep vein thrombosis events also has been raised. During PKA, the reduced amount of expected blood loss and the use of an intraoperative tourniquet reduces the benefit of hypotensive anesthesia. Our practice currently feels the risks outweigh the benefits in PKA.

Tissue Hemostasis

A more direct method to reduce intraoperative blood loss is obtained through improved tissue hemostasis within the operative field. Topically or locally active agents, including epinephrine, thrombin, collagen, and fibrin glues, have been used. These agents are efficacious in reducing postoperative blood loss and perioperative exposure to allogeneic blood transfusions.

At our institution, we advocate the use of a 30-ml lidocaine-with-epinephrine injection along the arthrotomy site prior to the arthrotomy. For a medial unicompartmental arthroplasty, a small midvastus split (1 cm) is performed. For patellofemoral or bicompartmental arthroplasty, a smaller quad-sparing incision in conjunction with the lidocaine-with-epinephrine injection is performed. This is based on our experience with TKA. When both the minimally invasive incision and the epinephrine injections were used, a decrease in blood loss was noted. In our series of 236 patients, the preoperative-to-postoperative drop in hemoglobin averaged 2.05 g/dl in the study group versus 3.37 g/dl in the control group ($p < .01$).[57]

Another option is fibrin tissue adhesives. The fibrin tissue adhesive is sprayed on the internal aspects of the operating field before skin closure. In addition to the direct mechanism of action, the fibrin sealants contain various amounts of antifibrinolytics, increasing their efficacy.[58] In several randomized controlled trials, fibrin sealants reduced the rate of exposure to allogeneic red blood cell transfusions by approximately 54%.[59] The use of fibrin tissue adhesive significantly reduced mean postoperative blood loss from 800 to 360 ml in a study of 58 patients undergoing joint surgery.[58] Molloy et al. compared three groups in a randomized, controlled trial of 150 patients undergoing TKA.[60] One group received a topical fibrin spray applied intraoperatively. One group received a tranexamic acid (TXA) bolus. The last group was the control. Both TXA and the topical fibrin spray were shown to be effective in decreasing blood loss compared to the control. There was no difference seen in the groups receiving TXA versus the fibrin spray. Everts et al. looked at utilizing an autologous platelet gel and fibrin sealant compared to a control group in 165 unilateral TKAs.[61,62] The hemoglobin following discharge was 11.3 g/dl for the platelet gel and fibrin sealant group versus 8.9 g/dl for the control group. They demonstrated a decrease in the rate of allogeneic transfusion, fewer wound complications, and a 1.4-day decrease in length of hospital stay with use of the platelet gel and fibrin sealant. Carless et al. published a meta-analysis looking at the benefit of fibrin sealant in minimizing perioperative allogeneic transfusion.[59] Although the analysis demonstrated an absolute risk reduction of 19%, conclusions were limited as the trials included were small, uncontrolled, and unblinded. Gardner et al. looked at platelet gels.[63] In a retrospective review of 98 TKAs, they found less narcotic use, better range of motion, and a shortened hospital stay with use of the platelet gel versus control. The decrease in hemoglobin was 2.7 g/dl with the platelet gel versus 3.2 g/dl in the control group.

Another option is the use of specialized cautery units that enhance operative hemostasis. An example of such technology includes the Aquamantys system (Salient Surgical Technologies, Portsmouth, NH), which improves hemostasis via collagen shrinking at cooler temperatures over broader fields and with less tissue destruction than standard electrocautery devices. Using bipolar radiofrequency energy combined with saline, high-risk areas for bleeding can be coagulated to obtain hemostasis with less tissue damage. These high-risk areas include exposed surfaces of bone, the posterolateral corner and posterior capsule, branches of the geniculate artery, and the synovium in the suprapatellar pouch. Rosenberg reviewed the orthopaedic literature and recommended bipolar sealing technology highly to decrease postoperative blood complications, pain, and swelling while possibly improving intraoperative visualization.[64] Marulanda et al. compared the use of bipolar sealing technology with conventional electrocautery in a randomized, prospective study of 50 consecutive patients undergoing primary unilateral TKA.[65] The authors report that patients in the bipolar sealing group experienced a significant reduction in mean total blood loss (296.0 vs. 424.5 ml; $p = .02$) and mean postoperative drainage (203.8 vs. 312.5 ml; $p = .05$) versus the control group. Isabell and Weeden recently reported on the results of a retrospective, controlled cohort study of 100 patients undergoing primary minimally invasive unilateral TKA, comparing the use of conventional electrocautery with bipolar sealing technology.[66] Patients in the bipolar sealing group had a significantly lower mean decline in hemoglobin compared with the control group (3.3 ± 1.1 vs. 3.9 ± 1.2 g/dl; $p = .0085$). The authors reported that the prevalence of autologous transfusion was significantly lower (16% vs. 44%; $p < .001$) for the bipolar sealing group compared with the control group. The prevalence of allogeneic transfusion was also reported to be significantly lower for the bipolar sealing group compared with the control group (8% vs. 22%; $p < .001$). Pierson et al. conducted a prospective, randomized, controlled study designed to evaluate the efficacy of a saline-coupled bipolar sealing device versus conventional therapy in patients undergoing unilateral TKA.[67] Ninety patients were randomized during the study, with the control and treatment groups each consisting of 45 patients. Preoperative hemoglobin levels were similar in both groups. The authors reported that the mean decline in hemoglobin was significantly lower for the bipolar sealing group compared with the control group (3.3 ± 1.0 vs. 3.8 ± 1.5 g/dl; $p = .01$). Further studies are needed to predict the device's effect on decreasing transfusion rates and maximizing postoperative blood values. The device costs approximately $500 per use; a cost-benefit analysis needs to be done to determine whether the increased expense is worthwhile for PKA. We currently employ the use of bipolar cautery and fibrin sprays in PKA due to our anecdotal experience of improved wound appearance and lower incidence of significant hemarthrosis.

Pharmacologic Strategies

Pharmacologic strategies to decrease transfusion requirements in patients undergoing surgery have been studied extensively.[51,68] One such drug class is the antifibrinolytics. Fibrinolysis is stimulated by surgical trauma and further augmented by the use of a tourniquet. Antifibrinolytics act to increase hemostasis within a surgical site by enhancing the clotting mechanism. A Cochrane review was performed to evaluate the use of antifibrinolytics to minimize perioperative blood transfusion.[69] Despite notable heterogeneity in the various trials, aprotinin seems to reduce the need for red blood cell transfusion and the need for reoperation because of bleeding. Mostly in cardiac surgery, aprotinin was found to reduce the rate of allogeneic blood transfusions by 30%. Similar trends in efficacy were seen with TXA and aminocaproic acid. Trials directly comparing TXA with aprotinin have been done, and no significant difference has been reported, though a trend toward an increased risk of transfusion with TXA over aprotinin was seen (relative risk increase of 21%).[70] However, aprotinin was withdrawn from the market in May 2008 due to concerns of complications and even death. It is now used restrictedly for research only.

Tranexamic Acid

Tranexamic acid inhibits fibrinolysis by blocking the lysine-bonding sites of plasminogen to fibrin. Numerous studies have documented the efficacy of TXA in reducing postoperative blood loss and transfusion requirements of TKA[70–76] and THA[1,77]; blood loss reductions of 25–50% have been noted.[70–76,78,79] In direct comparison studies, TXA has proved more efficacious than acute normovolemic hemodilution in patients undergoing TKA.[80,81] Optimal timing of administration and dosing are not yet defined. Several clinical studies have shown the efficacy of TXA boluses when given before surgery[74,78] at deflation of the tourniquet,[70,71,73] and for various times after surgery at variable doses.[9,81] Most frequently, dosing is 10–20 mg/kg. In our institution, we have had success with 10 mg/kg before surgery and at the time of the tourniquet deflation.

Some more recent studies of TXA are available. Rajesparan et al. looked at a standard bolus of 1 g of TXA in THA patients.[82] The bolus was given at anesthesia induction. With this protocol the TXA group demonstrated a significant decrease in early postoperative blood loss, total blood loss, and transfusion rate. Importantly, no increase in deep vein thrombosis was noted in the group receiving TXA.[82] Johansson et al. did a randomized, double-blind study in 100 THA patients using a 15-mg/kg dose of TXA.[83] Again, less bleeding was noted in the TXA group with no increase in venous thromboembolic events. Similar observations have been made in TKA patients. Camarasa et al. performed a double-blind, randomized study with 120 patients receiving TXA during TKA.[84] The transfusion rate was 7.5% in the study group compared to 38.3% in those not receiving TXA. The hemoglobin drop seen at the time of discharge was 2.5 g/dl in the study group compared to 3.4 g/dl in the control group. Kagoma et al. performed a meta-analysis of the 29 available prospective studies in orthopaedic surgery.[85] They concluded that patients receiving TXA demonstrate reduced transfusion need, reduced blood loss, and no increased incidence in DVT.[85]

Anaphylaxis has been noted to occur if the patient is given numerous doses of TXA. Caution should be used if the patient undergoes a procedure involving an infected TKA, where exposure can occur on two occasions within a 6- to 8-week period. By 6 months, the incidence of anaphylaxis decreases, but caution is still advised. Although the use of antifibrinolytics can reduce intraoperative blood loss, concerns about safety and cost remain. Further evaluation needs to be performed before their use can be routinely recommended. Their role now remains in the high-risk patient with significant concern for blood loss. Therefore, the role of antifibrinolytics in PKA is likely limited.

POSTOPERATIVE MANAGEMENT

Drain Usage

Drain usage has received little attention in the PKA literature. Confalonieri et al. have recently studied the necessity of closed-suction drainage following unicompartmental knee replacement.[86] In their prospective, randomized trial, 78 patients were divided into two groups based on the use of a postoperative drain. This series failed to show a clinical benefit of postoperative drain usage with regard to pain, wound healing, range of motion, or length of hospital stay. Despite limited numbers, this is the only available series in the literature. Our practice continues to use postoperative drains in our partial knee replacement patients. Anecdotally, we feel we have fewer wound complications with postoperative drainage. This has been supported in the TKA literature. Holt et al.[87] reported that blood loss was equal in patients with or without a postoperative drain. However, in the absence of a drain, the wounds exhibited greater ecchymosis and drainage. Niskanen et al.[88] also showed more wound drainage when a postoperative drain was not used.

Most blood loss in a knee arthroplasty procedure occurs in the postoperative period, and techniques have been developed to salvage this shed blood. Numerous types of drains exist and basically differ on whether the cells are washed or unwashed and whether red cells are used for reinfusion. Faris[31] studied the quality of shed blood and its reinfusion and found that shed blood was well tolerated, although a febrile reaction was noted in 2% of patients receiving the blood. Groh et al.[89] and Majkowski et al.[7] performed retrospective studies demonstrating the efficacy of postoperative drain usage. In a survey of American Association of Hip and Knee Surgeons members,[48] most respondents were found to use drains in the postoperative period; 62% always used a drain compared with 24% who never used a drain. Occasional use of a drain also was reported. The survey found that 47% of respondents used a reinfusion type of drain, which was removed in approximately 24–36 hours. Jones et al.[90] conducted a postoperative review of 43,000 hip replacements and 33,000 knee replacements performed in the United Kingdom. They evaluated the use of autologous salvage drains in hip and knee surgery patients. The authors concluded that reinfusion drains seemed to be a cost-effective means of reducing the requirement of allogeneic blood in hip and knee arthroplasty. In this series, allogeneic transfusion was required in 21% of patients with a reinfusion drain compared to 45.7% of patients with a suction drain. In another series, Grosvenor et al.[91] looked at the efficacy of postoperative blood salvage after hip arthroplasty in patients with and without deposited autologous blood. The results of this study showed that postoperative blood salvage significantly reduced the risk of allogeneic transfusions. The patients who were treated with postoperative blood salvage were approximately 10 times more likely to avoid allogeneic transfusions than patients who had a non-reinfusion drain. In a more recent randomized prospective review, Smith et al. demonstrated the benefit of reinfusion drains in THA.[92] In a series of 158 patients, reinfusion drains demonstrated fewer patients with a postoperative hemoglobin of less than 9 g/dl, a lower transfusions rate, and a slight overall cost savings. Friederichs et al. compared reinfusion drains with preoperative autologous blood donation in 200 consecutive joint arthroplasties.[77] In patients with a preoperative hematocrit of greater than 37%, the use of a reinfusion drain lowered the allogeneic transfusion rate to 1.2%. They concluded that perioperative blood salvage is safe and effective and makes it possible to discontinue the practice of predonating blood in arthroplasty patients with a preoperative hematocrit greater than 37%. This is the practice at our institution because PAD has been abandoned for patients with hemoglobin values greater than 13 g/dl.

If reinfusion is to be utilized, the decision must be made whether to use washed or unwashed cells. For our TKA patients, we switched to the OrthoPAT system (Zimmer Inc, Warsaw, IN) in an attempt to improve the quality of blood returned to the patient. Such a system has the benefits of a washed cell device without the additional costs of a cell-saver type system. We believe that a lower volume of better quality packed red blood cells is advantageous. Several studies have looked at the efficacy of the OrthoPAT system. Clark et al. evaluated the OrthoPAT system in 398 patients.[93] In this series, primary or revision hip arthroplasties with no preoperative autologous blood donation, knee arthroplasties with no preoperative autologous blood donation, and unilateral primary hip arthroplasties were 2.7, 2.3, and 2 times less likely ($p < .05$), respectively, to use allogeneic blood with OrthoPAT. Similarly, Del Trujillo et al. demonstrated a significant reduction in the allogeneic transfusion rate from 48% to 15% in 108 patients undergoing THA with the use of the OrthoPAT system compared to controls.[94]

Mont et al.[95] recommended a new approach, designing a study to evaluate the efficacy of an intraoperative surgeon decision to use a reinfusion drain. In the TKA group, 84% of the patients in the standard group had reinfusion, similar to the 85% in the reinfusion drain group. This demonstrated clearly that the surgeon could not predict intraoperatively whether a patient would require a reinfusion drain. However, in more than 94% of the cases, by 90 minutes postoperatively, a decision could be made as to whether a reinfusion drain was necessary based on early drain collection. This study concluded that a drain could be placed and converted to a reinfusion drain based on early postoperative blood loss. This approach may be reasonable in partial knee replacement patients, where fewer patients will actually benefit from a reinfusion drain.

Most surgeons use a drain after elective TKA. Although this practice can debated based on current literature, the studies about TKA show a significant decrease in the transfusion rates when postoperative salvage devices are used. It is likely that reinfusion drainage is not cost effective in partial knee replacement due to the reduced perioperative blood loss. Moonen et al. studied re-transfusion in 438 arthroplasty patients.[96] They concluded that re-transfusion of filtered shed blood following unicompartmental knee arthroplasty is doubtfully cost efficient due to the minimal bone resection required and the low risk of allogeneic transfusion.

CONCLUSION

The number one factor preventing allogeneic transfusion is the preoperative hemoglobin and hematocrit. To minimize transfusion, the surgeon must take a preemptive role and optimize patients prior to surgery. The practice of autologous blood donations should be questioned. Cushner et al.[43] highlighted orthopaedic surgery–induced anemia and questioned the autologous donation process. A patient-specific approach that identifies at-risk patients is likely most cost effective. Pierson et al.[67] reviewed a patient-specific approach based on the patient's preoperative blood status. Higher preoperative blood status not only reduces the risk of transfusion, but also improves patient outcome. For example, Keating et al.[97] assessed patient vigor after joint arthroplasty. Among the objective criteria studied, there was a significant correlation between vigor and hematocrit value: the higher the postoperative blood levels, the higher the vigor scale.

A multimodal, patient-specific approach is now utilized at our institution. This approach includes the preoperative optimization of hemoglobin levels with EPO in high-risk patients (hemoglobin < 13 g/dl), combined with meticulous intraoperative hemostasis utilizing lidocaine-with-epinephrine injection, special bipolar sealing units, and fibrin sprays. While reinfusion drains are used in our TKA patients, they may not be cost effective in PKA patients, but this is yet to be studied. In the highest risk patients, antifibrinolytics are considered. At our institution, PAD is now reserved for patients undergoing bilateral simultaneous TKA; it is combined with EPO to avoid orthopaedic-induced anemia, and is considered on a case-by-case basis. With this multimodal approach, allogeneic transfusion is minimized, while hemoglobin levels and postoperative vigor are improved, allowing a safe and quick recovery for our arthroplasty patients.

REFERENCES

1. Bierbaum BE, Callaghan JJ, Galante JO, et al. Analysis of blood management in patients having total hip or knee arthroplasty. J Bone Joint Surg [Am] 1999;81:2.

2. Keating EM, Ranawat CS, Cats-Baril W. Assessment of postoperative vigor in patients undergoing elective total joint arthroplasty: a concise patient- and caregiver-based instrument. Orthopedics 1999; 22:s119.

3. Brunson ME, Alexander JW. Mechanisms of transfusion-induced immunosuppression. Transfusion 1990;30:651.

4. Cascinu S, Fedeli A, Del Ferro E, et al. Recombinant human erythropoietin treatment in cisplatin-associated anemia: a randomized double-blind trial with placebo. J Clin Oncol 1994;12:1058.

5. Dodd RY. The risk of transfusion-transmitted infection. N Engl J Med 1992;327:419.

6. Goodnough LT, Skikne B, Brugnara C. Erythropoietin, iron, and erythropoiesis. Blood 2000;96:823.

7. Majkowski RS, Currie IC, Newman JH. Postoperative collection and reinfusion of autologous blood in total knee arthroplasty. Ann R Coll Surg Engl 1991;73:381.

8. Walker R. Transfusion risks. Am J Clin Pathol 1987;88:371.

9. Heck DA, Marmor L, Gibson A, Rougraf BT. Unicompartmental knee arthroplasty: a multicenter investigation with long-term follow-up evaluation. Clin Orthop Relat Res 1993;(286):154-159.

10. Jeer P, Cossey A, Keene G. Haemoglobin levels following unicompartmental knee arthroplasty: influence of transfusion and surgical approach. Knee 2005;12:358-361.

11. Mullaji AB, Sharma A, Marawar S. Unicompartmental knee arthroplasty: functional recovery and radiographic results with a minimally invasive technique. J Arthroplasty 2007;22(4 Suppl 1):7-11.

12. Zohar E, Fredman B, Ellis M, et al. A comparative study of the postoperative allogeneic blood-sparing effect of tranexamic acid versus acute normovolemic hemodilution after total knee replacement. Anesth Analg 1999;89:1382.

13. Alter HJ, Nakatsuji Y, Melpolder J, et al. The incidence of transfusion-associated hepatitis G virus infection and its relation to liver disease. N Engl J Med 1997;336:747.

14. Alter HJ, Purcell RH, Shih JW, et al. Detection of antibody to hepatitis C virus in prospectively followed transfusion recipients with acute and chronic non-A, non-B hepatitis. N Engl J Med 1989;321:1494.

15. Ammann AJ, Cowan MJ, Wara DW, et al. Acquired immunodeficiency in an infant: possible transmission by means of blood products. Lancet 1983;1:956.

16. Kleinman S, Busch MP, Schreiber GB. The incidence/window period model and its use to assess the risk of transfusion-transmitted human immunodeficiency virus and hepatitis C virus infection. Transfus Med Rev 1997;11:155.

17. Lackritz EM, Satten GA, Aberle-Grasse J, et al. Estimated risk of transmission of the human immunodeficiency virus by screened blood in the United States. N Engl J Med 1995;333:1685.

18. Schreiber GB, Busch MP, Kleinman SH, Korelitz JJ. The risk of transfusion-transmitted viral infections. N Engl J Med 1996;334:1685.

19. Stevens CE, Aach RD, Hollinger FB, et al. Hepatitis B virus antibody in blood donors and the occurrence of non-A, non-B hepatitis in transfusion recipients: an analysis of the Transfusion-Transmitted Viruses Study. Ann Intern Med 1984;101:733.

20. Buddeberg F, Schimmer BB, Spahn DR. Transfusion-transmissible infections and transfusion-related immunomodulation. Best Pract Res Clin Anaesthesiol 2008;22:503-517.

21. Biggerstaff BJ, Petersen LR. Estimated risk of West Nile virus transmission through blood transfusion during an epidemic in Queens, New York City. Transfusion 2002;42:1019.

22. Tang R, Chen HH, Wang YL, et al. Risk factors for surgical site infection after elective resection of the colon and rectum: a single-center prospective study of 2,809 consecutive patients. Ann Surg 2001; 234:181-189.

23. Kendall SJ, Weir J, Aspinall R, et al. Erythrocyte transfusion causes immunosuppression after total hip replacement. Clin Orthop Relat Res 2000;(381):145.

24. Pulido L, Ghanem E, Joshi A, et al. Periprosthetic joint infection: the incidence, timing, and predisposing factors. Clin Orthop Relat Res 2008;(466):1710-1715.

25. Shander A, Spence RK, Adams D, et al. Timing and incidence of postoperative infections associated with blood transfusion: analysis of 1,489 orthopedic and cardiac surgery patients. Surg Infect (Larchmt) 2009;10:277-283.

26. Murphy P, Heal JM, Blumberg N. Infection or suspected infection after hip replacement surgery with autologous or homologous blood transfusions. Transfusion 1991;31:212.

27. Pedersen AB, Mehnert F, Overgaard S, Johnsen S. Allogeneic blood transfusion and prognosis following total hip replacement: a population-based follow up study. BMC Musculoskel Disord 2009;10:167-179.

28. Boettner F, Altneu EI, Williams BA, et al. Nonanemic patients do not benefit from autologous blood donation before total hip replacement. Hosp Special Surg J 2010;6:66-70.

29. Canadian Orthopedic Peri-operative Erythropoietin Study Group. Effectiveness of peri-operative recombinant human erythropoietin in elective hip replacement. Lancet 1993;341:1227.

30. De Andrade JR, Jove M, Landon G, et al. Baseline hemoglobin as a predictor of risk of transfusion and response to epoetin alfa in orthopedic surgery patients. Am J Orthop 1996;8:533.

31. Faris PM. Unwashed filtered shed blood collected after knee and hip arthroplasty. J Bone Joint Surg [Am] 1991;73:1169.

32. Cushner FD, Friedman RJ. Blood loss in total knee arthroplasty. Clin Orthop Relat Res 1991;(269):98.

33. Nuttall GA, Santrach PJ, Oliver WC Jr, et al. The predictors of red cell transfusions in total hip arthroplasties. Transfusion 1996; 36:144.

34. Guerin S, Collins C, Kapoor H, et al. Blood transfusion requirement prediction in patients undergoing primary total hip and knee arthroplasty. Transfus Med 2007;17:37-43.

35. Cabibbo S, Garozzo G, Antolino A, et al. Continuous improvement of our autologous blood donation program carried out during 10

years in 1198 orthopaedic patients. Transfus Apher Sci 2009;40 (1):13-17.

36. Sculco TP, Gallina J. Blood management experience: relationship between autologous blood donation and transfusion in orthopedic surgery. Orthopedics 1999;22:s129.

37. Faris PM, Ritter MA, Ables RI; the American Erythropoietin Study Group. The effects of recombinant human erythropoietin on perioperative transfusion requirements in patients having a major orthopaedic operation. J Bone Joint Surg [Am] 1993;78:62.

38. Billote DB, Glisson SN, Green D, Wixson RL. A prospective, randomized study of preoperative autologous donation for hip replacement surgery. J Bone Joint Surg [Am] 2002;84:1299.

39. Cushner FD, Scott WN. Evolution of blood transfusion management for a busy knee practice. Orthopedics 1999;22:s145.

40. Stowell CP, Chandler H, Jove M, et al. An open-label, randomized study to compare the safety and efficacy of peri-operative epoetin alfa with pre-operative autologous blood donation in total joint arthroplasty. Orthopedics 1999;22:s105.

41. Hatzidakis AM, Mendlick RM, McKillip T, et al. Preoperative autologous donation for total joint arthroplasty: an analysis of risk factors for allogeneic transfusion. J Bone Joint Surg [Am] 2000; 82:89.

42. Etchason J, Petz L, Keeler E, et al. The cost effectiveness of preoperative autologous blood donations. N Engl J Med 1995;332:740.

43. Cushner FD, Hawes T, Kessler D, et al. Orthopedic-induced anemia: the fallacy of autologous donation programs. Clin Orthop Relat Res 2005;(431):145-149.

44. Green WS, Toy P, Bozic KJ. Cost minimization analysis of preoperative erythropoietin vs autologous and allogeneic blood donation in total joint arthroplasty. J Arthroplasty 2008;December 2. [Epub ahead of print]

45. Goldman M, Remy-Prince S, Trepanier A, Decary F. Autologous donation error rates in Canada. Transfusion 1997;37:523.

46. Cooper ES, Walker RH, Schmidt PJ, Polesky HF. The 1990 comprehensive blood bank surveys of the College of American Pathologists. Arch Pathol Lab Med 1993;117:125.

47. Pagnano M, Cushner FD, Hansen A, et al. Blood management in two-stage revision knee arthroplasty for deep prosthetic infection. Clin Orthop Relat Res 1999;(367):238.

48. Cushner FD, Scott WN, Scuderi GR, et al. Blood loss and transfusion in bilateral total knee arthroplasty. J Knee Surg 2005;28:102-107.

49. Moonen AF, Thomassen BJ, Knoors NT, et al. Pre-operative injections of epoetin-alpha versus post-operative retransfusion of autologous shed blood in total hip and knee replacement: a prospective randomised clinical trial. J Bone Joint Surg [Br] 2008;90: 1079-1083.

50. Keating EM, Callaghan JJ, Ranawat AS, et al. A randomized, parallel-group, open-label trial of recombinant human erythropoietin vs preoperative autologous donation in primary total joint arthroplasty: effect on postoperative vigor and handgrip strength. J Arthroplasty 2007;22:325-333.

51. Keating EM, Meding JB. Perioperative blood management practices in elective orthopaedic surgery. J Am Acad Orthop Surg 2002;10:393.

52. An HS, Mikhail WE, Jackson WT, et al. Effects of hypotensive anesthesia, nonsteroidal anti-inflammatory drugs, and polymethylmethacrylate on bleeding in total hip arthroplasty patients. J Arthroplasty 1991;6:245.

53. Niemi TT, Pitkanen M, Syrjala M, Rosenberg PH. Comparison of hypotensive epidural anesthesia and spinal anesthesia on blood loss and coagulation during and after total hip arthroplasty. Acta Anesth Scand 2000;44:457.

54. Sharrock NE, Beksac B, Flynn E, et al. Hypotensive epidural anaesthesia in patients with preoperative renal dysfunction undergoing total hip replacement. Br J Anaesth 2006;96:207-212.

55. Sharrock NE, Mineo R, Go G. The effect of cardiac output on intraoperative blood loss during total hip arthroplasty. Reg Anesth 1993;18:24.

56. Ho MC, Beathe JC, Sharrock NE. Hypotensive epidural anesthesia in patients with aortic stenosis undergoing total hip replacement. Reg Anesth Pain Med 2008;33:129-133.

57. Cushner FD, Kim R, Scuderi GR, et al. Use of lidocaine with epinephrine injection to reduce blood loss in minimally invasive total knee arthroplasty. Transfus Alternat Transfus Med 2007;9(Suppl 1):59.

58. Levy O, Martinowitz U, Oran A, et al. The use of fibrin tissue adhesive to reduce blood loss and the need for blood transfusion after total knee arthroplasty: a prospective, randomized, multicenter study. J Bone Joint Surg [Am] 1999;81:1580.

59. Carless PA, Henry DA, Anthony DM. Fibrin sealant use for minimising peri-operative allogeneic blood transfusion. Cochrane Database Syst Rev 2003;(1):CD004171.

60. Molloy DO, Archbold HAP, Ogonda L, et al. Comparison of topical fibrin spray and tranexamic acid on blood loss after total knee replacement: a prospective, randomized controlled trial. J Bone Joint Surg [Br] 2007;89:306-309.

61. Everts P, Devilee R, Mahoney B, et al. Platelet gel and fibrin sealant reduce allogeneic blood transfusions in total knee arthroplasty. Acta Anaesthesiol Scand 2006;50:593-599.

62. Everts P, Devilee R, Oosterbos C, et al. Autologous platelet gel and fibrin sealant enhance the efficacy of total knee arthroplasty: improved range of motion, decreased length of stay, and reduced incidence of arthrofibrosis. Knee Surg Sports Traumatol Arthrosc 2007;15:888-894.

63. Gardner MJ, Demetrakopoulos D, Klepchick PR, et al. The efficacy of autologous gel in pain control and blood loss in total knee arthroplasty: an analysis of the haemoglobin, narcotic requirement and range of motion. Int Orthop 2007;31:309-313.

64. Rosenberg AG. Reducing blood loss in total joint surgery with a saline-coupled bipolar sealing technology. J Arthroplasty 2007;22(4 Suppl 1):82-85.

65. Marulanda GA, Ragland PS, Seyler TM, et al. Reduction in blood loss with use of a bipolar sealer for hemostasis in primary total knee arthroplasty. Surg Technol Int 2005;14:281.

66. Isabell G, Weeden S. Hemodynamic efficacy of a bipolar sealing device in primary total knee arthroplasty [abstract]. In Proceedings of the Annual Meeting of the Texas Orthopaedic Association. Houston, TX: Texas Orthopaedic Association, 2006.

67. Pierson JL, Hellman EJ, Earles DR, et al. Randomized, prospective trial to examine the hemostatic efficacy of a bipolar sealing device in TKA [abstract]. Poster at AAOS, March 2006.

68. Porte RJ, Leebeek FWG. Pharmacological strategies to decrease transfusion requirements in patients undergoing surgery. Drugs 2002;2:2193.

69. Henry DA, Moxey AJ, Carless PA, et al. Anti-fibrinolytic use for minimizing perioperative allogeneic blood transfusion. Cochrane Database Syst Rev 2007;(3):CD001886.

70. Tenholder M, Cushner FD. Intraoperative blood management in joint replacement surgery. Orthopedics 2004;27(6 Suppl):s663.

71. Benoni G, Fredin H. Fibrinolytic inhibition with tranexamic acid reduces blood loss and blood transfusion after knee arthroplasty: a prospective, randomized, double-blind study of 86 patients. J Bone Joint Surg [Br] 1996;78:434.

72. Hiippala S, Strid L, Wennerstrand M. Tranexamic acid (Cyklokapron) reduces perioperative blood loss associated with total knee arthroplasty. Br J Anaesth 1995;74:534.

73. Hiippala ST, Strid LJ, Wennerstrand MI, et al. Tranexamic acid radically decreases blood loss and transfusions associated with total knee arthroplasty. Anesth Analg 1997;84:839.

74. Jansen AJ, Andreica S, Claeys M, et al. Use of tranexamic acid for an effective blood conservation strategy after total knee arthroplasty. Br J Anaesth 1999;83:596.

75. Tanaka N, Sakahashi H, Sato E, et al. Timing of the administration of tranexamic acid for maximum reduction in blood loss in arthroplasty of the knee. J Bone Joint Surg [Br] 2001;83:702.

76. Veien M, Sorensen JV, Madsen F, Juelsgaard P. Tranexamic acid given intraoperatively reduces blood loss after total knee replacement: a randomized, controlled study. Acta Anesth Scand 2002;46:1206.

77. Friederichs MG, Mariani EM, Bourne MH. Perioperative blood salvage as an alternative to predonating blood for primary total knee and hip arthroplasty. J Arthroplasty 2002;17:298.

78. Benoni G, Fredin H, Knebel R, Nilsson P. Blood conservation with tranexamic acid in total hip arthroplasty: a randomized, double-blind study in 40 primary operations. Acta Orthop 2001;72:442.

79. Ekback G, Axelsson K, Ryttberg L, et al. Tranexamic acid reduces blood loss in total hip replacement surgery. Anesth Analg 2000;91:1124.

80. Zohar E, Fredman B, Ellis M, et al. A comparative study of the postoperative allogeneic blood-sparing effect of tranexamic acid versus acute normovolemic hemodilution after total knee replacement. Anesth Analg 1999;89:1382.

81. Zohar E, Fredman B, Ellis MH, et al. A comparative study of the postoperative allogeneic blood-sparing effects of tranexamic acid and of desmopressin after total knee replacement. Transfusion 2001;41:1285.

82. Rajesparan K, Biant LC, Ahmed M, et al. The effect of an intravenous bolus of transexamic acid on blood loss in total hip replacement. J Bone Joint Surg [Br] 2009;91:776-783.

83. Johansson T, Pettersson LG, Lisander B. Tranexamic acid in total hip arthroplasty saves blood and money: a randomized, double-blind study in 100 patients. Acta Orthop 2005;76:314-319.

84. Camarasa MA, Ollé G, Serr-Prat M, et al. Efficacy of aminocaproic, tranexamic acids in the control of bleeding during total knee replacement: a randomized clinical trial. Br J Anaesth 2006;96:576-582.

85. Kagoma YK, Crowther MA, Douketis J, et al. Use of antifibrinolytic therapy to reduce transfusion in patients undergoing orthopedic surgery: a systematic review of randomized trials. Thromb Res 2009;123:687-696.

86. Confalonieri N, Manzotti A, Pullen C. Is closed-suction drain necessary in unicompartmental knee replacement? A prospective randomized study. Knee 2004;11:399-402.

87. Holt BT, Parks NL, Engh GA, Lawrence JM. Comparison of closed-suction drainage and no drainage after primary total knee arthroplasty. Orthopedics 1997;20:1121.

88. Niskanen RO, Korkala OL, Haapala J, et al. Drainage is of no use in primary uncomplicated cemented hip and knee arthroplasty for osteoarthritis: a prospective randomized study. J Arthroplasty 2000;15:567.

89. Groh GI, Buchert PK, Allen WC. A comparison of transfusion requirements after total knee arthroplasty using the Solcotrans Autotransfusion System. J Arthroplasty 1990;3:281.

90. Jones HW, Savage L, White C, et al. Postoperative autologous blood salvage drains—are they useful in primary uncemented hip and knee arthroplasty? A prospective study of 186 cases. Acta Orthop Belg 2004;70:466.

91. Grosvenor D, Goyal V, Goodman S. Efficacy of postoperative blood salvage following total hip arthroplasty in patients with and without deposited autologous units. J Bone Joint Surg [Am] 2000;82:951.

92. Sharrock NE, Mineo R, Urquhart B, Salvati EA. The effect of two levels of hypotension on intraoperative blood loss during total hip arthroplasty performed under lumbar epidural anesthesia. Analg Anesth 1993;76:580.

93. Clark CR, Sprat KF, Blondin M, et al. Perioperative autotransfusion in total hip and knee arthroplasty. J Arthroplasty 2006;21:23-35.

94. Del Trujillo MM, Carrero A, Munoz M. The utility of the perioperative autologous transfusion system OrthoPAT in total hip replacement surgery: a prospective study. Arch Orthop Trauma Surg 2008;128:1031-1038.

95. Mont MA, Low K, LaPorte DM, et al. Reinfusion drains after primary total hip and total knee arthroplasty. J South Orthop Assoc 2000;9:193.

96. Moonen AF, Thomassen BJ, van Os JJ, et al. Retransfusion of filtered shed blood in everyday orthopaedic practice. Transfus Med 2008;18:355-359.

97. Keating EM, Ritter MA. Transfusion options in total joint arthroplasty. J Arthroplasty 2002;17:125.

CHAPTER 31
Bilateral Unicompartmental Knee Arthroplasty

Erik P. Severson and Rafael J. Sierra

KEY POINTS

- Bilateral unicompartmental arthroplasty is a safe option for select patients with bilateral unicompartmental arthritis.
- A higher risk of DVT or PE must be discussed with patients.
- Those with previous history of DVT or PE and with cardiac history are not good candidates for the operation.

INTRODUCTION

Knee arthroplasty procedures have become a reliable, long-term solution for disabling knee pain, and have begun to be used in an increasingly younger patient population. The number of unicompartmental arthroplasties of the knee has increased at a rate of 32.5% annually over the last few years.[1,2] This procedure has emerged as an attractive alternative to total knee arthroplasty for many arthroplasty surgeons, when used in the proper surgical setting, as it spares more bone, is associated with better knee kinematics, provides a more rapid postoperative recovery, and potentially allows for an easier revision if needed.[3–7] Bilateral unicompartmental arthroplasty is an alternative in the patient with symptomatic bilateral knee arthritis isolated to one compartment of the tibiofemoral articulation (**Figs. 31–1 and 31–2**). This chapter discusses the indications and outcomes of bilateral unicompartmental arthroplasty as well as the surrounding controversies limiting its widespread use, followed by the authors' preferred method of treatment.

RATIONALE

There is a paucity of data on bilateral unicompartmental arthroplasties; therefore, the data on bilateral total knee arthroplasties (TKAs) could be extrapolated to the unicompartmental discussion, although clearly the morbidity and risks associated with TKA are quite different from those of unicompartmental arthroplasty. There are a myriad of studies investigating the safety of bilateral TKA. Although some authors have maintained that patient selection is quintessential to avoiding a higher complication rate, many other authors have reported an increased risk of cardiac and pulmonary complications as well as an increased postoperative 30-day mortality in the simultaneous bilateral total knee setting.[8–13] In a recent meta-analysis looking at the safety of bilateral TKA, the prevalences of pulmonary embolism (PE), cardiac complications, and mortality were higher after simultaneous bilateral total knee replacement.[11] In light of these known complications, some authors have stressed the importance of mitigating perioperative risk by screening for preexisting cardiac or pulmonary disease prior to proceeding with bilateral TKA.[9,12–17]

Although there are increased risks of complications associated with simultaneous bilateral TKA, there are certain advantages to undergoing both knee replacements under one anesthetic. Obviously, there is only one anesthetic risk and one hospital stay, which translate into a shorter cumulative stay and less overall cost. In addition, the patient undergoes symmetric rehabilitation, which may explain the better functional outcomes reported with simultaneous bilateral TKAs.[11–13,18–22] Zeni et al.[22] evaluated the functional outcomes of patients undergoing simultaneous bilateral TKA compared to those undergoing unilateral TKA and a healthy control group. These patients were matched for sex, age, and body mass index, and were observed prospectively for 2 years. Subjects in both surgical groups showed significant improvement in knee outcome scores, Short Form-36 physical component scores, timed up-and-go test, and stair-climbing tasks. No significant differences were seen in final outcomes between surgical groups. The authors of that study concluded that subjects medically appropriate for bilateral TKA should be given this option.

The cost-effectiveness of bilateral unicompartmental arthroplasty has not been reported in the literature, but it has been reported for bilateral TKA as well as unicompartmental arthroplasty on a single side.[23] Reuben et al.[21] used a hospital-based computer system to compare the inpatient costs of performing bilateral simultaneous sequential, staged, and unilateral TKAs. Bilateral simultaneous sequential TKA was 36% less costly than bilateral staged TKA. Prosthetic costs

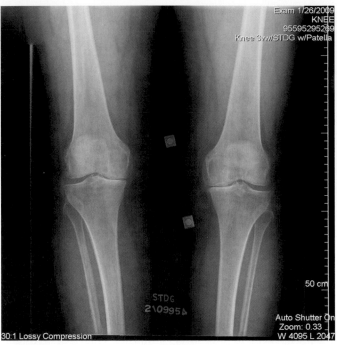

Figure 31-1 Preoperative radiograph of a patient with bilateral unicompartmental arthritis.

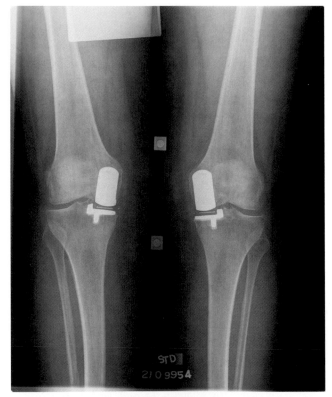

Figure 31-2 Postoperative radiograph of the same patient at most recent follow-up.

range between 28% and 43% of the total costs of hospitalization. There was a significant correlation between hospital length of stay, morbidity, and total costs, but no correlation with patient age and gender except in the unilateral knee surgery patients. The authors concluded that bilateral simultaneous sequential TKA can save more than $10,000 for each total knee replacement patient.[21] With the idea of looking specifically at overall cost of bilateral unicompartmental arthroplasties at the Mayo Clinic, we reviewed 20 patients who underwent bilateral unicompartmental arthroplasty on the same day as well as in a staged fashion and compared the two groups. The increase in overall costs for the bilateral unicompartmental arthroplasty performed in a staged fashion was 37% when compared to simultaneous bilateral UKA. For the staged procedure, the cumulative operating room costs increased 20%, hospital and nursing costs 28%, and the surgeon reimbursement was increased 25% when compared to the simultaneous bilateral knee group. However, the hospital net revenue was 39% more for the staged when compared to the simultaneous procedure.

OUTCOMES

Very little has been published reporting the outcome of patients who have undergone bilateral unicompartmental arthroplasties. The only available study in the published literature to date compares the immediate postoperative complications of single- versus two-stage bilateral unicompartmental knee replacement.[24] Chan et al. provided this retrospective look at the major complications occurring after simultaneous and staged bilateral unicompartmental arthroplasties by comparing 159 patients (318 knees) treated with one-stage and 80 patients (160 knees) treated with two-stage arthroplasty. The bilateral unicompartmental groups were comparable in age and in ASA grade. The major complications they tracked were death, PE, proximal deep vein thrombosis (DVT), and adverse cardiac events within 30 days of surgery. Major complications were seen in 13 patients (8.2%) with one-stage operations but none were encountered in the two-stage group, which reveals a statistically significant difference. The authors of that study concluded that the significantly higher risk of major complications associated with one-stage bilateral unicompartmental knee replacement should make surgeons take caution prior to undertaking such a procedure.

There were several limitations to this study that should be pointed out to the reader. No chemoprophylaxis was used in their protocol, and venous thromboembolism accounted for the majority of the complications. Ten different surgeons performed the cases, and the anesthetic protocol used was local wound infiltration in combination with general anesthesia.[24] These differences may not allow for the data to be translated to North America as chemoprophylaxis is routinely used and spinal anesthesia is typically used for anesthesia. At the closed meeting of the Knee Society in 2009, Berend et al. presented a large series of patients undergoing bilateral unicompartmental knee arthroplasty. They compared 141 patients (282 knees) treated with staged partial knee arthroplasty to 35 patients (70 knees) treated with simultaneous partial knee arthroplasty to evaluate perioperative complications and short-term functional outcomes. Patients in the study who underwent simultaneous unicompartmental knee arthroplasty had a significantly shorter cumulative operative time (109 vs. 122 minutes), a shorter cumulative length of stay in the hospital (1.7 vs. 2.5 days), higher Knee Society Functional scores at most recent follow-up (87.9 vs. 72.9), and higher Lower Extremity Activity Scale scores (12.0 vs. 10.2) without a difference in perioperative complications. In the study, the simultaneous cohort was significantly younger and less obese than the staged group, which could account for some of the differences encountered in the study. The lack of difference in perioperative complications is distinctly different from the findings by Chan et al. and is likely due to the disparity in anesthetic protocols and the changes in venous thromboembolism prevention. Berend et al. used a combined spinal and general anesthetic with local wound infiltration, and all of the patients received some form of chemoprophylaxis—either aspirin, low-molecular-weight heparin, or warfarin (Coumadin)—based on preoperative risk stratification.

The Mayo Clinic Joint Registry was searched to analyze for similar data. There were 487 unicompartmental knee arthroplasties performed in 415 patients dating back to January 2003. Seventy-two patients underwent bilateral unicompartmental knee arthroplasty. These 72 patients were divided into three distinct groups:

- Group 1: underwent unicompartmental arthroplasty under one anesthetic and consisted of 29 patients
- Group 2: underwent staged bilateral arthroplasty within 3 months and consisted of 13 patients
- Group 3: underwent staged bilateral arthroplasty after 3 months and consisted of 29 patients

The average age of the study group was 62 years (range, 42–88 years) and there were 39 males and 33 females. Both fixed-bearing and mobile-bearing designs were used. The only significant difference was that the anesthesia and operative times were higher in group 1, as would be expected. In group 1, two patients had major complications. One patient had bilateral atrial thrombi related to postoperative atrial fibrillation and the other patient had a deep infection. There were three complications in group 2: one patient had delayed wound healing, one patient had a deep infection, and one patient had tibial component subsidence. In group 3, three complications were noted. Two patients had delayed wound healing and one patient had tibial component subsidence. Except for the

patient in group 1 with the atrial thrombi, there were no major complications seen that were related to bleeding, cardiac, or thromboembolic disease in any of the three groups.

AUTHORS' PREFERRED METHODS

The medical risks associated with unicompartmental arthroplasty are likely less than for those patients undergoing TKA. The lesser invasiveness of the operation will likely place patients at less risk of developing pulmonary or cardiac complications after surgery. Lombardi et al.[25] have reported the complication rates associated with 1000 unicompartmental arthroplasties, with no patients requiring transfusions or developing cardiac complications, and one patient with a DVT. One could then possibly conclude that the risk of bilateral unicompartmental arthroplasty is likely less than that of bilateral TKA. In light of Chan et al.'s data,[24] however, the higher risk of DVT should be discussed with the patients, and those with a history of previous DVTs or PE are likely not good candidates for undergoing bilateral simultaneous unicompartmental arthroplasty. Patients with severe cardiac comorbidities are probably not good candidates either, and in those cases a staged approach might be a better option.

At our institution, patients undergoing bilateral simultaneous unicompartmental arthroplasties are given a multimodal anesthetic protocol.[26] The reader is referred to this reference for a complete description of the technique. The patient is placed supine and the legs are draped freely, or if the choice is bilateral mobile-bearing unicompartmental arthroplasty, then the patient is placed in bilateral stirrup leg holders with the extremities hanging over the distal aspect of the operating room table (**Fig. 31–3**). The table is broken distally to provide positioning for both legs. The surgeon can decide to prep both legs at the time of surgery and perform the arthroplasties in a staggered simultaneous fashion, or both legs can be prepped and draped separately and approached separately. After closure of the first knee, that knee can be extended on a Mayo stand (**Fig. 31–4**). Intraoperatively, our preference is to not elevate the tourniquet on both knees at the same time. The tourniquet is brought up for the first knee, and once the components are cemented, then the incision is made without tourniquet on the second side, and once the tourniquet has been released on the first side, it is elevated on the second side. An alternative to this technique would be to use the tourniquet only for cementing, and therefore knees could potentially be worked on by two teams simultaneously, taking care again not to cement at the same time. We typically use both chemical and mechanical DVT prophylaxis while the patient is in the hospital. Aspirin, 325 mg by mouth twice daily, is used for 6 weeks unless the patient has a medical comorbidity that requires long-term Coumadin. Mechanical prophylaxis is in the form of thromboembolic disease (TED) stockings and sequential

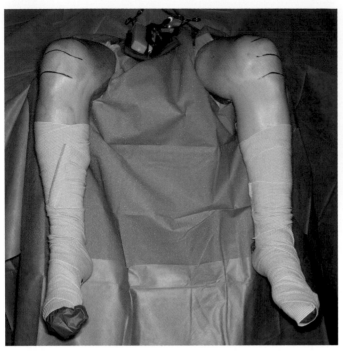

Figure 31-3 Intraoperative photograph of the bilateral knee setup.

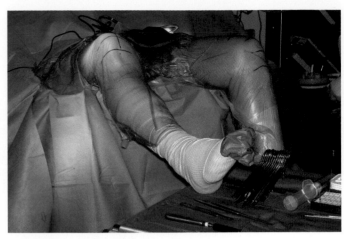

Figure 31-4 After closure of the first knee, that knee can be extended on a Mayo stand as shown in this intraoperative photo.

compressive devices, but these are used only while in the hospital. The postoperative rehabilitation protocol is very similar to that used for bilateral TKA. Patients are allowed to weight bear as tolerated routinely. Supine straight leg raises and flexion and extension exercises as tolerated are started on the day of surgery. Bilateral femoral nerve blocks help with postoperative pain but in some cases may hinder rehabilitation, and care must be taken to use knee immobilizers if these blocks are used. Femoral nerve blocks are usually removed 24–36 hours after surgery to allow for a more efficient rehabilitation.

SUMMARY

This chapter has discussed the indications and outcomes of bilateral unicompartmental arthroplasty as well as the surrounding controversies limiting its widespread use. After analyzing the available literature, it appears that the medical risks associated with unicompartmental arthroplasty are less than for those patients undergoing TKA; in addition, the lesser invasiveness of the operation places patients at less risk of developing pulmonary or cardiac complications after surgery. In light of the recent data presented, however, the higher risk of DVT should be discussed with the patients, and those with a history of previous DVTs or PE are likely not good candidates for undergoing bilateral simultaneous unicompartmental arthroplasty. Patients with severe cardiac comorbidities are probably not good candidates either, and in those cases a staged approach might be a better option. More data are needed on patient outcomes with regard to bilateral unicompartmental arthroplasty; however, the data available to date show that this technique can be safe and effective when done in the proper patient.

REFERENCES

1. Riddle DL, Jiranek WA, McGlynn FJ. Yearly incidence of unicompartmental knee arthroplasty in the United States. J Arthroplasty 2008;23:408.
2. Kurtz S, Ong K, Lau E, et al. Projections of primary and revision hip and knee arthroplasty in the United States from 2005 to 2030. J Bone Joint Surg [Am] 2007;89:780.
3. Dudley TE, Gioe TJ, Sinner P, Mehle S. Registry outcomes of unicompartmental knee arthroplasty revisions. Clin Orthop Relat Res 2008;(466):1666.
4. Kasodekar VB, Yeo SJ, Othman S. Clinical outcome of unicompartmental knee arthroplasty and influence of alignment on prosthesis survival rate. Singapore Med J 2006;47:796.
5. Laurencin CT, Zelicof SB, Scott RD, Ewald FC. Unicompartmental versus total knee arthroplasty in the same patient: a comparative study. Clin Orthop Relat Res 1991;(273):151.
6. Saito T, Takeuchi R, Yamamoto K, et al. Unicompartmental knee arthroplasty for osteoarthritis of the knee: remaining postoperative flexion contracture affecting overall results. J Arthroplasty 2003;18:612.
7. Scott RD. Three decades of experience with unicompartmental knee arthroplasty: mistakes made and lessons learned. Orthopedics 2006;29:829.
8. Leonard L, Williamson DM, Ivory JP, Jennison C. An evaluation of the safety and efficacy of simultaneous bilateral total knee arthroplasty. J Arthroplasty 2003;18:972.

9. Morrey BF, Adams RA, Ilstrup DM, Bryan RS. Complications and mortality associated with bilateral or unilateral total knee arthroplasty. J Bone Joint Surg [Am] 1987;69:484.

10. Parvizi J, Sullivan TA, Trousdale RT, Lewallen DG. Thirty-day mortality after total knee arthroplasty. J Bone Joint Surg [Am] 2001;83:1157.

11. Restrepo C, Parvizi J, Dietrich T, Einhorn TA. Safety of simultaneous bilateral total knee arthroplasty: a meta-analysis. J Bone Joint Surg [Am] 2007;89:1220.

12. Ritter MA, Harty LD, Davis KE, et al. Simultaneous bilateral, staged bilateral, and unilateral total knee arthroplasty: a survival analysis. J Bone Joint Surg [Am] 2003;85:1532.

13. Severson EP, Mariani EM, Bourne MH. Bilateral total knee arthroplasty in patients 70 years and older. Orthopedics 2009;32:316.

14. Borgwardt L, Zerahn B, Bliddal H, et al. Similar clinical outcome after unicompartmental knee arthroplasty using a conventional or accelerated care program: a randomized, controlled study of 40 patients. Acta Orthop 2009;80:334.

15. Borus T, Thornhill T. Unicompartmental knee arthroplasty. J Am Acad Orthop Surg 2008;16:9.

16. Bullock DP, Sporer SM, Shirreffs TG Jr. Comparison of simultaneous bilateral with unilateral total knee arthroplasty in terms of perioperative complications. J Bone Joint Surg [Am] 2003;85:1981.

17. Vince KG, Cyran LT. Unicompartmental knee arthroplasty: new indications, more complications? J Arthroplasty 2004;19(4 Suppl 1):9.

18. Lonner JH, Jasko JG, Bezwada HP, Booth RE Jr. Morbidity of sequential bilateral revision TKA performed under a single anesthetic. Clin Orthop Relat Res 2007;(464):151.

19. Malinzak RA, Ritter MA, Berend ME, et al. Morbidly obese, diabetic, younger, and unilateral joint arthroplasty patients have elevated total joint arthroplasty infection rates. J Arthroplasty 2009;24(6 Suppl):84.

20. Powell RS, Pulido P, Tuason MS, et al. Bilateral vs unilateral total knee arthroplasty: a patient-based comparison of pain levels and recovery of ambulatory skills. J Arthroplasty 2006;21:642.

21. Reuben JD, Meyers SJ, Cox DD, et al. Cost comparison between bilateral simultaneous, staged, and unilateral total joint arthroplasty. J Arthroplasty 1998;13:172.

22. Zeni JA Jr, Snyder-Mackler L. Clinical outcomes after simultaneous bilateral total knee arthroplasty comparison to unilateral total knee arthroplasty and healthy controls. J Arthroplasty 2010;25:541.

23. Soohoo NF, Sharifi H, Kominski G, Lieberman JR. Cost-effectiveness analysis of unicompartmental knee arthroplasty as an alternative to total knee arthroplasty for unicompartmental osteoarthritis. J Bone Joint Surg [Am] 2006;88:1975.

24. Chan WCW, Musonda P, Cooper AS, et al. One-stage versus two-stage bilateral unicompartmental knee replacement: a comparison of immediate post-operative complications. J Bone Joint Surg [Br] 2009;91:1305.

25. Lombardi AV, Berend KR, Tucker TL. The incidence and prevention of symptomatic thromboembolic disease following unicompartmental knee arthroplasty. Orthopedics 2007;30(5 Suppl):41.

26. Hebl JR, Dilger JA, Byer DE, et al. A pre-emptive multimodal pathway featuring peripheral nerve block improves perioperative outcomes after major orthopedic surgery. Reg Anesth Pain Med 2008;33:510.

Index

Note: Page numbers followed by f refer to figures; page numbers followed by t refer to tables; page numbers followed by b refer to boxes.

FLORIDA HOSPITAL
MEDICAL LIBRARY